D0787918

Oxford Medical Publications

BSE: risk, science, and governance

Oxford University Press makes no representation, express or implied, that the drug dosages in this book are correct. Readers must therefore always check the product information and clinical procedures with the most up to date published product information and data sheets provided by the manufacturers and the most recent codes of conduct and safety regulations. The authors and the publishers do not accept responsibility or legal liability for any errors in the text or for the misuse or misapplication of material in this work.

BSE: risk, science, and governance

Patrick van Zwanenberg
Research Fellow
Science and Technology Policy Research
University of Sussex
Brighton, UK

and

Erik Millstone
Reader in Science Policy
Science and Technology Policy Research
University of Sussex
Brighton, UK

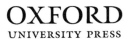

OXFORD
UNIVERSITY PRESS

This book has been printed digitally and produced in a standard specification
in order to ensure its continuing availability

OXFORD
UNIVERSITY PRESS

Great Clarendon Street, Oxford OX2 6DP

Oxford University Press is a department of the University of Oxford.
It furthers the University's objective of excellence in research, scholarship,
and education by publishing worldwide in

Oxford New York

Auckland Cape Town Dar es Salaam Hong Kong Karachi
Kuala Lumpur Madrid Melbourne Mexico City Nairobi
New Delhi Shanghai Taipei Toronto
With offices in
Argentina Austria Brazil Chile Czech Republic France Greece
Guatemala Hungary Italy Japan South Korea Poland Portugal
Singapore Switzerland Thailand Turkey Ukraine Vietnam

Oxford is a registered trade mark of Oxford University Press
in the UK and in certain other countries

Published in the United States
by Oxford University Press Inc., New York

© Oxford University Press, 2005

The moral rights of the author have been asserted

Database right Oxford University Press (maker)

Reprinted 2008

All rights reserved. No part of this publication may be reproduced,
stored in a retrieval system, or transmitted, in any form or by any means,
without the prior permission in writing of Oxford University Press,
or as expressly permitted by law, or under terms agreed with the appropriate
reprographics rights organization. Enquiries concerning reproduction
outside the scope of the above should be sent to the Rights Department,
Oxford University Press, at the address above

You must not circulate this book in any other binding or cover
And you must impose this same condition on any acquirer

ISBN 978-0-19-852581-3

Contents

Chapter 1

Introduction

The main themes

This book is about BSE (or bovine spongiform encephalopathy – also known as mad cow disease) but about a great deal more too. We will be describing and analysing the details of the BSE saga partly because it constitutes a fascinating and important series of events and developments, but also because the lessons to be learnt from this saga apply across a very wide range of policy challenges, not just in the UK but in all other countries; at multilateral jurisdictions such as the European Union and also in global bodies.

It has frequently been asserted that BSE policy-making in the UK, at least prior to the crisis of March 1996, was a catastrophic failure (or a series of failures). One purpose of this book is to assess that claim, and to explain what happened and why. We will eventually conclude that the UK government's BSE policy regime was profoundly flawed; that it had neither scientific nor democratic legitimacy. We will show how science was used tactically to pursue and disguise policy objectives that would not have been democratically sustainable if they had been explicit. We will also show how one of the consequences of those tactics was that policy-makers were not well-informed about the risks that BSE might pose, and therefore the policy failures were compounded and exacerbated. Our hypothesis is that the failure of BSE policy was not just a random or accidental phenomenon but that it was symptomatic of the inadequacies of a widespread and deeply ingrained approach to risk policy-making. We therefore seek to answer the question: How can policy-making processes of that kind can be understood? and to derive a general set of lessons on how science-based risk policy-making can and should be made in ways that can achieve both scientific and democratic legitimacy.

A crisis of governance?

The political cultures of the UK, the EU and industrial societies generally are confronted by a crisis in science and governance. Decisions frequently need to be taken even though facts are uncertain, values are in dispute, levels of trust are low, stakes are high, and decisions are urgent (cf. Funtowicz and Ravetz

1993). In some accounts of this crisis, the central problem is one of trust: the general public used to trust science, scientific experts and science-based policy decisions but that trust has been severely eroded, and needs to be re-established. Our view is that trust is important, but not the central issue. We assume that if the relationships between science and policy-making were legitimate, and seen to be so, then trust would be altogether less problematic. For us the central issue is not one of trust but of legitimacy. We assume that trust can be justified if policy-making is legitimate, the key issue is under what conditions can legitimacy be achieved, and it is from that perspective that we explore the lessons that can be learnt from the BSE saga.

All jurisdictions, such as nation states and multilateral bodies such as the European Union, are obliged to make policy to control a broad range of risk issues: they need to decide what is to be done, what is to be permitted and what is to be forbidden. Policy-makers face a crisis because there is a widespread recognition that the ways in which science-based risk policy decisions have been taken were inadequate, inappropriate and unsustainable. For obvious reasons, policy decisions regarding technological risks need to be taken in the light of advice from the scientific community, and often that advice is provided by official expert advisory committees. Our perspective on the crisis of science and governance will focus on the role of scientific considerations and advisors, and especially on their relationships with non-scientific factors such as economic, social, political and ethical considerations.

Historically many participants in, and commentators on, the policy-making process have feared that if scientific deliberations are influenced by political factors then the scientific legitimacy of those processes and their outcomes will be undermined, and if scientific experts drive political processes the democratic legitimacy of those processes will be compromised. The challenge therefore is to outline a way in which risk appraisal and decision-making can become both scientifically and democratically legitimate, that is to say to provide an account of how policy-making can be democratically legitimate without being anti-scientific, and how it can be scientifically legitimate without being anti-democratic.

Analyses of the crisis in science and governance

The crisis of science and governance has been described and represented in a range of different ways by different interests and groups of protagonists, but there is not yet even a shared description, let alone an agreed diagnosis. One (relatively complacent) approach has been to maintain that it is only a crisis of legitimation and not a crisis of substance. From this perspective, the policy-making processes have been, and remain, fundamentally sound but the main inadequacies have been in 'risk communication' which has been fragmented and partial amongst officials, and less than candid between officialdom and the outside world. Using this model, while there has been a failure, it has been a failure to enable the general public to understand and accept the wisdom of policy-makers, their advisors and their decisions.

An alternative approach, and one that we adopt, is to assume that we face a crisis of both legitimation and substance. In this respect, our analysis differs from that provided in the conclusions of the Public Inquiry chaired by Lord Phillips. The Phillips' Report portrays the failures in BSE policy-makers as having been no-one's fault; it argued that they were primarily a consequence of institutional failures of communication. The Phillips' Report concluded that the UK government's underlying policy objectives of trying to maintain market confidence and 'risk reduction' always were reasonable, and did not contradict each other. Problems arose, argued Phillips, because regulatory restrictions on what cattle and humans could consume could, and should, have been introduced slightly sooner, and enforced rather more effectively. We will argue that the report of the Public Inquiry under-estimates the extent and severity of the failures and doesn't adequately explain *why* those failures occurred.

What is distinctive about our approach?

One dominant traditional approach to science-based policy-making was to represent policy decisions as if they had been derived from, and solely from, scientific considerations. UK agriculture ministers frequently defended their policies on BSE to the House of Commons and with the media by insisting that they were doing what, and only what, their scientists told them to do. In subsequent chapters we will show why that rhetoric never was an accurate representation. To cut a very long story short, the science always was, and even now remains, highly uncertain and incomplete. Specific policy prescriptions never can be derived from uncertain and incomplete scientific knowledge, or even from all the available facts if *per improbabile* the uncertainties were eradicated. That traditional way of representing policy-making processes has become unconvincing. Official reassurances that some class of alleged risks have been proven to be unreal, or have now been entirely eradicated or are under perfect control, have also lost a large proportion of whatever plausibility they may once have had.

The BSE saga, and numerous other risk issues such as climate change, GM crops and the disposal and storage of radioactive wastes, have persuaded many that the ways in which policies have been made must be reformed, and the ways in which they have been justified and defended have to be enriched, but no one has yet provided a clear account of how this can be achieved. That is the gap that this book aims to fill. In this book, we will develop an analysis of the BSE saga and use that as a lens through which to examine, both critically and constructively, the main structural and procedural characteristics of science-based risk policy-making institutions.

Why BSE?

The BSE saga that began in the mid-1980s (and which continues to this day) represents the worst failure of UK public policy since the Suez adventure of 1956, when measured in terms of the economic, political and diplomatic harm it caused. The saga reached a critical juncture on 20 March 1996 when the British government acknowledged that a variant of Creutzfeldt-Jakob Disease (CJD) had emerged that was almost certainly attributable to the consumption of BSE-contaminated foods. The importance of the BSE saga for the overall narrative of this book does not lie in its uniqueness, but rather in the fact that many of the fundamental structural and procedural problems that characterised the way in which the British authorities dealt with BSE were also inherent in the ways in which the UK and other national and international jurisdictions dealt with – and perhaps still deal with – numerous other science-based risk policy challenges. A detailed analysis of the BSE saga of the sort that this book provides can therefore illuminate the general category of such problems, and that is how we propose to use it. We will use a discussion of the microscopic features of the interactions between scientific and political factors in BSE policy-making to illuminate a bigger picture and more general pattern, couple that analysis to a meso-level discussion about the institutions in which those deliberations took place, and locate that discussion in an overall analysis of the macroscopic political and economic context which framed the entire policy-making process. We will not argue that everything that occurred at the meso- and micro-levels can be explained macroscopically as direct consequences or expressions of wider political, economic and social interests, although we will document some of the ways in which the macroscopic context influenced microscopic processes and deliberations. But we will argue that at the micro- and meso-levels distinctive kinds of dramas were played out that contributed in important ways to the course and consequences of the BSE saga.

Was BSE a unique challenge?

The BSE saga was not, in many respects, an anomaly or an aberration, either domestically or internationally. Several senior officials in both France and Germany have had the wisdom and decency to acknowledge that if BSE had arisen in their jurisdictions, they would have made many of the same kinds of mistakes as were made by the UK. The British government's response to the report of the Phillips Inquiry makes it clear that it now assumes that the lessons of the BSE saga apply across the entire range of science-based risk policy challenges. All too often, however, national, international and even local policy-makers continue to reproduce some of the key mistakes for example by trying to hide behind the advice of scientific experts, and trying to misrepresent their policy judgements as if they were predominantly or entirely scientific. That suggests that many of the lessons of the BSE saga have yet to be learnt.

Two unique features of the BSE saga have been the severity of the consequences of the policy failure, and the fact that it has been subjected to a exhaustive public inquiry. The Phillips Inquiry was established partly because of the scale of the harm that BSE did to British agriculture, the food industry and consumer confidence in the integrity of food safety, but also because of the harm it did to public trust in official policy-making institutions. As the BSE saga unfolded, it became obvious, especially after March 1996, that the government, particularly the Ministry of Agriculture, Fisheries and Food (MAFF), had been less than frank and open with the British people. In response to the resulting sense of betrayal, the Phillips Inquiry was conducted, and had to be conducted, in as open and transparent a way as possible. All witness statements, the transcripts of all public sessions and cross-examinations, the resultant report, preliminaries to it and the entire archive of supporting documentation are available on the Internet, and were made available there at the earliest possible opportunity.

The structure of the building in which the Phillips Inquiry took place had to be reinforced to support the weight of documents that were gathered. It would be naive to assume that no documents had been discarded or even deliberately shredded before the Inquiry was formally announced, but the documentary archive assembled by the Phillips Inquiry team is stunningly comprehensive and freely available on the Internet. As a result, it provides a uniquely powerful research resource that facilitates finely detailed analyses of BSE policy-making, to a level of detail beyond that which has been possible on any other risk policy issue in any jurisdiction. Not even the provisions of the US Freedom of Information Act would have provided such a comprehensive archive.

The policy challenge posed by the discovery of BSE

When BSE was first recognised by researchers at MAFF's Central Veterinary Laboratory (CVL) in November 1986, and then brought to the attention of senior MAFF officials and ministers, the policy challenge was a very complex and difficult one, but not entirely exceptional. The question confronting them was: given that we are not sure whether the risks of BSE are vanishingly slight or potentially catastrophic, what steps if any should be taken to diminish or to eradicate the unknown risks? Policy-makers had to decide what risks and uncertainties were acceptable, and which forms and costs of intervention were necessary and appropriate given the fact that the more that is done to diminish the potential but unknown risks, the more disruptive and expensive those measures will be, both in terms of direct costs and opportunity costs.

The concept of 'precaution' and the phrase 'precautionary principle' were not in widespread use in MAFF in the autumn of 1986, but the policy challenge MAFF then faced could have been posed in terms of how precautionary a response was MAFF to take. Despite the way in which precaution has sometimes been misrepresented, it is not an 'all or nothing' policy: it is more helpful to think of precaution by analogy with a spectrum. A broad range of more or less precautionary responses could have been made by MAFF, extending from doing nothing at one end of the spectrum, to an attempt at total eradication at the other. Greater or lesser efforts could also have been expended trying to diminish the key scientific uncertainties.

The initial response in MAFF was to prevent any and all information from leaking outside of the ministry, to try to make sure that as few people as possible learnt about the existence of the disease. No steps whatsoever were taken (for some 18 months) to diminish possible risks to veterinary or public health. In particular, the initial insistence of the Secretary of State (John McGregor) that the meat industry should meet the costs of the separation and disposal of the carcasses of infected animals meant that they continued to enter the human food chain. That approach was the complete antithesis of precaution.

If it had adopted an extremely precautionary policy, MAFF might have required the slaughter and disposal of all and any animals that may have been exposed to any source of BSE infectivity, but that would have entailed the slaughter and careful disposal of almost the entire UK herd. Risk eradication would also have necessitated the destruction of all potentially contaminated feed, and the attempted decontamination of the entire feed chain.

We estimate that the cost of a full BSE risk eradication programme in the UK in the mid-1980s would have been in the order of £20 billion at 2000 prices. It is difficult to imagine any government, then or now, having been keen, or even willing, to devote such a huge sum to an entirely unknown and speculative risk. The question we are posing therefore is not 'Why did the British government not instantly eradicate all possible risks from BSE?' but rather 'How and why did the British government choose the policy on BSE that it adopted (namely as unprecautionary as they could possibly get away with), and what role did scientific considerations, expertise and advice play in decision-making processes?'

Why is science the focus of our analysis of BSE policy-making?

To a robust first approximation, the UK government consistently defended its policy on BSE (at least until March 1996) as having been based on, and only on, 'sound science' provided by expert scientific advisors. Science was, and remains, indispensable and crucial to policy-making but it never was, and never could be, sufficient. To understand how BSE policies were made, and why they were catastrophically misconceived, and how to conduct risk appraisal and decision-making in an altogether more scientifically and democratically legitimate fashion, we will describe and analyse both the scientific and political aspects of BSE, how they were constituted and how they interacted. Our approach will therefore take a sceptical view of the UK government's narrative that its policy was based on and only on 'sound science'. The UK government's representations of the science of BSE were not sound, and its policy decisions often did not reflect the scientists' understanding or advice. We will document, for example, the sharp disjunction between the cautious warnings of expert advisors and back-room officials and the confident ministerial reassurances that were articulated for public consumption.

We are not, however, going to argue that politicians should do what their scientists tell them to do. We also understand, and sympathise with, the concern that allowing politics to influence science risks may compromise the legitimacy of the science. Indeed we will argue that the science *was* so compromised in profoundly unsatisfactory ways. Similarly we also understand, and sympathise with, the concern that introducing scientific authority into policy-making can compromise the democratic legitimacy of decision-making. The objective therefore is to identify a way in which the demands for scientific and democratic legitimacy can be reconciled.

We are interested in delineating the proper roles of politics and science in the policy-making process, and in trying to design institutions and procedures through which both scientists and policy-makers can most effectively and legitimately contribute to decision-making. We will use the BSE saga to explore empirically and analytically the question of how far science and politics can and should be distinguished, separated and legitimated, and to indicate in what ways they can and should be coupled together so that policy-making can become both scientifically and democratically legitimate.

While the historical narrative that will unfold in the next few chapters is (all too often) a dismal one, the analysis we will build upon it will be predominantly optimistic, because our claim will be that our analysis of the past casts a positive and constructive light on the future, not just of food safety policy-making, but more broadly in relation to the entire range of science-based risk decision-making. If the analysis that we are going to provide is serviceable then it should be relevant to a very wide range of other issues of risk and public policy.

Those risk appraisal and decision-making challenges all have a great deal in common with the challenge of BSE policy-making, but the task of dealing with BSE has itself evolved over time. In the late autumn of 1986 so little was known about the disease that it was impossible to estimate the chances that BSE might be transmissible to humans. By the watershed of 20 March 1996 the evidence that it could do so had become very persuasive, and by the end of that year the evidence was almost as conclusive as it could be, short of deliberately experimenting on humans by exposing them, under controlled conditions, to BSE-contaminated materials (Collinge *et al.* 1996). In 1990, when a Bristol-based cat known as Max succumbed to a previously unknown feline spongiform encephalopathy, the grounds for MAFF's confidence that the risk of BSE transmitting to other species (especially humans) was 'remote' was undermined. We will document, moreover, how the plausibility of the UK government's reassuring narrative about BSE progressively unravelled as more information emerged, and as several of the key uncertainties were diminished.

The general class of risk policy challenges that we will be discussing, therefore, is not confined to those where the uncertainties are extensive and refractory, but will include those in which the knowledge base and uncertainties change over time. One key question will be concerned with how institutions respond to new information, especially information that contradicts the assumptions, expectations or wishes of the policy-makers and their advisors. Ironically, MAFF habitually argued that its policy-making systems had the great advantage of being very 'flexible'. Our analysis will indicate precisely the opposite, namely that it suffered from chronic rigidity. Our concern will be how policy-making institutions can become genuinely responsive both to uncertainties and new information and evidence.

This book is not intended to be an exhaustive account of all aspects of BSE policy-making. This is not a book that provides answers to questions such as: What were the origins of BSE? What is the nature of the pathogen? How many people will succumb to vCJD? Is British beef safe, or is the beef in other countries safe? If those are the questions to which you want answers, you must look elsewhere. If, however, you want an analysis of how we can diminish the chances of such problems and catastrophes from occurring again and again then read on.

Much of the work for this book was conducted as part of two European Commission supported multi-lateral research projects. One was entitled 'Building a common data base on scientific research and public decision on TSEs in Europe' (also known as the BASES project, or Commission project PL 976057). The second was called 'Public perceptions of BSE and CJD risk in Europe, their interplay with media, policy initiatives and surveillance issues. Drawing the lessons for information policy' (also known as the CJD Risk project, or Commission project PL 987028).

References

Collinge, J., Sidle, K. C. L., Meads, J., Ironside, J. and Hill, A. F. (1996) 'Molecular analysis of prion strain variation and the aetiology of "new variant" CJD', *Nature*, **383**, 685–90.

Funtowicz, S. and Ravetz, J. (1993) 'Science for the post-normal age', *Futures*, **25**, S.739–55.

Chapter 2

Analysing the role of science in public policy-making

Chapter 1 argued that contemporary industrial societies are now confronting a crisis in science and governance – decisions need to be taken about which technological practices and innovations to accept or encourage and which to discourage, restrict or prevent. Such decisions need to be made even though facts are uncertain, values are in dispute, levels of trust are low, stakes are high, and decisions are urgent. As Durkheim once remarked: 'Science is fragmentary, incomplete, it progresses slowly and is never finished; life cannot wait' (Durkheim 1912).

We aim to answer one central question: how can we understand the roles that science has played, can and should play in policy-making? In this chapter we will set out a range of theoretical ideas with which that question can be analysed, and their associated vocabularies. Two overlapping sets of ideas will be reviewed. One set includes the concepts that public policy-makers have themselves used to describe and justify their institutional practices and decisions. The second set includes the concepts that social science and science policy scholars have used to analyse and criticise institutional practices and policy decisions. What we are looking for, at this stage, are potentially useful ways of describing and analysing the relationships between scientific considerations and policy-making.

There is a substantial literature providing competing descriptions and analyses, but it does not provide anything resembling a single, coherent agreed framework: on the contrary, this is a fiercely contested domain. The literature contains a range of diverse, and often inconsistent, assumptions about the nature of scientific expertise and the role which scientific evidence and advice can and should play in the policy-making process. Our account of the theoretical, analytical and legitimatory literatures will be structured in historical terms, which will represent official and academic ideas interacting not just with each other but also with policy practices, challenges and experiences.

The evolution of ideas about science and governance

The idea that policy judgements can be based on uniquely correct and precise knowledge has a very long history, going back at least to Plato's *Republic* in which Socrates suggests that responsibility for government should be solely in the hands of those with the relevant expertise. In the late seventeenth and early eighteenth centuries, Leibniz had argued that if ever two scholars, advisors or rulers were confronted by apparent uncertainty or conflicting opinions they should settle the dispute with the words: 'Let us calculate' (Leibniz 1666).

For much of the nineteenth century, however, and the first half of the twentieth century, the role of experts in policy-making was rarely thought of as either essential or problematic. Policy had often been officially represented as emerging from the wisdom of the rulers, whose wisdom extended from time to time to seeking the advice of relevant experts. Policies were typically legitimated with narratives that simply insisted that all relevant considerations and information had been fully taken into account – a rhetorical tactic that continues to have some currency.

The Second World War and the crises of the Cold War created the conditions in which scientific expertise and policy-makers became entangled as never before. During and immediately after that period, the relationship between scientific expertise and public policy-making emerged as a topic of serious attention. Two important intellectual traditions strongly influenced the ways in which science and governance came to be understood in the twentieth century, and both have their roots in the late nineteenth century. One tradition can be traced back to the work of Max Weber and Emile Durkheim in Germany.

Weberian Decisionism

Weber and Durkheim recognised the radical historical novelty represented by the industrial society that evolved rapidly during their working lives. They argued that industrial societies could only function with increasingly bureaucratic forms of governance, and that industrial societies both required and developed new forms of organisation and administration. Weber was not, however, a neo-Platonist; he was not advocating technocracy, but warning against it. In response to what he perceived as the dangers inherent in governments becoming increasingly reliant on officials and experts, Weber argued that the proper role of bureaucrats should always be a subordinate one. The deliberations and judgements of bureaucrats (and by extension expert advisors) should always be framed by the policy goals and objectives that should be set by politically accountable representatives, rather than by unaccountable officials. Weber's model of the role of experts in policy-making has come to be known as a 'decisionist' model, because it stipulated that the deliberations and judgements of the bureaucrats should be framed by, and be secondary to, prior goal-setting policy decisions. A graphic representation of Weber's decisionist model is given in Figure 2.1.

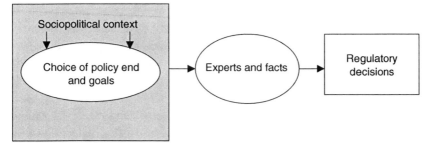

Figure 2.1 The Weberian decisionist model – 'Politics first, then experts'.

Both Weber and Durkheim argued that policy-making could be made more rational and scientific than it had been, but only partly, not entirely. The decisionist model presupposes a strict and clear division of labour between what Habermas referred to as ' . . . the objectively informed and technically schooled general staffs of the bureaucracy . . . '(including the experts) on the one hand and political leaders on the other (Habermas 1971, p. 83). Weber recognised the superficial attraction of the idea of assigning full responsibility for all aspects of policy-making to bureaucrats and technocrats, but argued that it was unrealistic. He argued that policy-making could never be decided solely by the facts since, although the choice of 'means' may be rationalised, the choice amongst the 'ends' and objectives of policy and the underlying values remain irredeemably subjective (Weber 1958, pp. 308ff).

On Weber's decisionist model there were two discrete set of deliberations, and correspondingly two distinct lines of accountability. Ministers should be responsible to elected representatives for their choice of policy goals, and through them to the electorate. Bureaucrats and experts, on the other hand, should be accountable to ministers for effectively pursuing the goals set from above, and to other experts for the knowledge and judgements that they bring to bear in the discharge of their responsibilities.

Weber correctly anticipated that, in industrial societies, official decision-making would increasingly appeal to judgements based on ostensibly accurate observations and calculations, and that expert advisors would play increasingly important roles in decision-making in bureaucratic institutions. While industrial societies certainly did become more bureaucratic in the nineteenth and twentieth centuries, it was not until the twentieth century that scientific experts came to make more than very marginal contributions policy-making deliberations. Bureaucracies are, of course, not always rational or scientific.

The division of labour envisaged in the decisionist model was not without its difficulties. In a relatively static pre-industrial society, political goal-setting might be relatively independent of up-to-date scientific knowledge, but in a rapidly changing and technologically dynamic society, those responsible for goal-setting may need a great deal of scientific and technical advice about the potential benefits and risks arising from new technologies and knowledges. Without that advice, policy-makers might not even know which areas of policy to develop. Under those conditions, the division of labour between those that choose the ends of policy and those that select the means for attaining those ends breaks down. If, however, expertise has to contribute to the deliberations on goal-setting, the question can arise: how can scientists legitimately perform that role and what role remains for policy-makers?

Weberian decisionism was also predicated on the assumption that the relevant experts are adequately knowledgeable, and unified, fully to meet their responsibilities. If the information and knowledge available to the experts is incomplete, uncertain or equivocal, and if different groups of experts make conflicting judgements, then the deliberations of the bureaucrats and experts will be inconclusive, and the decision-making process cannot reach closure without some arbitrary decisions by the bureaucrats, or without the reintro-duction of some downstream political deliberations.

The idea of a 'technocracy'

In France, a competing vision of expertise and policy-making was developed by the positivist theorists Henri de Saint-Simon and Auguste Comte; they were not warning against technocracy but enthusiastically recommending it. They adopted especially optimistic assumptions about the progress, accuracy and adequacy of science and argued that public administration by impartial experts should replace governance by those with partial biases, ignorance and vested interests.

The technocratic model of policy-making, as it is widely termed, has often been encapsulated in the claim that policy should be based on, and only on 'sound science'. As Peter Weingart explained 'In this "technocratic" model . . . the politician becomes fully dependent on the expert. Politics is replaced by a scientifically rationalised administration' (Weingart 1999, p. 154). The assumption of technocracy, that scientific and technical consider-ations are not just necessary but also sufficient for policy decision-making, implies that policy-making can and should be delegated to scientific and tech-nical experts, because they and they alone are in possession of the relevant facts. Elected representatives' and government ministers' responsibilities might then be confined to recruiting the elite experts.

The technocratic idea that emerged in the theoretical writing of Saint Simon and Comte had been not just articulated, but caricatured, earlier in the nineteenth century by Charles Dickens. At the start of his novel *Hard Times*, Dickens introduced us to the educational philosophy of Mr Gradgrind with the words:

> Now, what I want is, Facts. . . . Facts alone are wanted in life. Plant nothing else, and root out everything else. You can only form the minds of reasoning animals upon Facts: nothing else will ever be of any service to them . . . Stick to Facts, sir!

(Dickens 1854)

The technocratic model of policy-making can be thought of as a political analogue of Mr Gradgrind's educational philosophy.

Technocratic ideas began to acquire some currency in policy circles in the first half of the twentieth century, especially in the USA. In 1926, Leonard White wrote about the role of technical experts in the US political system, saying: 'These men are not merely useful to legislators overwhelmed by the increasing flood of bills; they are simply indispensable. They are the government' (White 1926).

The conceptual structure of the technocratic model is given in Figure 2.2. It presupposes that the science and the facts are entirely objective and socially and politically neutral and that all the facts can readily be gathered. Technocratic rhetoric is therefore potentially very vulnerable to criticisms that the evidential base and the understanding of experts is incomplete, unreliable or equivocal. Scientific uncertainty and disputes amongst the experts undermine the plausibility and credibility of the technocratic model.

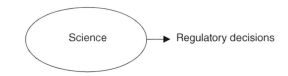

Figure 2.2 The technocratic model.

Rhetoric of policy justification, and the structure of science-based policy-making after 1945

During the Second World War science-based innovations in decisive military technologies, especially radar and the atom bomb, transformed the relationships between scientists and governments as expert scientific advisors came to play an increasingly important role in public policy-making (Rose and Rose 1969). The crises of the Cold War, and the perceived importance of technological innovations and competition, also reinforced the tendency for scientific expertise and policy-makers to become ever more closely entangled.

Politics and science have subsequently influenced each other in important ways, but their relationship has been both complex and problematic.

By 1990, Jasanoff was able to represent scientific advisors as the 'Fifth Branch' of the US policy-making establishment, after the Executive and Legislative Branches, the Judiciary and the Media. As Jasanoff said: 'The proposition that science-based decisions should be reviewed by independent experts strikes us today as hardly more controversial than the proposition that there is no completely risk-free technology' (Jasanoff 1990, p. 1).

In was in the post-1945 period, in the context of an expanding regulatory state, that policy-makers found themselves increasingly under pressure to make decisions about the acceptability of newly emerging technologies or in response to newly emerging evidence of risks from technologies that were already in use, especially in relation to matters of health, safety and the environment. Policy-makers were, however, poorly prepared and equipped to respond to those challenges. They could accept the general argument that some kinds of restrictions needed to be placed on the products and processes of, for example, the food, chemical and pharmaceutical industries, but they had no basis for judging which products and processes needed to be restricted, nor the extent of those restrictions. To make those judgements, they turned to selected scientific experts to provide advice on those matters.

The scientific community was also ill-prepared for those roles. Very few scientists understood how to make themselves and their knowledge useful to policy-makers, and scientific knowledge of what was, and was not safe, was very limited. By the mid-1950s, scientists only had the ability to identify materials that caused severe harm that occurred either rapidly or frequently, or both. The disciplines of epidemiology, toxicology and ecology were rudimentary and the available evidence was fragmentary, incomplete and equivocal. If asked, many scientists then would have said either 'we do not know what is and is not safe' or 'there are risks everywhere', but that was not much help to policy-makers.

A set of alliances then developed between, on the one hand, a fraction of the scientific community that found that it could gain an increasingly important role in, and influence over, policy-making processes, and on the other hand the officials and elected representatives responsible for administering those aspects of policy-making. One distinctive feature of those alliances was that they coalesced around a premise that thresholds of exposure to potentially hazardous materials could be readily identified, below which adverse effects would not occur. Scientists could help policy-makers by indicating what those threshold levels might be, then the policy-makers could take responsibility for deciding the most appropriate way of trying to ensure that those designated levels were not exceeded. A second distinctive feature of that group of scientists was that many of them worked for, or with, the industries whose products they were assessing. That was typically justified officially by arguing that the relevant expertise was bound to reside within that particular group of experts.

There always were problems with the assumption that the presumed thresholds were real and especially with the assumption that they could accurately be identified, but the scientists who claimed to be able to identify those thresholds were providing policy-makers with what they wanted, and policy-makers chose for their expert advisors only those from the minority of scientists who were then confident of being able to identify such thresholds.

In the 1950s and early 1960s, policy-makers, powerful stakeholders and their chosen expert advisors developed a new vocabulary of scientific-seeming concepts to refer to those presumed thresholds. Concepts such as 'an acceptable daily intake', 'a recommended daily allowance', 'a maximum residue level', 'a maximum tolerated dose' and 'a threshold limit value' were coined and regularly invoked, especially in the USA. As the US National Research Council has indicated:

> The threshold hypothesis has been criticized as inadequate to account for some toxic effects, and it has not been accepted by [US] regulators as applicable to carcinogens, but it remains a cornerstone of other regulatory and public health assessments.
>
> (US NRC 1994, p. 31)

In the UK, and in some Continental European countries, prior to the mid-1990s, there was less focus on quantitative targets, but rather the adoption of the vocabulary of 'safe' or 'acceptably safe'.

Habermas provided a provocative analysis of these types of developments. He argued that technocratic arguments undermined Weber's nineteenth-century version of decisionism. Instead of scientists working to a policy agenda set for them by the politicians:

> The dependence of the professional on the politician reversed itself. The . . . [politician] becomes the mere agent of a scientific intelligentsia, which, in concrete circumstances, elaborates the objective implications and requirements of available techniques and resources as well as of optimal strategies and rules of control . . .
>
> (Habermas 1971, p. 63)

Habermas's account is, however, ambiguous and invites two contrasting interpretations: one is that technocracy displaced decisionism, and the other is that technocracy transformed decisionism by inverting it, placing the scientists at the heart of the policy-making process, and the policy-makers taking a secondary role. Our reading of the history of the post-war period is that both of those processes occurred, but that the extent to which they occurred varied as between countries, policy topics and across time. In the UK, and in many but not all Continental European countries, the dominant official post-war model of science-based policy-making became a technocratic one, and remained that way until after the BSE crisis of March 1996. In the USA, and in other continental countries, a new (post-1945) model of science and governance emerged in their official discourse, which we are calling 'inverted decisionism'.

Post-1945 technocratic narratives

Food, chemical and environmental policy-making in several European countries, including the UK, during the period from 1945 to the late 1990s was legitimated by a technocratic rhetoric, and embodied in a set of institutional arrangements that corresponded to that model of policy-making. Typically, policy decisions on what to permit and under what conditions emerged from (ostensibly) scientific advisory bodies. Expert committees did not just summarise scientific evidence and judgements, they routinely advised governments to adopt particular policies. Those decisions were represented, however, as if they had been decided solely by reference to robust and unequivocal scientific considerations. Typically, though not invariably, those recommendations were endorsed and adopted by ministers, who often provided little more than the proverbial 'rubber stamp' to decisions that they had not taken, but which had been taken for them by their expert advisors. Whenever policy-makers said, in effect, 'we are just doing what our expert advisors tell us should be done' they implicitly appealed to technocratic assumptions.

Sometimes a slightly subtler version of technocratic thinking could be discerned. Rather than trying to argue that all the facts were accessible and known to the chosen experts, policy-makers and their expert advisors would occasionally acknowledge that some uncertainties remained. In those circumstances, the rhetoric could be modified; rather than asserting just that policy was based on sound science, the narrative would be that advice has been obtained from the best available scientific experts and that all other relevant considerations had been fully taken into account. Sometimes officials and ministers might acknowledge that policy-making involved making discretionary judgements, but then they would argue that scientists, and other experts, were the most appropriate groups to decide policy precisely because their expertise and professionalism (and in some cases academic autonomy) diminished their biases, enabling them to provide judgements that were more objective and fair than those of any other group. On that version of technocracy, technocrats may not be perfect, but they are less imperfect than all their compatriots and competitors.

Technocratic structures and rhetorics of legitimation can be very attractive to politicians, civil servants, expert advisors and the industries whose products and processes are being controlled, because they can serve to insulate the policy-making system from scrutiny and criticism. An assertion that policy has been based solely on objective and reliable facts often served to diffuse, deflect or discourage scrutiny or challenge. Without some sort of counter-expertise it was often extremely difficult for organisations or individuals to participate in or to challenge either scientific or policy deliberations.

Inverted decisionism

It would be a mistake to pretend that technocracy was absent from the rhetoric and practices of policy-making in the USA, but even by the late 1950s technocratic representations of policy-making processes became increasingly difficult for US regulators. The US Federal government is inherently plural, composed as it is of the executive, the legislative and the judicial branches. The utility of technocratic narratives to the executive branch in the USA was undermined by the separate and contrary interventions of Congress and the courts. As early as 1958, Congress passed legislation that explicitly imposed a political framework upon the interpretation of science for policy; an arrangement that directly undermined the suggestion that policy derived from science alone. Under the provisions of what was called the Delaney Amendment, Congress stipulated how incomplete and uncertain scientific evidence about possible cancer risks should be interpreted by federal government advisors and public officials (US Congress, 1958). Congress recognised that evidence about the possible carcinogenicity of a compound is often fragmentary, incomplete and equivocal and it deliberately deprived the US Food and Drug Administration (FDA) of a considerable portion of its scope to exercise discretion over how to respond to such uncertainty. The Delaney Amendment stipulated that if there was any evidence suggesting that a chemical could induce cancer 'when ingested by man or animal' then it must not be permitted for use as a food additive (Food Drug and Cosmetic Act, Section 409 C-3-A). For those compounds, the only acceptable threshold was zero.

Under those conditions, technocratic accounts of policy-making lost their plausibility. Policy is self-evidently a product of both political and scientific judgements, so an alternative account was imperative. The alternative account was a version of decisionism, but one that, in response to a technocratic critique, had been inverted. Policy-making was once again represented as a two-stage process, but now science is in the lead and policy-makers follow and respond. US, and subsequently other government, officials retained their understandable attachment to the slogan 'policy is based on sound science' only now the narrative became: first the scientists gather and interpret the scientific evidence that enables them to identify the relevant thresholds, and then policy-makers develop measures to ensure that those thresholds are not (often) exceeded.

The kinds of issues that policy-makers need to address at the second stage are not difficult to discern. There is typically a range of different means by which a given target could be reached. Some might be more or less expensive, more or less speedy and/or effective, and they are likely to be more or less acceptable to the constituencies that will be affected by any measures taken. Policy-makers will typically need to make judgements about what kinds of risks and measures are acceptable in exchange for some anticipated benefits. A graphic representation of the structure of the inverted decisionist model is given in Figure 2.3.

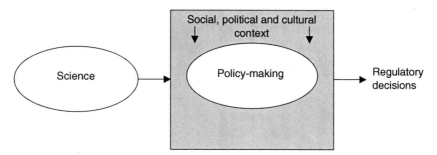

Figure 2.3 Inverted decisionism.

This new narrative of policy legitimation was curious in at least one key respect. In Weber's version of the model, political deliberations identified the goals of public policy, while technocrats then identified and utilised the best available means to those ends. In this inverted model, it is the scientific deliberations that are presumed to identify the goals that should be reached, while policy-makers are confined to deciding the most appropriate means with which to reach the science-derived targets.

It is not difficult to see why policy-makers need to have regard, for example, to the costs of alternative courses of action and their likely effectiveness: what is harder is to understand is how scientific deliberations can be sufficient to choose amongst alternative and competing policy goals. That is where the introduction of concepts such as the 'maximum tolerated dose', and an 'acceptable daily intake' was not just useful but probably also essential to give the inverted decisionist model its plausibility. That was partly because if you could convey the impression that a product can be used in ways that are entirely safe several otherwise vital policy questions can be discounted as irrelevant. For example, no one need ask: 'Given that this technology or product is associated with possible risks that may be hard even to anticipate, is there a clear social purpose or benefit to the technology which would mean that taking those potential risks was worthwhile?' The fact that a new product might have no significant social benefit, or provide benefits that only accrue to particular sections of the population, might not really matter; no one would be harmed. A promise of 'safety' could render a prior policy question of 'do we need or want this product' irrelevant. A decisionist regime that provides confident reassurances concerning public and environmental safety can provide particular encouragement to the private sector to develop and adopt technological innovations.

Inverted decisionism was adopted not just as a form of rhetoric, but also as a design principle for the structure of policy-making institutions. Scientific advisory committees were established, sometimes on a statutory basis, and given terms of reference indicating that they should provide scientific advice on policy matters. That scientific advice would then be passed to, and received by, a separate part of the bureaucracy which would be responsible for conducting and completing the second and final stage of the policy-making process.

On this model, public policy-makers are responsible, through normal processes of democratic political accountability (including for example the legislature and the courts) for obtaining and being guided by the advice of the scientific experts, and for their subsequent downstream discretionary policy judgements. Expert scientific advisors, on the other hand, can be accountable, but only to their scientific peers. In this model, non-experts have no standing as judges of, or contributors to, the deliberations of the experts. In particular, that restriction is supposed to apply to the policy-makers for in this model, the experts are presumed to provide scientific advice that is entirely independent of, and not influenced by, the policy-makers or other interested stakeholders. It is the neutrality and objectivity of the science that is presumed to justify the role of scientific advice as providing the foundations upon which a legitimate policy regime can be constructed. Official accounts of the role which scientific evidence and expertise played in public policy-making therefore tended to emphasise the objectivity and reliability of scientific advice, and to insist upon and exaggerate the independence of science from politics and its ability fully to understand and predict the risks posed for example by chemicals, nuclear radiation and diseases such as BSE.

Problems with the plausibility and adequacy of the inverse decisionist model emerged soon after the model was first deployed. For understandable reasons, those difficulties were most conspicuous in the USA. A key factor was the introduction of Freedom of Information legislation in 1966 during the Vietnam War. A Congressional majority for the legislation was a product of the anger that erupted in response to the emergence of what at the time were known as The Pentagon Papers. These were documents officially designated as secret but which reached the public domain and revealed that the US government had been actively misleading Congress and citizens about its bombing campaigns in Vietnam and Cambodia. The initial legislation was only partly effective, and numerous complaints emerged about official obstruction of the disclosure process, and about officials having excessive discretion when deciding what to disclose. The legislation was revised in 1974 and considerably strengthened in 1976 in the immediate aftermath of the Watergate scandal when irrefutable evidence emerged of a complex web of official concealment, dishonesty and conspiracies to mislead.

Once US government agencies were compelled to place in the public domain large portions of the scientific evidence by reference to which regulatory decision were being made, the extent to which the evidence was incomplete and equivocal became increasingly conspicuous. The inverted decisionist model is able to cope with some marginal uncertainties in the science, especially if their magnitude can be estimated, because policy-makers can make allowances, for example by introducing a corresponding margin of safety. If, however, the uncertainties are profound, extensive and difficult to diminish then policy-makers face far greater difficulties, and the decisionist model becomes harder to invoke. Once such uncertainties were recognised, it was obvious that a multiplicity of different policies could be consistent with the available scientific knowledge. Scholars and representatives of commercial and/or public interest stakeholders were then able to question and challenge the legitimacy of the policies that were being selected, and the ways in which policy-makers were interpreting the available scientific evidence.

Starting in the early 1970s, and taking advantage of the provisions of the Freedom of Information regime, a series of books and papers started to emerge in the USA that challenged what purported to be the secure scientific foundations of risk policy-making. Books such as Turner's *The Chemical Feast* (1970), Jacobson's *Eater's Digest* (1972) and Verrett and Carper's *Eating may be hazardous to your health* (1974) contributed to that corpus of work. Those authors reviewed a broad range of food safety policy issues and argued that the science was not clear cut, that officially convened groups of experts had provided oversimplified and over-optimistic representations of the evidence and the risks. They argued that both the expert advisory bodies and the policy-making bureaucrats understated the uncertainties, and awarded the benefit of the doubt in favour of corporate interests rather than the interest of consumers and/or the protection of the environment.

In response, an alternative set of critiques emerged from representatives of corporate interests arguing that, contrary to what the consumer and environmental campaigners were arguing, the uncertainties and the risks were being overestimated, and that control measures were unduly restrictive and not scientifically justified. A classical example was provided by Edith Efron in her 1984 book *The Apolcalyptics*. Efron argued that US government agencies had chosen to adopt the agendas of the consumer and environmental campaign groups without acknowledging that they were doing so, and consequently interpreting unreliable and partial fragments of evidence as pessimistically as possible.

The decisionist orthodoxy of US policy-makers was also challenged by senior members of the US scientific community who began to see controversies over risk policy issues as a serious political threat to the autonomy and reputation of the scientific community. In an influential paper, published in 1972, Alvin Weinberg argued that many of the policy issues that arose in the course of the interaction between science and public policy, such as the identification of acceptable levels of exposure to ionising radiation:' . . . hang on the answers to questions which can be asked of science *but yet which cannot be answered by science*' (emphasis in original) (Weinberg 1972).

Weinberg argued that the existing intellectual and/or financial resources were insufficient to answer such politically important questions. He noted, for example, that no fewer than 8 billion experimental mice would be needed to establish, at 95 per cent confidence levels, whether the dose–response relationship between the incidence of spontaneous mutations in mice and exposure to ionising radiation was linear, down to the levels of exposure that humans might realistically encounter. Such issues were key to public policy debates at the time, but could not be practically answered. The only honest answer that the scientific community could provide to the question was 'we don't know'. Weinberg called those kinds issues 'trans-scientific', and he argued that judgements on trans-scientific matters required resolution and decisions by the use of non-scientific methods, such as legal adversarial procedures, where contrary sets of evidence could be juxtaposed and evaluated. Weinberg's agenda seems to have been driven as much by a concern to protect the autonomy and integrity of the scientific community as by a concern to help policy-makers resolve their dilemmas. The concept of trans-science suggested that what was happening in regulatory disputes lay beyond science proper, and that with such challenging problems, science could not provide (and therefore was not providing) a secure foundation on which policy decisions could be constructed and by reference to which they could be legitimated.

A series of studies emerged from the academic science policy community that did not consistently endorse the perspectives of either the consumer or the industrial pressure groups, but which provided indirect support for the more general argument that scientific representations of risk were profoundly influenced by conflicting values, and therefore that science did not and could not provide neutral and objective foundations to which policy-making could be anchored.

As early as 1971, Dorothy Nelkin published a compelling analysis of the scientific and policy debates surrounding a proposal to build a nuclear power plant on Cayuga Lake in Central New York State (Nelkin 1971). In 1967 the New York State Electric and Gas Corporation announced its intention to build an 830 megawatt plant on the shore of Cayuga Lake, but five years later the plans for that plant were abandoned because of the opposition of the local community, environmental campaigners and scientists: the site was just 12 miles from Cornell University. Nelkin found that different factions of the scientific community gave different answers to the question: 'Will the plant be acceptably safe?' There was no consensus about which possible changes to the environment were the ones on which scientific deliberations should focus. There was not even a consensus on the question of whether the *status quo ante* of the lake should be presumed to be unpolluted or already polluted. As a consequence, it was not possible for compelling arguments to be marshalled for any single perspective, and the project ran into a quagmire of hearings and endless disputes.

Nelkin, and other scholars in both the USA and Europe, reviewed numerous other science-based risk debates and argued that controversies about risk policy did not arise only because of irreducible uncertainties in the scientific knowledge base, but also because competing economic, political and social interests and commitments influenced scientists' definitions of what it is that might be at risk, the questions that needed to be asked, the range of policy options that needed to be assessed, the criteria by which those options should be evaluated, the data considered relevant and the standards used to produce and interpret those data (cf. Nelkin 1979; Epstein 1978; Robbins and Johnston 1976; Gillespie *et al.* 1979; Wynne 1982).

That body of work, of which just a few examples have been cited, represented a severe challenge to those who were responsible for legitimating both policy-making institutions and specific policy decisions. If, in the context of regulatory disputes, all scientific representations of risk and safety are in some way influenced by non-scientific judgements and commitments, and if those commitments are concealed, deliberately or tacitly, then policy-making may have no scientific legitimacy and may possess no political legitimacy either.

Those intellectual challenges were reinforced, moreover, by several judicial decisions, some of which overturned US governmental regulatory decisions on the grounds that they were arbitrary and insufficiently supported by the available scientific evidence. One of the most important of those court cases was a landmark judgement in the 1980 decision of the Supreme Court in Industrial Union Department, *AFL-CIO* v. *American Petroleum Institute*, 448 U.S. 607 (1980) (also known as the 'benzene' decision). In the 1970s the Occupational Safety and Health Administration (OSHA) had lowered its standard for the maximum permitted airborne concentration of benzene from 10 parts per million (ppm) to 1 ppm after evidence emerged indicating that occupational exposures to benzene were linked to increased rates of leukaemia. OSHA's view was not that 1 ppm was a level below which the risk was negligible, but rather that 1 ppm was the lowest level that was then achievable, and close to the minimum level of detection with the monitoring equipment then available.

The Court ruled that OSHA had 'exceeded its authority by reducing permissible exposure limits to benzene at industrial worksites without making a threshold determination that a significant risk was present at the original level' (Mounts 1980, p. 53). The court overruled OSHA because it had failed to provide an adequate scientific case to justify the proposed standard. The court introduced, moreover, a particular expression, namely a scientific 'risk assessment', arguing that the analysis on which the proposed regulation was based did not constitute such a risk assessment.

From that judgement onwards, the decisionist model was recast into a new vocabulary. Within the US, at any rate, the process by which science-based risk policies were decided came to be described as a two-stage process the first of which was called 'risk assessment' and the second of which came to be known as 'risk management'. This revised model is represented graphically in Figure 2.4.

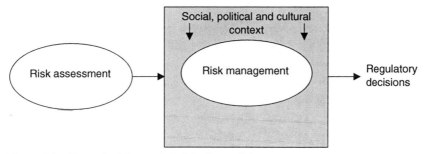

Figure 2.4 The revised inverted decisionist model.

The invocation of this version of a decisionist model served not only to meet a minimum requirement indicated by the Court but also provided some resources with which to respond to the earlier criticisms of the inadequacies and partiality of official representations of risk and of the risk policy-making process.

An important step in that process came with the publication by the US National Research Council of a hugely influential book called *Risk Assessment in the Federal Government: Managing the Process* (US NRC 1983). In what came to be known as the 'Red Book' the US National Research Council (NRC) examined the feasibility of separating the scientific aspects of risk decision-making from the policy aspects (US NRC 1983). The NRC had been asked by the Federal government to review these issues partly because the authorities felt besieged, attacked as they saw it from all sides, by representatives of consumer and environmental organisations on the one hand and by the US food, chemical and energy industries on the other. The Red Book has been widely interpreted as asserting that science-based risk policy-making can and should be entirely legitimate, but only if it is conducted in ways that ensure a proper separation of science from policy in precisely the same way as had been envisaged in the science-first (or inverted) version of decisionism.

A curious irony is that the Red Book came to be seen as setting out most clearly a science-first version of decisionism, despite the fact that a careful reading of the text suggests that it adopted a more complex and nuanced model. The Red Book was misinterpreted partly because the text is itself ambiguous, partly because key protagonists, including public officials, scientific advisors, and representatives of some powerful stakeholder groups had an interest in representing scientific deliberations on risk as entirely independent of political considerations, and partly because of the binary contrast of the 'take-home sound bite' provided by the distinction between 'risk assessment' and 'risk management'. Although the Red Book argued strongly that the division of labour between scientific expert advisors and policy-makers needed to be far more carefully and clearly delineated than had previously been the custom, it did not argue that risk assessment was a purely scientific enterprise. In ways that fundamentally undercut the decisionist model, the Red Book emphasised that subjective value judgements are typically present, though often implicitly, in what are ostensibly scientific risk assessments (US NRC 1983, p. 28). Consequently the NRC recommended against an institutional separation of risk assessment from risk management because the report's authors saw risk assessment as a hybrid (Jasanoff 1990, p. 33).

Despite what the text of the Red Book actually said, it has widely been interpreted and cited as providing a secure inverted decisionist rationale for organising and understanding the process of appraising risks and deciding policies. This model, often supplemented marginally with a third stage known as 'risk communication', has been adopted by almost all of the most powerful policy-making institutions; it became the new orthodoxy. In the 1990s, it spread from the USA to several multilateral bodies such as the OECD and the Codex Alimentarius Commission which, under the rules of the World Trade Organisation, sets global baseline standards for all internationally traded food and agricultural products.

The European Commission, along with the UK government and the governments of most other European countries (with very few exceptions) resisted the Red Book model and clung on, instead, to versions of the technocratic model until after the BSE crisis of March 1996. One of the long-term effects of the BSE crisis upon public policy-making in the UK and EU has been that it forced a reconceptualisation and an institutional reorganisation of science-based risk policy-making. To a good first approximation, most British and other European policy-making systems have been reorganised by reference to the 'Red Book model'. For example, as from 2003, EU food safety policy-making will be decided at the Commission by the Directorate General for Health and Consumer Protection which is responsible for 'risk management' but acting on the advice provided in the scientific 'risk assessments' that a new separate body called the European Food Safety Authority will provide. Curiously, that is not exactly what has happened in the UK. The UK Food Standards Agency is, in effect, responsible for both risk assessments and risk management decision-making. The UK has adopted the rhetoric, but without a formal separation of scientific from policy deliberations that most other jurisdictions have thought necessary. Why that happened, and what the consequences may be, are issues to which we shall return.

Many scholars have argued explicitly, or implied, that regulatory policy-making institutions have only been able to continue to represent their policy-making processes with technocratic or decisionist models because they contrived to construct representations of the scientific aspects of risk in narrow consensual terms. To achieve this they had to very carefully select their expert advisors from a narrow fraction of the scientific community, and by excluding those who, in the cricketing metaphor, might not provide a 'safe pair of hands'. The suggestion, therefore, has been that policy-makers have carefully selected those scientists to serve as their expert advisors who can be relied upon to provide advice that is broadly consistent with the pre-existing policy objectives and commitments of the regime and who are likely to acquiesce with a technocratic or decisionist portrayal of decision-making.

Edward Shils argued, for example, that:

> Advisors are too frequently chosen not so much because the legislators and officials want advice as because they want apparently authoritative support for the policies

they propose to follow. It is obvious that in complying with these desires, the legislators and officials are in collusion with scientists to exploit the prestige that scientists
have acquired for objectivity and disinterestedness.

(Shils 1987)

Sheila Jasanoff, on the other hand suggested a rather more subtle analysis
when she argued that: '... scientific advice is merely a thin disguise for the
transfer of policy authority to experts' (Jasanoff 1990, p. 230). On that account,
rather than policy-makers using decisionism as a veil for covertly recycling
preferred policies through carefully selected scientists, policy-makers may use
decisionist rhetoric to sidestep their proper responsibilities, by handing them
over to expert advisors.

While much of the academic science policy community has, in effect,
ridiculed and abandoned both the technocratic and decisionist models as useful
representations of how policies actually have been and are being made, orthodox decisionist policy-makers continue to argue that science and policy need
more effectively to be separated from each other. Many scholars, by contrast,
have argued that science and policy need to be more explicitly and effectively
interrelated.

The co-evolutionary model of science and policy-making

Key elements of a co-evolutionary model of science and policy-making were
already present in the 1983 text of the US NRC's Red Book since it did not
represent risk assessments as if they were purely scientific; the report's authors
saw risk assessments as hybrid constructs. Moreover, numerous regulatory policy
analysts and sociologists of science have documented ways in which social,
economic, political and cultural considerations have influenced the agendas,
deliberations and conclusions of official scientific advice on risk issues (Levidow
et al. 1997; Jasanoff and Wynne 1998; Millstone et al. 1999; Abraham 1993;
Castleman and Ziem 1998; van Zwanenberg and Millstone 2000; Huff 2002).

As Jasanoff has remarked:

Although pleas for maintaining a strict separation between science and politics
continue to run like a leitmotif through the policy literature, the artificiality of
this ... can no longer be doubted. Studies of scientific advisors leave in tatters the
notion that it is possible, in practice, to restrict the advisory process to technical issues
or that the subjective values of scientists are irrelevant to decision making.

(Jasanoff 1990, p. 230)

Accepting that premise entails abandoning both the technocratic and
decisionist models (in both versions) and indicates an alternative approach.

That alternative, which we call a 'co-evolutionary model' of science in policy-making is graphically represented by Figure 2.5.

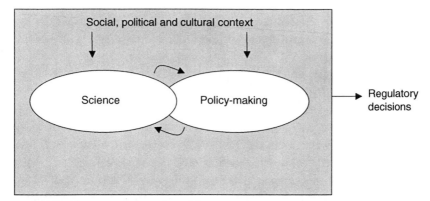

Figure 2.5 The co-evolutionary model.

The key features distinguishing this model from its antecedents are that it represents scientific deliberations as located in particular contexts, which may have both policy and broader social dimensions. The model is predicated on the assumption that those contexts can affect the content and direction of those deliberations. Consequently representations of risks are assumed to be hybrid judgements constructed out of both scientific and non-scientific considerations, even if they may be presented as if they were purely scientific.

The suggestion that the social, economic, political and cultural contexts in which scientists work could influence the content and outcome of their researches and deliberations has a long history, going back especially to scholars including Marx, Durkheim, Weber and Mannheim, but that idea only became popular with British and American scholars since the mid-1980s. An important step forward was taken when scholars provided a general characterisation of some of the more important ways in which non-scientific considerations influenced the content and outcome of scientific work. Advocates of this model, such as Wynne and Jasanoff, have argued that one of the main ways in which non-scientific considerations influence scientific deliberations is by providing framing assumptions that shape the ways in which science is conducted and constructed; moreover those framing assumptions are often taken for granted and unacknowledged.

The concept of a 'framing assumption' was introduced by the sociologist Erving Goffman, who used it to characterise the implicit underlying features of the world view of individuals or social groups (Goffman 1974). Many science policy analysts and sociologists of science have subsequently developed and applied that concept more broadly. It is often used to refer not just to underlying beliefs about the world but also to a broader set of what might be called framing conditions that influence the production of scientific claims and results. In what remains an exciting vital topic of empirical research they have tried to explore how far it is possible to identify and explicate various framing conditions, and the commitments and practices that flow from them.

One of the ways in which framing conditions influence scientific delibera-tions concerns the scope of those scientific deliberations. There are compelling a priori arguments implying that the deliberations of scientific advisors must always be circumscribed within some boundaries defined, in effect, by assumptions about the extent and limits of their agenda. A considerable body of empirical evidence also demonstrates that, in science-based risk debates, one of the main reasons why different groups of experts reach different conclusions is because they adopt or are subjected to different framing assumptions about the categories of risks that they address and those that they discount or ignore.

For example, in the USA, risk assessments of the commercial cultivation of genetically modified crops, in the mid- to late-1990s, only counted as an adverse effect those environmental changes that could harm the commercial prospects of US farmers, whilst in Europe, the scope of risk assessments of the same crops also included effects on flora and fauna that could disrupt the non-agricultural environment. (House of Lords 2000). A few years later, the scope of scientific deliberations in both jurisdictions had widened, in response to pressure from environmental and scientific groups, for example, to include not just direct and short-term effects but also some indirect and long-term effects.

Other ways in which framing conditions influence scientific deliberations include the shape of regulatory institutions' research agendas (and thus the kinds of evidence available and unavailable for subsequent risk assessments), the choice of benchmarks against which risks are measured, choices about the definition and selection of the policy options that are subject to scientific assessment, and choices about the criteria against which those options are evaluated, (Levidow et al. 1997; Stern 1991; Stirling 1999) Such choices are not in themselves issues that scientific information can resolve, although they do shape the conduct of subsequent scientific deliberations and risk assessments.

Scholars have also argued that framing conditions and assumptions can and do influence what frequently appear to be, and are almost always represented as, solely evidence-based decisions. Brian Wynne (1995) has argued that when expert advisors make indicative assertions about the existence and magnitude of certain types of risks, their claims typically depend on, usually tacit, assumptions about the behaviour of the social institutions within which those risks are manifest. For example, expert assessments of nuclear reactor safety are predicated on the assumption that the quality of manufacture, maintenance, operation and regulation are high and will persist long into the future. While those kinds of commitments might sometimes be justified, they are not always so, and they are conditional social commitments rather than scientific premises.

Similarly, choices about which kinds of disciplinary specialities are used in a scientific assessment, the kinds of models that are invoked, the ways in which evidence is selected or discounted and the manner in which research is reported and challenged may not be purely scientific (Jasanoff 1987a; van Zwanenberg and Millstone 2000). For example, during a scientific assessment assumptions are typically invoked about the kinds of knowledge claims that are taken for granted and assumed to be correct, and those that are candidates for a critical assessment. The fact that some claims are taken for granted does not mean that they too can never be the subject of critical assessment. For instance, expert advisors often make judgements about the magnitude and significance of possible risks by relying on extrapolative or quantitative models. Historically it has been observed that scientific risk assessors have often treated their models as if they were unproblematically reliable. Toxicologists often assume, for example, that laboratory mice and rats can provide reliable models of the possible effects of chemicals on humans. The established experimental methods and extrapolative models are, however, based on a host of assumptions, for example, about the differences and similarities between small groups of genetically homogenous rodents exposed to large quantities of a single chemical and a large heterogeneous population exposed to far smaller doses of multiple compounds. Occasionally those groups of experts have acknowledged some of the assumptions inherent in the predictions that they derive from their models, and thus make explicit uncertainties that would otherwise remain implicit, and less frequently they acknowledge the assumptions arising from the differences between their chosen models and alternative possible models.

The issue of how explicit or implicit such assumptions are is important for policy-makers, but in this context we want to emphasise that whenever experts are trying to judge the extent and significance of particular types of risks, a line has to be drawn somewhere between what is to be subject to critical assessment and what is assumed to be true, and consequently it may often be possible, and sometimes appropriate, to ask why that line was not drawn elsewhere. In all cases, knowledge claims about risks are always dependent on the truth value of the underlying knowledge claims and assumptions.

Commentators have also argued that framing conditions and assumptions influence the ways in which scientists interpret and respond to *explicit* uncertainties. For example, different groups of experts may make different assumptions about how much (or how few) data are required before specific kinds of inferences can be drawn and conclusions reached. Scientific evidence about risks can also be more or less indirect, and often direct evidence is not available and the only evidence that is available is indirect. Different groups of advisors can make different assumptions about how much reliance to place on different kinds of indirect evidence. Evidence is often equivocal, with different fragments pointing in different directions. Experts therefore often have to make assumptions about how much reliance to place on contrasting types of evidence, some for example qualitative and others quantitative, and some positive and others negative. In each case, those different kinds of assumptions may influence the content and outcome of scientific deliberations, although the judgements that determine the selection of those assumptions may not be purely scientific.

In addition to documenting the multitude of different ways in which framing conditions can affect scientific deliberations (as indicated in the discussion above) scholars have also attempted the – often more difficult – task of explicating the sources of those framing conditions. Some scholars have sought explanations in terms of the social and political interests of individuals and institutions and some in terms of more tacit cultural practices and assumptions, for example as reflected in disciplinary subcultures or in the structure, history and mandates of policy-making institutions. (Gillespie *et al.* 1979; Abraham 1993; Jasanoff 1987b; Wynne 1982) Some accounts have sought to identify framing conditions within the immediate policy and institutional contexts in which scientific activities have taken place, whilst others have emphasised the influences of more general political, social, institutional or cultural phenomena.

Co-evolutionary approaches in practice

Even though, to the best of our knowledge, no country or international jurisdiction has yet operated a science-based risk appraisal and decision-making system that is structured and organised explicitly and overtly in accordance with a co-evolutionary model, remarks that have directly or implicitly endorsed a co-evolutionary approach have emerged in official statement and documents and to some extent in practice too.

We have already noted that the US National Research Council's 1983 Red Book invited a co-evolutionary interpretation. Prior to the publication of that text, in the late 1970s, several US regulatory institutions had developed a series of inference principles that could be used to identify and evaluate potential carcinogens (Interagency Regulatory Liaison Group 1979). The principles were an explicit reflection of the fact that numerous social judgements were inevitably deployed in the production of policy-relevant scientific advice. In the political context of public and occupational health and safety regulation in the United States, those social judgements had been rendered both visible and highly contested (Jasanoff 1987a). With every important regulatory decision subject to legal challenge on the grounds that the regulators had discriminated against the products of the chemical industry, regulatory institutions responded by specifying a number of generic inference principles that they hoped would not be later contested in court (Albert 1994).

Many years later, in 2001, a working party of the Codex Alimentarius Commission, which is the body that, under the auspices of the World Trade Organisation (WTO) and the agreements by which it was constituted sets baseline regulatory standards for food commodities and products that are traded internationally, released a document that attempted something very similar. It developed and articulated the concept of a 'risk assessment policy' to refer to decisions about how scientific advice should be obtained and used and the scope of the agenda that risk assessors are expected to address. The working party defined 'risk assessment policy' in the following terms:

> Risk assessment policy consists of documented guidelines for policy choices and related judgements and their application at appropriate decision points in the risk assessment such that the scientific integrity of the process is maintained. Risk assessment policy should be established by risk managers in advance of risk assessment, in consultation with risk assessors and all other interested parties in order to ensure that the risk assessment process is systematic, complete and transparent . . . The mandate given by risk managers to risk assessors should be as clear as possible. Where necessary, risk managers should ask risk assessors to evaluate the potential risk reduction resulting from different risk management options.

> (Codex Alimentarius Commission 2001, paras 13–17)

Both the draft Codex definition, and the inference guidelines produced many years earlier by US regulatory institutions, are interesting because they implied that risk assessment policies may be either explicit or implicit, although the documents suggest that it is preferable for risk assessment polices to be explicit and documented rather than implicit, and set out by risk managers in advance of expert deliberations on risk assessment.

The legitimacy of broader public views about the definition of risk problems, as well as an acknowledgement that typically risk assessment and risk management decision-making mutually inform each other, has been reflected in a number of other official reports. In the UK the Royal Commission on Environmental Pollution's 1998 *Report on Setting Environmental Standards* adopted a model that had some striking resemblances to a co-evolutionary model (RCEP 1998) and in the USA, the National Research Council's 1996 document entitled *Understanding Risk: informing decisions in a democratic society* argued that risk policy-making should not be understood as a science-driven enterprise but rather as a reciprocal 'analytic-deliberative' process in which all relevant stakeholders negotiate over how the risks are to be defined and dealt with (US NRC 1996). Both documents acknowledged that scientific appraisal is predicated on unacknowledged and non-scientific policy-sensitive assumptions.

The closest to an explicit endorsement of a co-evolutionary model in an official UK policy document came in the report of the Agricultural and Environment Biotechnology Commission entitled *Crops on Trial* (AEBC 2001). This report emerged in the context of a debate about the acceptability of genetically modified crops and its explicit focus concerned how the UK government might respond to the findings of the farm scale trials of several GM crops that were then under way. The AEBC pointed out that previous official statements had suggested that the results of those experiments would provide 'the final piece of the jigsaw' puzzle. The AEBC was partly arguing that the results of the farm scale trials could not by themselves settle all the relevant possible scientific questions, but also that not all the outstanding questions about the acceptability and safety of GM crops were scientific. The AEBC recommended a process of public debate and deliberation, which eventually evolved into the tripartite debate known as GM Nation. The debate had three ostensibly separate sets of deliberations: one was a review of the available scientific knowledge, a second assessed the likely possible economics costs and benefits of cultivating GM crops, and a third stream was public debate. The AEBC's argument was, in effect, that the public debate could, and should, in part constitute a review of the framing assumptions that were guiding the scientific and economic evaluations. The AEBC's approach was therefore in effect predicated on a co-evolutionary model, even if it did not explicitly invoke or endorse such a model.

Our approach

In this book we want to explore in detail whether, and how, the science and politics of BSE were interacting with each other, and how those interactions might have contributed to the problems and crises that ensued. We also want to build on that analysis to indicate more generally which kinds of institutional and procedural changes might be required to provide policy-making structure and processes with greater scientific and democratic legitimacy than hitherto.

We shall approach those issues by drawing on a co-evolutionary understanding of the relationship between science and politics, but in doing so we have chosen to focus on a particular set of questions. First, whilst we have been careful not to overlook significant possible sources of alternative framing conditions, in this book our focus is on the putative links between the deliberations of the scientists who actively participated in the BSE policy-making system and the policy agendas, considerations, structures and practices of the government departments that they worked in and advised. We will also examine the links between those departments and the government's broader policy framework. We have given less attention to the ways in which more diffuse social and cultural considerations may have influenced the appraisal of risks from BSE.

Although a co-evolutionary model suggests that scientific assessments of risks are in practice likely to be hybrid judgements, constructed out of complex mixtures of both scientific and non-scientific considerations, some sociologists of scientific knowledge have suggested that in practice, scientific and non-scientific considerations become so thoroughly intertwined that it may not be possible to disentangle them and it may be that they become ultimately indistinguishable. That is not our approach. One intellectual ambition of this book is to explore the extent to which it is possible, in practice, to disentangle scientific from the non-scientific considerations and to track and document their interactions in the history of BSE policy-making. A further ambition is to identify some of the mechanisms by which non-scientific considerations couple with scientific considerations. While many commentators have argued that scientific deliberations on risks are influenced by their contexts, how those influences operate in practice often remains unclear.

Another intellectual objective is to explore the implications of a co-evolutionary analysis for the credibility of scientific risk assessments and for public policy-making. Given the kinds of interactions envisaged between scientific deliberations and political considerations, what were (and are) the implications, if any, for the reliance that can or should be placed upon the conclusions of expert scientific advisors? If scientific deliberations and assessments are routinely framed by non-scientific considerations what implications does this have for the suitability of scientific advice for specific kinds of policy goals? Do the existence and character of those links compromise the reliability of the scientific risk assessments, and what consequences do those links have for the suitability of the scientific advice for policy-making? Do those links imply that policy-making can never be scientifically or democratically legitimated, or do they indicate that under some conditions those two forms of legitimacy could coexist and maybe even reinforce each other? Those questions are not purely abstract or speculative ones: they have direct policy implications.

Bibliography

Abraham, J. (1993) 'Scientific standards and institutional interests: carcinogenic risk assessment of Benoxaprofen in the UK and US', *Social Studies of Science*, **23**, 387–44.

AEBC (2001) *Crops on Trial* : Agriculture and Environment Biotechnology Commission, London.

Albert, R. E. (1994) 'Carcinogen risk assessment in the U.S. Environmental Protection Agency', *Critical Reviews in Toxicology*, **24** (1), 75–85.

Barnes, B., Bloor, D. and Henry, J. (1996) *Scientific Knowledge: a sociological analysis*: Athlone Press London and University of Chicago Press.

Castleman, B. I. and Ziem, G. E. (1998) 'Corporate influences on threshold limit values', *American Journal of Industrial Medicine*, **13**, 531–59.

Codex Alimentarius Commission (2001) *Draft Working Principles for Risk Analysis in the Framework of the Codex*, 2001, CL 001/24-GP CX/GP 02/3. UN Food and Agricultural Organisation, Rome.

CEC (2000) *Science, Society and the Citizen in Europe*, SEC(2000) 1973, Brussels: Commission of the European Communities.

Dickens, C. (1854) *Hard Times*. London: Chapman and Hall (1868 corrected edn).

Durkheim, E. (1912) *The Elementary Forms of Religious Life*. George Allen and Unwin, London.

Efron, E. (1984) *The Apolcalyptics: how environmental politics controls what we know about cancer*. New York: Simon and Schuster.

Epstein, S. S. (1978) *The Politics of Cancer*. Sierra Club Books, San Francisco.

Gerhardt, C. J. (ed.) (1890) *Die philosophischen Schriften von Gottfried Wilhelm Leibniz*, vol. 7. Weidmann, Berlin.

Gillespie, B., Eva, D. and Johnson, R. (1979) 'Carcinogenic risk assessment in the United States and Great Britain: The case of Aldrin/Dieldrin', *Social Studies of Science*, **9**, 265–301.

Goffman, E. (1974) *Frame Analysis: an essay on the organization of experience*, Harper and Row, New York, reprinted 1986, Boston, Mass: Northeastern University Press.

Gummer, J. (1990) *Hansard* 21 May 1990, Volume 173, No. **110**, column 82.

Habermas, J. (1971) 'The scientization of politics and public opinion', first published in *Technik und Wissenschaft als Ideologie*, Suhrkamp Verlag, Frankfurt am Main 1968, and translated in English in *Toward a Rational Society*, Beacon Press, Boston Mass 1971, pp. 62–80.

House of Lords (2000) Science and Technology Committee, Third Report, HL **38**, *Science and Society*, February 2000, London: The Stationery Office.

Huff, J. (2002) 'IARC monographs, industry influence, and upgrading, downgrading, and under-grading chemicals', *International Journal of Occupational and Environmental Health*, **8** (3), 249–70.

Interagency Regulatory Liaison Group (1979) 'Scientific bases for identification of potential carcinogens and estimation of risks: Report of the Interagency Liaison Group, Work Group on Risk Assessment', *Journal of the National Cancer Institute*, **63** (1), 241–68.

Jacobson, M. F. (1972) *Eater's Digest*. New York: Doubleday.

Jasanoff, S. (1987a) 'Contested boundaries in policy-relevant science', *Social Studies of Science*, **17**, 195–230.

Jasanoff, S. (1987b) Cultural aspects of risk assessment in Britain and the United States. In B. B. Johnson and V. T. Covello (eds) *The Social and Cultural Construction of Risk: Essays on Risk Selection and Perception*, pp. 359–397. Dordrecht and Boston: D. Reidel.

Jasanoff, S. (1990) *The Fifth Branch: Science advisors as policy-makers.* : Harvard University Press.

Jasanoff, S. and Wynne, B. (1998) Science and decision-making. In S. Rayner and E. L. Malone (eds) *Human Choices and Climate Change: Volume 1 – the societal framework.* Ohio: Battelle Press.

Leibnitz, G. W. (1666) Dissertio de Arte Combinatoria. In C. J. Gerhardt (ed.) *Die philosophischen Schriften von Gottfried Wilhelm Leibniz*, p. 200, vol. 7, 1890 p. 2000. Berlin: Weidmann.

Levidow, L., Carr, S., Wield, D. and von Schomberg, R. (1997) 'European biotechnology regulation: framing the risk assessment of a herbicide-tolerant crop', *Science, Technology and Human Values*, **22**, 472–505.

Millstone E., Brunner E., and Mayer, S. (1999) 'Beyond substantial equivalence', *Nature*, **401**, 525–6.

Mounts, G. J. (1980) 'OSHA Standards: the burden of proof', *Monthly Labor Review*, **103** (9), 53–6.

Nelkin, D. (1971) *Nuclear Power and its Critics: the Cayuga Lake controversy.* Cornell University Press, Ithaca, New York.

Nelkin, D. (ed.) (1979) *Controversies: the politics of technical decision-making.* Sage Publications Sage, Beverley Hills.

Robbins, D. and Johnston, R. (1976) 'The role of cognitive and occupational differentiation in scientific controversies', *Social Studies of Science*, **6**, 349–68.

Rose, H. and Rose, S. (1969) *Science and Society.* Harmondsworth: Penguin Books.

Shils, E (1987) Science and the Scientist in the public area, *The American Scholar*, vol **65**, 185–2020

Stern, P. C. (1991) Learning through conflict: A realistic strategy for risk communication. *Policy Sciences*, **24**, 99–119.

Stirling, A. (2003) Risk, uncertainty and precaution: some instrumental implications from the social sciences. In F. Berkhourt, M. Leach and I. Scoones (eds) *Negotiating Environmental Change: new perspectives from social science.* Cheltenham: Edward Elgar.

Turner, J. S. (1970) *The Chemical Feast: the Ralph Nader study group report on the Food and Drug Administration.* New York: Grossman.

US Congress (1958) Food Additive Amendments to the 1938 Federal Food, Drug and Cosmetic Act. Section 409-C-3-A.

US NRC (1983) *Risk Assessment in the Federal Government: Managing the process.* US National Academies Press.

US NRC (1983) *Risk Assessment in the Federal Government: Managing the process.* Washington DC: National Research Council.

US NRC (1994) *Science and Judgment in Risk Assessment.* Commission of the Life Sciences, Washington DC: US National Research Council.

van Zwanenberg P. and Millstone E. (2000) 'Beyond skeptical relativism: evaluating the social constructions of expert risk assessments', *Science, Technology and Human Values*, **25** (3), 259–82.

Verrett, J. and Carper, J. (174) *Eating may be Hazardous to Your Health.* New York: Simon and Schuster.

Weber, M. (1958) *Gesammelte Politischen Schriften,* 2nd edn. J. C. B. Mohr, Tübingen.

Weinberg, A. (1972) 'Science and trans-science', *Minerva,* **10**, 209–22.

Weingart, P. (1999) 'Scientific expertise and political accountability: paradoxes of science in politics', *Science and Public Policy,* 151–61.

White, L. (1926) *Introduction to the Study of Public Administration.* New York: Macmillan; cited in Jasanoff 1990, p. 10.

Wynne, B. (1982) *Rationality and Ritual: The Windscale Inquiry and Nuclear Decisions in Britain,* British Society for the History of Science, 1982.

Wynne, B. (1995) Public understanding of science from S. Jasanoff *et al.* (eds.) Handbook of Science and Technology Studies, pp. 361–388 Sage, Thousand Oaks, California USA.

Chapter 3

The evolution of the UK's agriculture and food policy regimes

This chapter looks back over the last two centuries of British (primarily English) agricultural and food policy-making, to provide a context within which the Ministry of Agriculture, Fisheries and Food's (MAFF) responses to BSE can be comprehended. From many point of view, MAFF's BSE policies might seem puzzling or even bizarre, but from MAFF's perspective they had a recognisable logic to them. To understand MAFF's logic, and in turn the logic of the UK government, it is necessary to understand the historical processes that led to the creation of MAFF, and the development of its internal policy-making culture. BSE policy-making in the UK was always a difficult and complex challenge, but some of the complexity was of the government's own making or it was, at any rate, internal to the institutional structure and culture of policy-making.

BSE, when it first appeared and when it was officially recognised, represented an obvious risk to animal health and a potential risk to human health, but it also represented a threat to the economic interests of the cattle, meat and food industries, and to the reputation of the British government. MAFF, which was responsible for BSE policy-making, was supposed to take account of, and to balance, all of those different and often conflicting policy goals. To understand the institutional and policy context within which the BSE challenge was addressed by MAFF therefore necessitates outlining the historical and institutional evolution of both agriculture and food safety policy-making in the UK, as well the development of MAFF itself.

This chapter cannot provide a detailed history of food safety and agricultural institutions and policies in the UK over the last 200 hundred years, let alone analogous histories for other European countries. It will be sufficient, in this context, to describe the main characteristics of the British policy-making regimes, and the main stages in their evolution. The discussion will deal separately with agricultural and food safety policy until 1955 when MAFF was created, after which their interactions within MAFF will be reviewed.

This chapter's central purpose is to provide an explanation of why MAFF developed into an institution that was committed to intervening in agricultural and food markets to support the economic interests of producers while also aiming to adopt as laissez faire an approach as possible to the protection of consumer interests and public health. Our account will also indicate how MAFF routinely used science in support of those commitments.

The evolution of UK agricultural policy-making – 1846–1955

The Repeal of the Corn Laws in 1846 – a watershed

The watershed that marked the start of modern British agricultural policy is the repeal of the Corn Laws in 1846. At least since the Norman Conquest of 1066 there had, from time to time, been restrictions on the import and export of staple grains to and from England, and similar restrictions were imposed by many other jurisdictions. The purpose of those statutes had been to try to stabilise grain prices in what were otherwise chronically volatile markets.

The Corn Laws of Britain also served to protect British producers of staple crops against competition from foreign imports, particularly from France. The rules typically stipulated that imports were permitted only when the domestic price for grain rose to particularly high levels. Similarly exports were permitted only when the domestic price fell below a designated threshold. The abolition of those protectionist measures in 1846 has been widely and plausibly interpreted as a political and economic victory for industrial and mercantile interests over the landed gentry (Woodward 1962; Winter 1996, p. 72).

Burnett has explained that in the period from 1850 to 1874:

> The gloomy prognostications [from agricultural interests] about the effects of the repeal of the Corn Laws were not fulfilled . . . England was not swamped with foreign corn, but in expectation of fierce competition landlords were compelled to introduce improvements which, for a time, made English farming the model for Europe and the world. Improvements in seeds, manures, tools, machinery and breeds of cattle, the introduction of rational methods of land drainage and the application of new methods of communication and the new knowledge of science all contributed to the intensity and efficiency of farming practice.
>
> (Burnett 1979, p. 152)

The more open market for agricultural products that prevailed after 1846 facilitated increasing levels of agricultural imports. In the late nineteenth century, cost-saving technological developments, especially in North America, reduced the costs of producing and transporting food. The introduction of refrigerated ships after 1882, for example, allowed sheep meat from New Zealand to be imported at prices that were competitive with British producers. The increasing importation of foodstuffs exerted downward pressure on food prices.

Even though the final 20 years of the nineteenth century witnessed a severe depression in British agriculture, after 1846 'Agricultural protection was at an end, and for the remainder of the century few mainstream politicians gave any serious thought to its reintroduction' (Winter 1996, p. 72). The interval from the mid-1870s to the outbreak of the First World War was a period of great volatility in the British agricultural economy. To understand why the UK government eventually reintroduced policies to control prices and the production of staple agricultural commodities, the causes and consequences of that volatility need to be understood.

The volatility of unregulated agricultural markets

The market for staple foods is, in several important respects, an untypical market. Historically, unregulated food markets have been more prone to volatility and instability than the markets for most other types of commodities. The supply of foods can vary sharply from season to season, especially in response to the weather. The demand for basic foodstuffs is, however, notoriously inelastic. If the price of potatoes halves, very few people will eat twice as many potatoes. If the price of basic foodstuffs doubles, many people will choose to pay those higher prices and forego expenditure on other commodities or services, especially luxuries. Exactly the opposite applies, for example, to the market for fashion clothes, books and recorded music. If the price of books is halved, people might well buy twice as many books than before, while if prices were to double, sales would decline sharply. Many markets can reach saturation, but food markets are more readily saturated than most, and suggestions of an imminent scarcity of foodstuffs have often provoked panic buying.

In the late nineteenth and early twentieth centuries, unregulated agricultural markets in the UK, US and much of Europe were prone to what economists understandably call the 'bunching' of investment. That phenomenon can be illustrated with what in US agricultural history is known as the 'corn-hog cycle'. If each individual farmer tries to decide which commodities to concentrate on, and invest in, for next season, e.g. by planting seeds or breeding and buying stock, they will typically select that (or those) commodities which then command the highest price(s). When the price of hogs rose, many US farmers moved out of corn and into hogs, only to find by the time their animals were ready for market the price of hogs had fallen and the price of corn had risen. When the subsequent set of investment decisions were taken they were consequently bunched in the opposite direction, driving the cycle round again.

Given the price inelasticity of demand for staple foodstuffs, and the instabilities in supplies, the net result was sharp fluctuations in both prices and supplies, to the distress of both urban consumers and rural producers. The magnitude and consequences of the fluctuations in food supplies and prices have, however, been reinforced and exacerbated by the impact of the high rates of technological change that have characterised the agricultural and food sectors.

With the possible exception of the micro-electronics industry from the late 1970s to the late 1990s, over the past 200 years it has been the agricultural sector that has seen the fastest and most sustained rate of growth in productivity compared to all other major productive sectors. Since the early eighteenth century, technical improvements in, for example tools, seeds, breeds, methods of cultivation and husbandry, harvesting and processing, preservation, storage and distribution have been pervasive and sustained. On average, and over the long-term, the relative prices of agricultural commodities have consequently fallen more rapidly than those of the goods and services for which agricultural commodities are exchanged; the terms of trade have deteriorated from the farmers' point of view. The combination of the long-term deflationary effects of technological change on agricultural prices, in combination with the instability of prices and supplies, meant that unregulated agricultural markets in the late nineteenth and early twentieth centuries were exceedingly volatile.

Even though the dominant policy assumption of government ministers and officials was that intervention would be inappropriate and counterproductive, there often were economic and social pressures on governments to intervene and take responsibility for stabilising agricultural markets. The main events that transformed UK agricultural policy in the twentieth century from a laissez faire regime to an interventionist one were the two World Wars, the inter-war depression and joining the Common Market. The outcome of that process was that by the 1980s, UK agricultural policy, like that in all industrialised countries, was predicated on the assumption that the state had an indispensable role to play in stabilising agricultural markets, food prices and food supplies. Beyond that, however, they still favoured laissez faire.

Agricultural policy in war time

Historians have explained in considerable detail how the exigencies of the First World War brought about an abrupt shift in the framework for UK agricultural policy (e.g. Beveridge 1928; Barnett 1985; Dewey 1989; Cooper 1989). The war disrupted the agricultural economy in Britain in an unsustainable fashion. Army recruitment drew a significant proportion of some of the most productive labourers off the farms, while imports fell because prices on the

Continent were rising sharply and because the risks and costs of marine transportation rose sharply following the outbreak of submarine warfare. By 1915, average food prices had risen by 35 per cent compared to the pre-war level (Beveridge 1928, p. 23).

Initially the Board of Trade, which was an anti-interventionist institution, was given responsibility for ensuring that an adequate food supply was available but in 1916 Lord Devonport was appointed 'Food Controller', an extraordinary title for a regime historically wedded to a policy of non-intervention. Coller and Hammond agreed in their description of the creation of the post of Food Controller 'as a reluctant sacrifice on the altar of industrial unrest' (Coller 1925, p. 1; Hammond 1951, p. 3). The government took the radical step of establishing a Ministry of Food in 1916, although its did not start to have a significant impact on supplies or prices until 1917. (BIFHS-USA Guide 2003).

The new regime, that after 70 years effectively reversed the repeal of the Corn Laws, combined several key elements including:

- a guaranteed minimum price for domestically produced wheat
- a guaranteed minimum wage for agricultural workers
- a freeze on rents for farm workers
- controls on the acreage that could be used for cultivating crops and for livestock, and
- the elaboration of a bureaucracy for the administration of those controls.

In the immediate aftermath of the armistice, the British government kept those controls in place but the post-war depression, which afflicted the economies of Europe and North America, produced abrupt declines in agricultural prices on international markets, and consequently the costs of maintaining the guaranteed minimum price for domestically produced staples rose sharply. That increase in the costs of intervention coincided with a perception in government circles that, in response to the economic recession, government expenditures should fall rather than rise. Under those conditions, the Ministry of Food was abolished and a policy of laissez faire was reintroduced. The kinds of instability that had characterised the 30-year period prior to 1917 rapidly reappeared.

The full panoply of wartime interventions were not reintroduced in the UK until the Second World War, but during the Great Depression the British government was persuaded to intervene partially. The Depression affected farming particularly severely and raised serious questions about the long-term viability of laissez faire agricultural policies (cf. Smith 1990, p. 58). The UK government established several cooperative marketing organisations such as the Potato and Milk Marketing Boards to try to help farmers. The government reasoned that, since the retail price of foodstuffs had declined far less than farm gate prices, a solution could be to try to ensure that the proportion of the eventual retail price that accrued to farmers would rise (Hammond 1954, p. 5). They argued that by enabling individual farmers to co-operate as well as to compete, the decline in their incomes could be halted or partly reversed.

Under Roosevelt's New Deal in the US a complex set of interventions in agricultural markets were introduced to support American farmers, and to sta-bilise food supplies and prices. The Nazis in Germany and Austria did not hes-itate to tell the farmers what they should and should not be producing, nor shrink from imposing price controls. Protectionism was contagious, and so in the run-up to the Second World War, and during that war, food markets came to be managed and directed by the governments of most industrialised countries.

The case for intervention was, however, two-sided. Not only were farmers suffering, so too were urban consumers, especially the unemployed and other poor households. In 1939 Lord Horder, the President of the British Medical Association, explained that:

> A short time ago I was so bold – even so impertinent – as to express the wish that the Ministers of Health, of Agriculture and of Transport, with the governor of the Bank of England, might be locked in a room together and kept there until they had solved the problem of food production and food distribution in this country. This was only another way of saying that I believed the problems of malnutrition, of food, and of poverty in the midst of plenty – that is surely not an overstatement – could never be solved if dealt with compartmentally, but that they could be solved if taken together and dealt with by a long-term policy.

> (BMA 1939, p. 5)

Winter has estimated that at the outbreak 'of the Second World War British agriculture supplied less than one third of its domestic food requirements' (Winter 1996, p. 88). The government recognised the urgent need to intervene in agricultural markets as early as 1939, introducing the Emergency Powers (Defence) Act. The government was able to intervene rapidly because plans had been prepared several years earlier. Burnett estimated that: 'In 1939 the operational structure of rationing was already complete, and plans had been drawn up to create what was probably the greatest state trading organization in the world' (Burnett 1979, p. 323). The system was effective:

> By 1944 there had been, compared with pre-war production, a 90 percent increase in wheat, 87 percent in potatoes, 45 percent in vegetables and 19 percent in sugar-beet: moreover the output of barley and oats had doubled. All this made possible the halv-ing of imported food, from a total of 22,026,0000 tons before the war to 11,032,000 tons in 1944.

> (Burnett 1979, pp. 322–3)

Given the efforts of the German Navy to blockade Great Britain and attack convoys of food shipments from the US, and the shift of labour from farm work to military forces and arms production, that increase in agricultural productivity, and reduced reliance on imports, was both impressive and indispensable.

As Smith has explained:

> As soon as the war started the Minister of Agriculture promised farmers prices which would allow them to respond to the need for increased output . . . Such was the importance [to the UK government] of increasing production that many other aspects of wartime agricultural policy followed from this end. If production was to be increased the confidence of the farmers had to be maintained, and financial incentives had to be provided in order to encourage investment and to change production patterns. The need to increase production also greatly changed the economic importance of agriculture . . . The consequence was that farmers became more important . . . The NFU's [National Farmers Union's] political power was increased in relation to the government because of their centrality which led to changes in the Union's institutional position.
>
> (Smith 1990, pp. 88–9)

In the aftermath of the Second World War UK agricultural policy, like that of many continental European countries, was dominated by a concern to diminish reliance on imported staple foodstuffs and to support farm incomes. Policy-makers were eager to avoid a return to the economic chaos of the Great Depression and governments of all parties enthusiastically embraced the kinds of interventionist policies that had been repeatedly rejected (except in wartime) in the century following 1846. As Smith says:

> It was agreed that a permanent policy was necessary to prevent a return to the instability and depression of the 1930s. The war also created the belief that there would be an even greater strategic necessity for agriculture when the Second World War ended.
>
> (Smith 1990, p. 98)

Since 1945, all governments of all industrialised countries have implemented highly interventionist agricultural policies. The objectives of agricultural policy, and the policy instruments used, have evolved considerably, but the dominant themes of agricultural policy have been the maintenance of farm incomes, and ensuring stability of supply to consumers.

In 1945 UK food and agricultural policies were the responsibility of two separate ministries: The Ministry of Food and the Ministry of Agriculture. The former department was responsible for food rationing and nutrition policy while the latter was responsible for supporting and managing farming. The Agriculture Act of 1947 then formalised the relationship between the Ministry of Agriculture and the National Farmers' Union by providing the latter with an almost unique statutory right to be consulted over agricultural policy. As Carter has argued:

> The British [agricultural] policy community... primarily involves the Ministry of Agriculture, Fisheries and Food and the National Farmers' Union (NFU). It first emerged in the late 1930s and was formalised in the Agriculture Act 1947 when farmers were given a statutory right to be consulted over policy. The members were bound together by the shared belief that farmers should maximise the output and efficiency of their land.
>
> (Carter 2001, p. 176)

In 1955 the two Ministries were merged to form the Ministry of Agriculture, Fisheries and Food (MAFF) (Smith 1990, p. 145, fn 1; Butler and Butler 2000). A defining characteristic of MAFF was that it assumed responsibility for simultaneously promoting the economic interests of agricultural, fisheries and food companies, while also being responsible for protecting consumers and public health. Not only was MAFF confronted by two conflicting sets of objectives, it also addressed them from contradictory perspectives. It approached its responsibilities for agricultural and industrial sponsorship with a fundamental commitment to subsidies, support and an alliance, while it addressed its consumer protection mandate from a premise of laissez faire.

Before exploring in detail how those tensions were managed in MAFF, however, we will first outline the historical evolution of food safety policy-making in the UK, up to the point at which MAFF was established.

The evolution of food safety policy-making in the UK: 1815–1955

For our purposes, the first stage in the evolutionary history of food safety policy-making in the UK could be designated as the pre-industrial period that came to an abrupt end in the second decade of the nineteenth century, in the aftermath of the Napoleonic Wars, with the repeal in 1815 of what were known as the 'Assize of Bread' (Webb and Webb 1904). From 1266 until 1815

> The price and quality of bread and ale were nationally controlled by the system of Assizes, while local inspectors, often acting in conjunction with the guilds, kept watch over other foods. Offenders might find themselves pilloried, imprisoned, dragged on hurdles through the streets, and if still recalcitrant, finally banished from the town.
>
> (Burnett 1979, p. 101)

In pre-industrial Britain the adulteration of food had been extensively, but locally and unevenly, regulated.

The industrial revolution resulted in substantial movements of people from the countryside into the cities. Urban populations provided the embryonic food processing industry with a market, and with incentives and opportunities for increasing innovation (and adulteration) of food products. Nonetheless in the early nineteenth century Parliament decided to dismantle traditional restrictions on both the production of, and trade in, agricultural and food products, giving unrestricted rein to market forces.

A committee of the House of Commons reported in 1815 that it was:

> Distinctly of [the] opinion that more benefit is likely to result from the effects of free competition . . . than can be expected to result from any regulation or restriction under which [the bakers] could possibly be placed.

(House of Commons 1815)

In 1815 Parliament consequently abolished the last remaining residue of medieval food regulations when they repealed the Assize of Bread (Filby 1934; Paulus 1974). From 1815 until 1875 the quality and safety of food marketed in Britain was effectively unregulated. Consumer protection was left to the less-than-tender mercies of the marketplace and there was a marked deterioration in the quality and safety of the British food supply. A new regulatory regime was eventually introduced, however, sixty years later, but only after a lengthy struggle between health professionals on the one hand and industrial interests on the other.

The adverse consequences for public health of de-regulating food rapidly became evident. In 1820 a landmark publication emerged when Frederick Accum published his *Treatise on Adulterations of Food and Culinary Poisons.* The cover of the first edition of Accum's book was illustrated with a skull and crossbones and a biblical quotation to the effect that 'There is Death in the Pot' (2 Kings iv, 40). Accum used chemical analyses to demonstrate the extent and significance of food adulteration. He showed that a large fraction of the industrially processed food and drink products were seriously adulterated (Paulus 1974). For much of the mid- to late-nineteenth century British governments showed great reluctance to accept any responsibility for controlling the actions of the food industry; while representatives of the industry campaigned effectively to discourage governments from doing anything more than the minimum necessary to assuage public outrage.

Eventually, however, local authorities in London concluded that they had to impose restrictions on the food trade, following a long series of scandals involving the fraudulent and toxic adulteration of foods, and in response to a sustained and eventually effective public campaign from the citizenry and from the medical profession. The British government did not act, however, until after leading sections of the food industry had themselves taken voluntary initiatives to provide food products that were significantly more wholesome than their competitors. The Co-operative Movement, which started in Rochdale in 1844, aimed to provide safe and reasonably priced foods that would not otherwise have been available.

In 1860 an *Adulteration of Foods Act* was eventually introduced, but the regulatory regime it established had such a light touch as to be ineffective. It empowered local authorities to appoint public analysts, but did not oblige them to do so, and stipulated that the cost of the analyses should be met by the people making a complaint (MAFF 1976, p. 5). It was not until 1875 when the Sale of Food and Drugs Act became law that local authorities were eventually required to appoint public analysts and local inspectors were empowered to obtain samples for analysis. With those powers, the provisions of the 1860 Act could be enforced. The consequent regime needed, however, to be supplemented progressively to deal with novel features arising from subsequent industrial innovations, but it set a framework that was used for all UK food safety regulations into the late twentieth century (MAFF 1976). The legislation empowered ministers to set regulations, and enabled them to act on such advice as they saw fit, but there was nothing in the legislation compelling them to obtain advice or to take action.

At various stages in the twentieth century, the post-1875 food safety control regime was strengthened and reorganised. In 1925, for example, statutory controls on food additives were introduced, to supplement the controls on adulteration and contamination. Legislation to control the use of industrial chemicals in agriculture and pharmaceutical products in livestock farming was incorporated in the 1938 Food and Drugs Act. The practice of requiring that ingredients be subject to testing and evaluation before being permitted in the food supply was only introduced in 1955 when MAFF was created.

The official regulatory regime controlling food safety in the UK, that developed in the 110 years after 1875, served to partially protect some of the interests of consumers and of the food trade, but mainly in those areas where they coincided. It was in the interests of neither producers nor consumers for food products to be so severely contaminated that they caused adverse effects that occurred rapidly, or were sufficiently widespread and distinctive, that they could be traced back to the products and producer(s) responsible. The scientific understanding of microbiological food poisoning and acute toxicology was sufficient to enable some problems, such as botulism and acute lead poisoning, to be identified and controlled.

What emerged was a regime that focused on controlling those food-borne risks that could reliably be attributed, using available scientific techniques, to identifiable causes. In the absence of scientific proof of a causal link to a specific risk, the regime typically declined to regulate. In such circumstances, the laissez faire approach prevailed. The contemporary notion of 'precaution' was antithetical to that regime. MAFF was a reluctant public health regulator; it imposed as few controls as possible and only in the face of compelling evidence. How that regime developed will be outlined in the next section on MAFF's institutional evolution.

MAFF's policy-making culture and its evolution

Within the structure of MAFF, when it was established in 1955, the agricultural policy division and its concern to promote the interests of UK farming was dominant. By the 1960s MAFF's policy focus expanded to include the promotion of the economic interests of the increasingly powerful food processors, and in the 1970s and 1980s it expanded further to address the interests of the increasingly powerful food retailers, but the interests of consumers were consistently marginalised and subordinated to those of producers (Cannon 1987).

The record of the celebration MAFF organised for its twentieth birthday, and for the centenary of the 1875 Act, is noteworthy for the frequency with which representatives of the food industry celebrated their close working relationships with MAFF. It also reveals that once senior MAFF officials and industrialists had congratulated themselves on producing an optimally safe food supply, a representative of the Consumers Association was allowed to make a brief contribution (MAFF 1976, pp. 219–28). His modest suggestions, such as ensuring that the consumers should be in a position to know what was in the foods they were buying and eating, that pre-packed foods should be date-marked and that novel ingredients and processes should not be allowed unless they had been shown to be acceptably safe, were promptly dismissed by industrialists, led by a representative of Birds Eye Foods Ltd (MAFF 1976, pp. 228–30). The Birds Eye representative instead issued a passionate warning about the dangers inherent in increased collaboration between 'consumerists' and the media who would publish food safety scare stories instead of reassuring the public about how safe their food really was. In his defence, the representative of the Consumers Association explained that he was a member of the Conservative Party, and that from the point of view of the consumer movement he was not adopting a radical perspective. Although he had drawn attention to the limitations of the available scientific knowledge, he had not even suggested that consumer representatives should be included in the membership of expert advisory committees, nor that all the scientific evidence should be in the public domain.

By the mid-1970s MAFF had become a department that saw its primary role as helping British farmers, food processors, distributors, retailers and commercial caterers to thrive economically. In 1993, the Secretary of State for Agriculture,

Fisheries and Food (Mrs Gillian Shephard) addressed the Guild of Agricultural Journalists. She emphasised the fact that 'MAFF is a trade department ... our usefulness depends crucially on the practical support we can give to our industries' (MAFF 1993). She was not articulating a novel approach but merely acknowledging a fact that had obtained for forty years.

MAFF ministers and officials routinely worked very closely with representatives of the National Farmers Union, and the trade associations representing the food industry, and with representatives from companies in the food and chemical sectors. MAFF's relations with consumers and their representatives were, however, never close. The close relationship between MAFF and its client industries was conducted, not just discreetly, but covertly.

The policy-making culture that prevailed in MAFF in the mid-1980s when BSE emerged was one that saw its primary responsibilities as focussed towards the Department's agricultural and industrial clientele. MAFF and its client industrial sectors almost invariably saw themselves as jointly and severally providing consumers with a food supply that was not just 'acceptably safe' but unproblematically safe. Consumers and their representative organisations were seen either as irrelevances or as irritants but not as constituents or as collaborators. MAFF and its client industries became increasingly dependent upon each other their to legitimate their activities and decisions.

A reluctant and minimalist regulator

One of the key characteristics of the tightly knit, producer-oriented, food policy community was a general reluctance to regulate or to tighten existing controls. If controls were unavoidable, the preferred option was for self-regulation on the part of the industry. If state regulation was inevitable, the preference was always to regulate in ways that involved as little disruption to commerce and industry and the use of as few internal resources as possible.

The reluctance to regulate affected a very wide range of policies, but in this context the evolution of pesticides policy can provide an illustration (van Zwanenberg 1996). Before the Second World War, pesticide products could be sold without any prior approval. The post-war period saw a rapid expansion in the use of new synthetic chemicals in both industry and agriculture and this provoked a scientific and public debate about the safety of those compounds. Several agricultural workers had been killed using herbicides during the 1940s and numerous instances of non-fatal poisonings had also been reported (Bidstrup 1950; Gilbert 1987). Questions about the safety and toxicity of pesticides were being asked, both by scientists and by consumers and their representative organisations (Mellanby 1951; Crouch 1988, pp. 111–15).

As early as 1952, a working party of the Ministry of Agriculture and Fisheries (MAF) reported that the pesticide industry was willing to move to a mandatory form of regulation (PRO MAF 130/61). It recommended: '. . . [t]hat Departments should take statutory powers to call for the registration and licensing of all chemicals that are introduced and offered for sale as substances which protect agricultural products from disease and pests' (PRO MAF 130/61). That proposal alarmed the Department's officials. Some argued that statutory registration was unjustified while others insisted that 'it has not been necessary to take [statutory] powers in this country because trade organisations have a highly developed sense of social responsibility' (PRO MAF 130/61). Ministry of Health officials shared MAF's view, arguing that a statutory body would be 'embarrassing' (PRO MH 55/1069). Officials realised that the introduction of a statutory regime might reveal how little was known about the toxicity of those compounds.

Although a majority of members of the working party felt that 'a clear case for statutory powers had been made' the chairman agreed to amend the conclusions after consultation with the officials, so that by April 1953 the working party's draft report included a compromise (PRO MH 55/1069). It recommended merely that a voluntary notification scheme should be established (PRO MH 55/1069). This provides an illustration of a more general pattern: it is an example of the department persuading an expert committee to provide the kind of advice it had already decided it wanted to receive.

Little action was taken until after MAFF had been established in 1955. It took until 1957 before a voluntary notification scheme – later known as the Pesticides Safety Precautions Scheme (PSPS) – was introduced by the leading firms in the sector. In 1985, statutory controls were eventually introduced at the insistence of the European Community but during the 28 years prior to that date, pesticide regulation relied on the voluntary compliance of the industry. The PSPS's non-statutory basis meant that there were no legally based procedures, standards, requirements or criteria for decision-making, thus ensuring unrestricted administrative discretion and no interference from Parliament or other forms of oversight (van Zwanenberg 1996). In practice, small groups of officials in the technical secretariat decided the vast majority of cases, and did so rapidly, in confidence, on the basis of very small amounts of data from few studies that were relatively insensitive. MAFF also depended on the good will of the industry to provide the data the officials requested and to ensure compliance with the scheme. An unsuccessful attempt was made by the government's expert advisory committee on pesticides in the 1960s to ask the Government to put the scheme on a statutory footing, and the reasons why the committee did so was because evasions of the scheme by the pesticides industry could not be controlled (Department of Education and Science 1967).

MAFF's reluctance to regulate was evident in numerous other fields, but in this context one further example might suffice. On 5 March 1996, just 15 days before the BSE crisis of 20 March 1996 exploded, the Secretary of State at MAFF, Douglas Hogg issued a press release to assert that the agricultural and food biotechnology industries must not be 'over-regulated' (MAFF 1996). When that statement was issued, however, there was no requirement that food products sold in the UK containing ingredients derived from genetically modified sources should be labelled to indicate their presence, no toxicological or immunological impact studies had been conducted and studies of possible environmental impacts had been few, rudimentary and superficial.

Senior officials in MAFF, and other UK government departments, often claimed that the main advantage of the British approach, when compared for example to that in the US, was that it was 'flexible' and could consequently be far more responsive to new information than would be possible in a more open, accountable and rule governed regime (MAFF 1976). We will be subjecting this claim to a careful and detailed empirical assessment.

Industrial and commercial bias

Under British legislation it was often unlawful for the public, independent analysts or scholars to know, even less to document, how regulatory decisions were reached. What evidence does exist indicates that regulatory processes and outcomes were very congenial to the farming, agriculture and food industries, but far less so to consumer and occupational interests (Lang *et al.* 1988). Again, the evolution of pesticides policy can provide an illustration.

All important decisions taken under the PSPS, for example, were negotiated between the pesticide companies and the ministry. Representatives of consumer, environmental or public health groups were not involved. The PSPS scheme was not government regulation of the pesticide industry, it was industrial self-regulation under the sympathetic gaze of government officials who obligingly administered the scheme. There is very little evidence that considerations of the occupational health and safety of those manufacturing and handling pesticides, or protecting the environment or public health had much influence (van Zwanenberg 1996).

One important feature of the PSPS that was especially congenial to the pesticide companies was the understanding between the government and the companies that all the information that the companies supplied would remain confidential, unless the companies chose to publish their data. Another was that the information requirements were not too onerous. As James Bates, a senior member of MAFF's pesticide division, said in 1978: 'Unreasonable demands [for product and toxicological data] could lead to a break in the *essential mutual trust* between government and industry' (Bates 1978, p. 174, emphasis added). That remark indicates the closeness and interdependence that prevailed between MAFF and its client industries.

The approach adopted by MAFF towards the regulation of pesticides was not untypical. MAFF saw itself as working primarily for, and closely with, UK producers and distributors of food and food products. In 1975, MAFF officials could persuasively insist that, along with the USA, the UK food and agricultural policy system was 'as liberal as any . . . in the world in encouraging new technology . . . [and that its expert advisory committees were] . . . far from wanting to inhibit new developments' (MAFF 1976, p. 17). There is a substantial body of literature documenting in detail the process by which the National Farmers Union came to play a forceful role in MAFF's policy-making processes, but MAFF also became extraordinarily close to the leading representatives of the British food processing, retail and chemical and agricultural supply industries (Smith 1990; Winter 1996; Cannon 1987).

When celebrating with MAFF the centenary of the 1875 Act, a representative of the Food Manufacturers' Association emphasised the longstanding close working relationship between the food industry and senior MAFF officials (Lawton 1976, p. 14). The Products Director of Rowntree Mackintosh Ltd, one of the UK's leading manufacturer of confectionery, remarked that he had spent 'many happy hours' with MAFF officials and that 'By and large my particular sector of the food industry is happy with our relation with the ministry' (Colquhoun 1976, p. 19). An Under-Secretary at MAFF explained that 'the consultation we [MAFF] have with the food industry . . . is in almost permanent session' (Giles 1976, p. 19) which suggests that policies were being negotiated between MAFF and the food industry rather than being decided by MAFF following consultation with all interest parties. The close alliance of MAFF and industry routinely, jointly and severally represented its agreed regime as both science-based and good for consumers. From that perspective, any one who dissented from that consensus could be discounted as unscientific and unhelpful.

The food and agricultural policy regime into which BSE emerged in the mid-1980s was therefore a seemingly robust alliance between the productive sector and the public policy-makers, ostensibly stabilised by sound science. The policy community, and the networks of which it was comprised, saw themselves as serving a common set of interests. They also shared a common set of beliefs, including many about the nature and acceptability of possible risks from routine practices, and most of the participants in that community routinely represented their beliefs and judgements as sound science. That community, and the policy regime that it produced and sustained, took full advantage of the rules of official secrecy to ensure that it remained unaccountable and shielded from public scrutiny. Parliamentary scrutiny was consequently insubstantial and judicial oversight was non-existent.

Food hygiene: a role for the Department of Health (DoH)

While MAFF took direct responsibility for almost all food and agricultural policy issues, the Department of Health had an abiding responsibility for some important aspects of food hygiene and microbiological food safety. The DoH was the lead department with responsibility for public health, and therefore for dealing with bacterial and viral contamination of the food supply that posed a risk to human health.

The relationships between MAFF and the DoH involved drawing some fine and problematic lines. The term 'zoonosis' is used to refer to animal diseases that can be transmitted to humans; to a first approximation the DoH was responsible for protecting public health from zoonoses. Zoonoses include familiar pathogenic microbial contaminants such as *salmonella, botulism, listeria,* and *E.Coli.* If an infection afflicts agricultural livestock but not human beings then it is not a zoonosis, but is categorised rather as a 'veterinary disease', which entailed that the responsibility for its control fell on MAFF, not the DoH. BSE was problematic precisely because when it emerged there was no way of being sure if, or reaching agreement as to whether, it could afflict human beings as well as cattle. With a small number of diseases that could be passed from animals to humans, but without provoking any symptoms in humans, their categorisation was problematic, and the locus of departmental responsibility was correspondingly ambivalent.

The arrangements between MAFF and the DoH were not always clear or friction-free. MAFF had responsibility for all aspects of the production and supply of milk as well as on-farm aspects of meat production and meat hygiene in slaughterhouses, but responsibility for monitoring and enforcement of meat hygiene standards in meat cutting and processing plants was assigned to local authority public health departments, which until 1974 were led by medical officers of health who were in turn employed by and accountable to the DoH. The DoH's Public Health Laboratory Service (PHLS) provided a national network that was responsible for diagnosing outbreaks of food poisoning, and public health doctors were responsible for disease control, but DoH had no control over agricultural hygiene.

The lines of responsibility were blurred, in part because until April 1995 when the Meat Hygiene Service was established, the local authorities' enforcement officials were subject to monitoring by the State Veterinary Service (SVS), which in turn was part of MAFF, and which was supposed to provide advice to the local authority officials on how the standards were to be interpreted. The Meat Hygiene Service was created in part to diminish the ambiguities in the lines of responsibility, but also to facilitate compliance by the UK with European Community rules on hygiene and inspection.

Science and expertise

MAFF and the DoH drew on two sources of scientific expertise: their internal scientific resources and a network of external advisory committees. The former were members of what was then deemed to be a distinct category namely the 'scientific civil service' (Gummett 1980). The scientific civil servants were, in the UK, employed on a separate, and subordinate, set of grades to the remainder who comprised the 'administrative civil service'. During the 1950s and 1960s this group of officials operated at some remove from their administrative colleagues, with relative autonomy. One of the most senior scientific civil servants in MAFF was the Chief Veterinary Officer (or CVO).

During an outbreak of Foot and Mouth Disease in 1967–68 MAFF faced its most severe agricultural policy crisis, prior to the emergence of BSE. It is ironic that although the Committee of Inquiry, which retrospectively evaluated MAFF's response to the crisis, was critical of many aspects of MAFF's handling of the crisis, it was seen within the Department as having been a major triumph for the CVO (*Report of the Committee of Inquiry on Food and Mouth Disease* 1969). The institutional memory within MAFF came to assume that the CVO had, by drawing on scientific tests and advice, taken appropriate decisions, mobilised the necessary resources and implemented those decisions effectively. The CVO consequently was able to play a central role in veterinary disease policy within MAFF's livestock division and to exercise a degree of authority that many other parts of MAFF found extremely difficult to contest or challenge.

As we explained in Chapter 2, technocratic ideas provided the official rhetoric of much of UK regulatory policy-making. MAFF was no exception – the Department routinely failed to acknowledge that it was taking any political decisions in relation to food safety, but preferred rather to represent itself as a technocratic institution which, in the public interest, made optimal decisions on the basis of a good knowledge of agricultural and industrial science and practice. Since policy-making was dominated by a technocratic rhetoric, and a set of institutional arrangements that embodied that model of policy-making, many policy decisions were represented as emerging from (ostensibly) scientific expert advisory committees.

MAFF invariably portrayed its expert advisory committees as entirely independent of the department and the government. Those committees were typically expected not only to review and evaluate scientific information but also to provide policy advice and specific policy recommendations. Many advisory committees were expected to help the department decide which substances and processes became subject to regulatory control, and they were expected to recommend which products, practices and processes should be permitted and which forbidden. Although the recommendations of the expert committees only constituted advice to Ministers, official accounts routinely assumed that committee recommendations were accepted by policy-makers as providing the necessary and sufficient conditions for decisions.

The scholarly literature on, and evidence about, the role of expert advisory committees in British food safety policy-making (and regulatory policy-making more generally) is surprisingly thin. Most, although by no means all, commentators appear to agree with official claims that advisory committees had a powerful role in regulatory decision-making or they at least assumed that this was the case. For example, Brickman, Jasanoff and Ilgen's classic cross-national study of chemical regulation policy emphasised the role advisory committees played in British policy-making, whilst Irwin noted, referring to a 1983 study of British policy for the control of carcinogens, that 'an almost total reliance was found on expert advisory committees to direct policy' (Brickman, Jasanoff and Ilgen 1985; Irwin 1995, p. 66). While that may have been the official orthodox account, the extent to which policy really was directed by expert committees, and the relative independence of expert committees from government and the immediate political process was, and is, quite difficult to examine, and part of what we want to do in this book is shed light on the ways in which expertise was used within MAFF.

British expert committees historically have lacked transparency and public accountability, proceedings were often not published and the committees were not subject to requirements of due process. None of the scientific analyses undertaken by expert committees in MAFF were subject to peer review. Expert advisory committees often judged dossiers of information that were mainly or entirely assembled by the companies whose products were being judged. Much of the information was the property of the companies concerned, and if the companies chose not to publish it, then the UK authorities would not require publication. Furthermore, the publication of the advice from expert advisory committees to Ministers was entirely at the discretion of the Ministers. Ministers did not always accept the advice of their experts, but when they did not do so, hardly anyone, other than the firms concerned, knew what had happened.

Those practices have hindered documentation and research into the role of science and expertise within MAFF. There is, however, some evidence that expert committees did not always have an influential role in policy-making, nor that they operated in relative isolation from the pressures and influences from government and other stakeholders. For example, in the field of pesticide policy, analyses of pesticide toxicity data and draft regulatory recommendations were provided by MAFF's civil servants rather than its Advisory Committee on Pesticides (House of Commons 1987, p. 61). A senior official in MAFF's Pesticide Safety Division has indicated that the ACP's role was largely one of legitimating the work of MAFF civil servants. In 1998, the official said that:

> I speak with knowing what happens with the Advisory Committee on Pesticide, when they consider all the evidence that had been put up to them by individual civil servants going through a great deal of work. Those civil servants individually are experts in their field, they are top people on toxicology and so forth, but they have to have their findings gone over by an independent body of people and they give essentially a stamp of approval.
>
> (Hollis 1998)

Similar arrangements were reported from other MAFF advisory committees too, such as the Veterinary Products Committee (Lacey 1997).

Hollis acknowledged that it was therefore important to MAFF and its client companies that the members of advisory committees were chosen carefully, and he explained that

> The key decisions are who you put on which committee. Once you have set the Committee up and running, then there is very little you can do about it, because as you know people do not believe what Ministers say, inherently they do not believe what they say, therefore you have to turn to external bodies to try to give some credibility to public pronouncements, you are very dependent therefore on what the Committees then find. . . . Really the key to it is setting up the Committee, who is on it, and the nature of their investigations.
>
> (Hollis 1998)

In practice, there was little to prevent government departments like MAFF from selecting their expert advisors from those groups that shared their assumptions about the desirability of tempering concern for consumer protection with a concern to promote industry, commerce and industrial innovation. The extent to which expert advisors shared those assumptions was very difficult to examine. So too was the extent of the financial links between expert advisors and the industries whose products and processes were being evaluated because it was standard practice not to require expert advisors to declare their interests publicly, and in some case there was no requirement that individual conflicts of interest should be disclosed to other members of expert advisory committees or even to the civil servants who provided the secretariats to those committees.

One of the very few occasions on which light was cast on those links came in July 1987 when The *Guardian* carried a report by James Erlichman of an interview with a senior advisor to the UK government on food and chemical safety (Erlichman 1987). Francis Roe was a member of the Committee on Toxicity (CoT) who also acted as a paid consultant to many of the companies whose products the CoT evaluated. Roe insisted that he was not beholden to any of the companies because he took money from so many of them. Roe explained that 'At any one time I am involved with 30 to 40 companies. I don't feel I need to defend one, to be truthful' (ibid.). When asked why he did not step aside when a topic on which he had an interest arose on the agenda he replied: 'I asked the chairman whether he wanted me to leave the room or not, but the fact is that on many occasions . . . I would have to declare an interest on every item on the agenda' (ibid.).

Powerful evidence that a close relationship routinely existed between industrial companies, civil servants and members of expert advisory committees was provided by Richard Lacey, professor of microbiology at the University of Leeds. Before Lacey became an active critic of MAFF's food safety policy regime, he had been a member of the Veterinary Products Committee that reviewed veterinary medicinal products and productivity boosters such as growth and lactation promoters. Lacey said:

> With major products, everything is geared for the benefit of the company, therefore they [MAFF] organise the people who are on the committee, they are vetted very carefully . . . I recall very clearly about 8 years ago on one occasion a lawyer from MAFF threatened us. She said that if anyone leaked information about this product . . . to any other party, we would be prosecuted using the Medicines Act of 1968, with a likely prison sentence of two years . . . I can't tell you about the safety data that worry me because that would be breaking the law. I should be able to tell you . . . It is in the public interest. But . . . the Minister of Agriculture puts the interests of the drug companies and the farmers before that of the public. The consumer is there for the benefit of the drug companies and the farmers, therefore there is a conflict and the Ministry puts the drug company and the farmers first and the consumer second.

> (Lacey 1997)

Lacey's account reinforces the claim that the tensions within MAFF's policy objectives, and the contradictions in the Department's approach to those objectives, penetrated into the conduct of scientific deliberations on the risks to public health from industrial practices and innovations.

From entrenched complacency to abolition

By the mid-1970s MAFF, and its client industries, had became very complacent about the safety of the UK's food supply. In 1975, when MAFF celebrated the hundredth anniversary of the 1875 Act, and the twentieth anniversary of the creation of MAFF, the Under-Secretary for Food Standards and Subsidies outlined the highlights of the Department's history. On MAFF's behalf, he claimed lineage back to the earliest consumer protection legislation in Britain, in 1266, to control short weight in loaves of bread and the sale of unsound meat. He failed, however, even to mention the 1815 Acts repealing all the medieval controls or the crises that ensued. His simplified representation of history was one that pretended that the adulteration of food had always been a chronic problem before 1875, but never again after that date (Giles 1976, p. 4). He confidently asserted in 1976 that 'Food is now purer and safer than it has even been before' (Giles 1976, p. 14).

By 1975 some senior MAFF officials and many representatives of its client industries believed that food safety regulation had reached what they referred to as 'the point of diminishing returns' (MAFF 1976, p. 16 and p. 229). They took the view that the British food supply was then so safe that any further efforts to tighten regulations to diminish what were already vanishingly slight and therefore negligible risks would impose costs entirely out of proportion to any extra benefit that could possibly be anticipated (MAFF 1976, p. 16). That view was enthusiastically endorsed, indeed it was seen as self-evident, by the incoming Conservative Administration of 1979, under the premiership of Margaret Thatcher. The characteristics of MAFF's approach to food safety policy-making, and its contradictions and tensions, if anything, intensified under the Thatcher administration. Twenty-three years later, however, after BSE and numerous other food safety crises, responsibility for food safety policy-making was taken away from MAFF and given to the newly established Food Standards Agency. Two years later, after the food and mouth disease crisis of 2001, MAFF was abolished.

Food safety policy after the 1979 general election

When the Conservative government came into power in 1979, one of the first decisions taken in MAFF was to abandon a set of draft regulations the Department had prepared under the previous regime to try to prevent the spread of infectious diseases to livestock through the animal feed chain. In the UK, as in many countries, slaughterhouse waste, consisting of those parts of the carcass that could not be used directly in the food chain, was routinely transferred to rendering plants, where the material would be heated and processed to separate out a stream of fat from a solid residue known as 'meat and bonemeal' or MBM. MBM was relatively high in protein and for several decades had routinely been incorporated into animal feedstuffs, especially for dairy cows, pigs, poultry and sheep.

During the 1970s changes had been introduced to the technology used in rendering plants. The traditional method was a batch process that involved heating the material to relatively high temperatures for relatively long periods, and then using organic solvents to separate the fat from the solids. The new processing method was a continuous flow process that used less heat and lower temperatures, kept the material hot for a shorter time, and avoided the use of organic solvents. In 1979 the Royal Commission on Environmental Pollution (RCEP) discussed the possibility that these technological innovations might result in pathogens that had previously been destroyed by the more severe methods surviving the newer and less severe processes (Royal Commission on Environmental Pollution 1979). In response, the Labour government proposed regulations setting minimum process conditions in the rendering industry, referring in particular to temperatures and minimum cooking times. Before that decision could be implemented, the 1979 general election occurred and the new Conservative government took office.

The incoming government decided that MAFF's draft regulations were unnecessarily restrictive, explaining that 'in the *present economic climate* the *industry should itself determine how best to produce a high-quality product*, and that the role of Government should be restricted to prescribing a standard for the product and to enforcing observance of that standard' (MAFF 1980, emphasis added). In retrospect, many commentators have suggested that that decision may have played a significant part in enabling BSE to enter the UK cattle herds, and to spread as widely and rapidly as it did. It is not possible to tell, at this stage, whether or not that decision was crucial, but it does indicate that under the Thatcher government MAFF was even more reluctant to regulate than had previously been the case.

The Thatcher government's approach to food safety and food science can also be discerned from several other key decisions that were taken in the years immediately before the emergence of BSE. In September 1982 the Cabinet Office's Advisory Council for Applied Research and Development (ACARD) published a report on *The Food Industry and Technology* (ACARD 1982). That report was prepared by a carefully selected group of food industrialists and technologists. They argued that the food processing industry represented a crucial national strategic economic asset and they argued for increased public investment in research into food technology, to support industrial innovation and competitiveness, and that it should be paid for by a corresponding reduction in expenditure on research into food safety. The proposals of the ACARD Report were accepted and implemented. That decision was in line with MAFF's general policy of trying to raise the profitability of farming and the food industry, without increasing subsidies.

The resulting reorganisation of food safety research included closing the Institute of Food Research's laboratory in Bristol and dismantling its specialist team that had been working on ways of predicting and controlling the transmission of pathogens in meat products (Roe 1989). In the mid-1980s MAFF also proposed to close the UK's only research laboratory specialising in scrapie, namely the Neuropathogenesis Unit (NPU) based in Edinburgh. The only reason the NPU survived is because BSE emerged just before the closure decision could be implemented. In the event, scientists at the NPU played a vital role in identifying BSE as a scrapie-like TSE (Transmissable Spongiform Encephalopathy), and in subsequent research into the disease, because the requisite expertise and resources were not available at MAFF's Central Veterinary Laboratory in Weybridge.

The decisions taken by MAFF not to set minimum conditions on the industrial rendering of abattoir wastes and to reduce expenditure on food safety research were not isolated or aberrant decisions; they were consistent with, and intrinsic to, what came to be called 'Thatcherism'. Mrs Thatcher's political philosophy was predicated on the assumption that, other things being equal, the state should intervene less in market transactions and that the proportion of the gross national product spent by the State should be reduced. The Thatcher government argued that human welfare would be increased if people retained more of their own money and decided for themselves how it should be spent and if the state diminished its interference in the marketplace. Thacherite policy favoured a laissez faire approach to consumer protection, while reluctantly tolerating MAFF's traditional role as protector and promoter of Britain's farmers. It also insisted that the best way to protect consumers was not to impose regulations but by encouraging competition. Stigler, for example, argued similarly that

> The leading protector of the exploited classes is the businessman's competitors. I need not be well informed, because if anyone seeks to profit by my ignorance, his efforts will merely arouse his rivals to provide the commodity at a competitive price.

(Stigler 1975, p. 12)

When John Gummer was Secretary of State of MAFF he insisted that: 'Market forces play a major part in winnowing out what people do not want and what they know is not good for them. The common sense of the consumer should never be underestimated' (MAFF 1989b). The approach of the Thatcher government was to avoid introducing new regulations and, as far as possible, to dismantle existing regulatory controls and to reduce public expenditure. Shortly after Thatcher came to power Hencke reported that 'The Ministry of Agriculture wants to curb the "excessive zeal" of work monitoring food standards and no longer be responsible for standards in food hygiene' (Hencke 1979). Those aspirations were not just consistent with, but an intentional expression of, the Prime Minister's political philosophy.

Food scandals in the 1980s

During this period, and throughout the entire food sector from the agricultural supply trades to the food retailers and caterers, the introduction and diffusion of technological innovations continued apace. Consequently the amounts of fertilisers, insecticides, herbicides, fungicides, hormones and antibiotics used in farming rose rapidly alongside the rise in the frequency and severity of bacterial infections. Similarly the scale and sophistication of food processing increased, with ever-greater quantities of food additives, as well as increases in the opportunities for, and consequences of, cross-contamination. Food supplies and diets changed rapidly, and in ways that made them less, rather than more, healthy. Increasing quantities of fats and sugars were consumed, as the food processing industry responded to opportunities provided by the ready availability of subsidised fats, sugars and proteins from the surpluses generated under the Common Agricultural Policy.

Starting in the early 1980s, a series of concerns were raised about the adverse effect of those changes in farming, food processing and retailing on public health (Lang 1997). Nutritionists, public health clinicians, toxicologists, microbiologists and science policy specialists as well as consumer and environmental campaigners were increasingly focusing on issues of nutrition, chemical food safety and microbiological contamination. They articulated a set of arguments concerning both the scientific and political aspects of food quality and safety. They argued that the quality and safety of both food and diets in the UK had deteriorated, and was deteriorating, and that more rather than less regulation was appropriate. They often argued that the main reason why policies needed changing was because MAFF had subordinated the health and well-being of consumers to the economic interests of farmers, the agricultural supply trade, and to the food processing and retail industries.

The first food scandal of the 1980s in the UK concerned nutrition and erupted in 1983 (Walker and Cannon 1984; Lang 1997, pp. 239–40). In 1979 the outgoing Labour government had convened a body that came to be known as the National Advisory Committee on Nutrition Education – NACNE. NACNE was set up as a hybrid body consisting of nutritionists and epidemiologists, as well as civil servants from MAFF and the Department of Health, plus representatives of the food and beverage industries. NACNE was supposed to reach a consensus but agreement amongst the entire group was never reached. As Walker and Cannon explained:

> The 'conflicting advice' offered within NACNE at its first meeting was not because doctors and scientists of the committee were in basic or scientific disagreement. Rather the causes of disagreement and conflict were of a political and commercial nature . . . some members of NACNE whose jobs involved protecting the interests of farmers and of the food industry did not readily accept that the British public should eat – and drink – a lot less fat. Fats, sugar and salt are profitable commodities; fresh cereals, vegetables and fruit less so.

(Walker and Cannon 1984, pp. x–xi)

By 1983 the deliberations in NACNE had reached stalemate, although all the independent scientists on the Committee agreed that advice should be issued recommending a marked reduction in the consumption of fats, sugars and salt. Despite the efforts of the food industry and the government, the recommendations from NACNE emerged in *The Lancet* in the autumn of 1983, and were then issued somewhat reluctantly by the Health Education Council as a discussion document (Robbins *et al.* 1983). In the subsequent twenty years British governments have taken very few steps to implement NACNE's recommendations. The policy has hardly changed, but the political and economic price that has had to be paid for that failure has grown considerably.

In 1984 a vigorous public debate on the safety and acceptability of chemical food additives was initiated by two coincidental publications. Hanssen provided the first easily understandable list of some 300 food additives that could be listed on food product labels, and provided a brief résumé of their safety or toxicity (Hanssen 1984). Millstone provided an overarching analysis and critique of the technology, science, and politics of food additives (Millstone 1984). The impact of those publications was far greater than either of those authors had anticipated. The British supermarkets and food manufacturers were besieged with requests from their customers for products that contained fewer, or better still no, food additives. MAFF tried to persuade the food industry not to respond by changing the composition or labelling of their products, but instead to reiterate alongside MAFF that all the additives then in use were both necessary and safe. Large parts of the food industry, especially the retailers, recognised that it was in their interests to respond substantively and not merely rhetorically to changing patterns of consumer demand. Firms responded by relaunching some of their food products after re-formulating them and by relabelling other products with so-called 'negative claims' – proclaiming for example that they were free of artificial colourings and preservatives. MAFF's response was merely to reiterate its orthodox reassuring narrative that nothing was being used that was not both technologically necessary and scientifically safe.

In April 1985 the London Food Commission (LFC) was launched (*London Food News* 1985). The LFC was launched with funding provided by the Greater London Council, and it aimed to raise the quality of the food supply in London and the UK, and to provide a voice and representative organisation for consumers on issues of food and health (Lang 1997).

One of the first documents issued by the LFC was a review of UK food legislation, and it argued that the prevailing legislative regime was too weak to provide consumers with an adequate level of protection (LFC 1985). The LFC argued that food laws were then already out of date, that the resources available to local authorities were insufficient to enable them effectively to discharge their responsibilities and that the government's proposals to diminish the regulatory burden on food processing companies would diminish already weak levels of protection for public health. The LFC also called for the abolition of what was termed 'Crown immunity', which meant that the government exempted publicly owned property such as hospitals and prisons from the scope of the rules that it imposed on others. That exemption was not abolished until 1 April 1992 (MAFF 1990, p. 3).

The LFC, and a penumbra of organisations that crystallised around it, found a ready outlet for their arguments and analyses in the print and broadcast media and they had a considerable impact by raising the salience of issues of food safety and quality on the public policy agenda, even before the first appearance of BSE in 1986. From the mid-1980s onwards, MAFF frequently found itself having to respond to crises about food safety. MAFF then lost the policy initiative, and never regained it.

One of the first television documentaries to examine food safety issues in depth were two hour-long programmes entitled *Good Enough To Eat* – from Thames Television – and shown on the ITV network in October 1985. Amongst other things, the programmes showed film of the production of mechanically recovered meat (also known as MRM) and its use in sausages and meat pies. Within two weeks of the transmission of those programmes a 35 per cent reduction in the sales of sausages occurred. That response was powerful evidence of a lack of confidence in the safety and acceptability of the food supply, and of MAFF's policy regime.

Evidence that there were significant problems with not just the composition of food products but also the microbiological safety of foods, emerged repeatedly during the 1980s. One particularly serious outbreak of food poisoning occurred in August 1984 at the Stanley Royd Psychiatric Hospital in Wakefield, Yorkshire. As Pennington has explained, at the time, 'in 1984 the hospital . . . had

830 patients. Over a third were aged 75 of older and more a quarter had been there for over 29 years' (Pennington 2003, p. 45). In other words, many of the hospital residents were long-stay elderly patients who were especially vulnerable to bacterial food poisoning. The outbreak was eventually ascribed to *Salmonella* contamination in some roast beef that was served cold to the patients and staff. The outbreak led directly to the deaths of 19 elderly patients and acute illness for another 300 patients and staff who survived.

The standards of hygiene in the hospital's kitchen and food distribution system were very poor, and the consequences so serious that an inquiry was held. As Deer reported:

> As the inquiry heard . . . Rats and cockroaches thrived in the hospital's cavernous kitchen. Food was sent to patients mouldy and open drains were left to fester. On wards, patients were left at night with no nursing supervision. And such was the record-keeping that doubts were raised last week over how many inmates there were. For years, environmental health officers had been warning the hospital that its kitchen and staff practices posed a threat to patients. But managers either took no notice or felt that they were unable to act. Nobody appeared to accept responsibility and, during 32 days of hearings, the phalanx of lawyers representing them each contrived to blame someone else.

(Deer 1985)

In that case, regulations had been set and rules should have been followed, but they were not complied with or enforced, partly as a consequence of lack of resources on the part of the hospital and the enforcement authorities. Moreover, the legislation that then prevailed stipulated that, like other government premises such as ministries and prisons, hospitals were subject to 'Crown immunity' meaning that the government's own food rules could not be enforced on those premises. It is not surprising that under those conditions, kitchen hygiene was not a high spending priority in many hospitals.

Problems with the microbiological safety of food were not confined, however to government-owned premises. In 1987 an outbreak of *Salmonella* contamination in a milk processing plant located in Kendal in Cumbria, and owned by Farley, caused food poisoning in at least 63 infants that had received contaminated milk powder. In June 1989, evidence emerged of botulism poisoning caused by contamination of hazlenut purée used to flavour yoghurts that infected 27 people, one of whom died as a consequence (Anon, 1989c). Outbreaks of food-borne infections from *Listeria moncytogenes* in England and Wales more than doubled between 1983 and 1998, carried mostly in soft cheeses and so-called 'cook–chill' products, and the overall incidence of outbreaks of food poisoning was estimated by the Committee on the Microbiological Safety of Food to have risen from fewer than 15,000 outbreaks in 1982 to almost 40,000 by 1988 (Richmond *et al.* 1990, pp. 8–9).

Of all the food scandals of the late 1980s, the one that commanded most public and political attention concerned not toxicological or ecological hazards but the risks posed by the presence of *salmonella* bacteria in eggs and poultry. That became a cause célèbre in part because it resulted in a severe economic crisis for the egg industry and the resignation of the flamboyant junior minister in the Department of Health – Edwina Currie.

On 3 December 1988 Edwina Currie was asked by a journalist to comment of the growing incidence of *salmonella* in eggs. She said, correctly, that the majority of egg-producing facilities in the UK were contaminated with *salmonella*. She did not say that the majority of eggs were contaminated, but that was how her remarks were widely interpreted and reported. Her comment provoked a tempestuous debate during which MAFF and the food industry (especially the egg producers) insisted that their products were entirely safe and wholesome, but it rapidly became evident that British consumers found those arguments unpersuasive; the demand for eggs fell rapidly. Within two weeks Mrs Currie had been forced to resign, mainly because of threats from the food industry that if she failed to resign it would take legal action against the Department of Health for their loss of revenue.

In the wake of the eggs-*salmonella*-and-Currie affair, MAFF was reluctantly driven to review its policy-making arrangements. To discourage the Prime Minister from abolishing the department, and to respond to the criticism that its contradictory remit undermined its ability to meet its responsibilities, ministers decided to introduce a new Food Safety Act and to establish a new Food Safety Directorate within MAFF, ostensibly separated from other divisions with responsibility for sponsorship (Phillips *et al.* 2000, vol. 16, paras 7.12–7.14; *Hansard*, 8 March 1990, cols 1023–32).

On 25 September 1989, the then Secretary of State at MAFF, John Gummer, announced that a new Food Safety Act would be introduced, and argued that once the legislation had come into force there would be 'no compromise on food safety . . . [and] . . . no cosiness with vested interests' (MAFF 1989a). The bill was introduced to Parliament in November 1989, and had received Royal Assent by 5 July 1990 (Arnold 1990).

The Act marginally increased the powers of local authority enforcement officers, for example by enabling them to intervene before unfit foods were offered for sale rather than having to wait until they reached their final point of sale, and to impound entire consignments of food rather than merely overtly unfit portions of those consignments. Otherwise it was mainly a tidying up exercise supplemented by extending the power of Ministers to impose new regulations and to authorise the introduction of technological novelties such as food irradiation and genetically modified foods (MAFF 1989c, p. 5; Anon 1989).

Colin Spencer argued that the main effect of the Food Safety Act was to impose crippling restrictions and costs on traditional niche producers, and do very little to large installations, but also that: 'it [did] nothing to tackle food contamination at its source' (Spencer 1991). It also had no impact on the levels of under-investment in enforcement activities and failed to abolish the exemption for agricultural products from the general product liability laws. In other words, it maintained the arrangement under which farmers were insulated from legal obligations not to harm their customers that applied to all other productive sectors (Lang, Lobstein and Miller 1989).

At a seminar to review the provision of the Food Safety Act 1990, organised by Bradford University's Food Policy Unit, Richard Lacey also argued that the Act would make no difference whatsoever to BSE policy-making, and asserted that his calculations suggested that there was a 60 per cent probability that human cases of BSE would emerge in 1996 – a remarkably prescient calculation (Spencer 1991).

When those internal changes were made in MAFF, Gummer, then the Departmental Secretary of State was challenged to explain how the new Directorate would differ from the predecessors, and to indicate what difference it would make. Gummer's response, given to the Guild of Food Writers in February 1990, was to assert that the consequences of the institutional changes in MAFF would rapidly become obvious, and that henceforth food safety crises would occur less frequently, and the problems would be less severe. It was remarkable that in July 1990, the then President of the National Farmers' Union, Simon Gourlay, called for the creation of a new food safety agency separate from MAFF, because the Department had lost all credibility (Erlichman 1990). The events of the 1990s and the subsequent abolition of MAFF suggest that Mr Gummer's perspective was then over-optimistic.

The main changes brought about by the 1990 Food Safety Act were to increase the powers the Ministers had to impose regulations; it was in the jargon primarily an 'enabling act'. Giving Ministers greater powers could only make a difference, however, if those powers were then exercised. In subsequent chapters, evidence will be provided showing that the passage of the 1990 Food Safety Act, and the ostensible separation of consumer protection (in the Food Safety Directorate) from industrial sponsorship made no noticeable difference to BSE controls.

In the wake of the eggs-*salmonella*-and-Currie affair MAFF and the entire government was determined that nothing should be said or done that might further undermine the confidence of UK consumers in the safety of the food supply, and Ministers in particular were mindful of the political price they might have to pay if they were to make an injudicious comment about food safety. It was in those circumstances that MAFF found itself needing to make decisions about how to respond to a new problem: one that came to be known as mad cow disease.

Bibliography

ACARD (Advisory Council for Applied Research and Development) (1982) *The Food Industry and Technology*. Cabinet Office HMSO, London.

Adam Smith Institute (1988) *A Change of Government*. London.

Anon (1989c) 'The Food Bill', *Which?*, November 1989, 536–7.

Arnold, N. (1990) 'Are you ready for the Food Safety Act?', *Catering*, August, 10.

Barclay, C. (1996) *Bovine Spongiform Encephalopathy*, Commons Library Research Paper No 96/62, House of Commons Library.

Barnett, L. M. (1985) *British Food Policy in the First World War*. London: Allen & Unwin.

Bates, J. A. R. (1978) 'The control of pesticides in the United Kingdom', *Biotrop, Special Publication* 7, 165–79.

Bernstein, M. H. (1955) *Regulating Business by Independent Commission*. Princeton, NJ: Princeton University Press.

Beveridge, W. (1928) *Food Control*. Oxford: Clarendon Press.

Bidstrup, P. L. (1950) 'Poisoning by organic insecticides', *BMJ*, vol 2, 548–51.

BIFHS-USA Guide British Isles Research (2003) http://www.rootsweb.com/~bifhsusa/admhist.html

Boyd Orr, J. (1936) *Food, Health and Income: a report on a survey of Adequacy of Diet in relation to income*. London: Macmillan.

Brickman, R., Jasanoff, S. and Ilgen, T. (1985) *Controlling Chemicals: The Politics of Regulation in Europe and the USA*. Ithaca, NJ: Cornell University Press.

BMA (1939) *Nutrition and Public Health: proceedings of a national conference on the wider aspects of nutrition*. London: British Medical Association.

Bufton, M. (2001) 'Coronary heart disease versus BSE: characterising official British expert advisory committees', *Science and Public Policy*, **28** (5), 381–8.

Burnett, J. (1979) *Plenty and Want: a social history of diet in England from 1815 to the present day*. London: Scolar Press.

Butler, D. and Butler, D. (2000) *Twentieth Century British Political Facts*. Palgrave Macmillan, London.

Cannon, G. (1987) *The Politics of Food*. London: Century.

Carter, N. (2001) *The Politics of the Environment: ideas activism, policy*. Cambridge: Cambridge University Press.

Coller, F. H. (1925) *A State Trading Adventure: an account of the Ministry of Food, 1917–21*. Oxford: Oxford University Press.

Colquhoun, J. W. (1976) The development of food legislation in the UK. In *MAFF, Food Quality and Safety: a century of progress*, p. 19. HMSO.

Cooper, A. F. (1989) *British Agricultural Policy 1912–36: a study in conservative politics*. Manchester: Manchester University Press.

Crouch, D. (1988) *A Political Sociology of Toxicology*, unpublished DPhil thesis, University of Sussex, Brighton.

Deer, B. (1985) 'The stark lessons of a scrapheap hospital', The *Sunday Times*, 19 May 1985.

Department of Education and Science (1967) *Review of the Present Safety Arrangements for the Use of Toxic Chemicals in Agriculture and Food Storage*, Report by the Advisory Committee on Pesticides and Other Toxic Chemicals. London: HMSO.

Dewey, P. E. (1989) *British Agriculture in the First World War*. London: Routledge.

Erlichman, J. (1987) 'Food watchdog denies conflict of interest', *Guardian*, 20 July 1987, p. 4.

Erlichman, J. (1990) 'NFU seeks independent food agency', *Guardian*, 3 July 1990, p. 4.

Filby, F. A. (1934) *A History of Food Adulteration and Analysis*. London: Allen & Unwin.

Gilbert, D. G. R. (1987) *Pesticide Safety Policy and Control Arrangements in Britain*, Unpublished PhD thesis, University of London.

Giles, R. F. (1976) 'The development of food legislation in the UK'. In MAFF, *Food Quality and Safety: a century of progress*, pp. 4–21. HMSO.

Gummett, P. (1980) *Scientists in Whitehall*. Manchester: Manchester University Press.

Hammond, R. J. (1951) *Food – Volume I: The Growth of Policy*. London: HMSO.

Hammond, R. J. (1954) *Food and Agriculture in Britain: 1939–45*. Stanford University Press.

Hansard (1990) 8 March 1990, cols. 1023–1032.

Hanssen, M. (1984) *E for Additives: the complete E number guide*. Wellingborough: Thorsens.

Hencke, D. (1979) 'Rolling back the frontiers of government', *Guardian*, 3 Sept 1979, p. 4.

Hollis, G. (1998) Comments to BSE public inquiry. Transcript, day 38 (29 June 1998): 80–1. Available: *http://www.bse.org.uk*

House of Commons (1815) Report from the Committee of the House of Commons on the Laws relating to the Manufacture, Sale and Assize of Bread (1815): Minutes of Evidence, reprinted in *The Pamphleteer*, vol. VI, 1815, p. 162. Cited in Burnett 1979, p. 111.

House of Commons (1987) *The Effects of Pesticides on Human Health*, vol. III, Second special report of the Agriculture Committee, Session 1986–87. London: HMSO.

ILGRA (1998) *Risk Communication. A Guide to Regulatory Practice*, Interdepartmental Liaison Group on Risk Assessment. London: Health and Safety Executive.

Irwin, A. (1995) *Citizen Science: a study of people, expertise and sustainable development*. London: Routledge.

Lacey, R. (1997) Interview with BBC Social Affairs Unit, Broadcast BBC TV, 15 April 1997.

Lang, T. (1997) Going public: food campaigns during the 1980s and early 1990s. In D. F. Smith (ed.) *Nutrition in Britain: science, scientists and politics in the twentieth century*. London: Routledge.

Lang, T. (1999) 'The complexities of globalization: the UK as a case study of tensions with the food system and the challenges to food policy', *Agriculture and Human Values*, **16**, 169–85.

Lang, T. *et al.* (1988) *Food Adulteration and how to Fight it*. London: Unwin.

Lang, T., Lobstein, T. and Miller, M. (1989) *Food Legislation: time to grasp the nettle*. London Food Commission, October 1989.

Lawton, F. J. (1976) The development of food legislation in the UK. *MAFF, Food Quality and Safety: a century of progress*, p. 14. HMSO.

Le Gros Clarke, F. and Titmuss, R. M. (1939) *Our Food Problem and its Relation to our National Defences*. Harmondsworth: Penguin Books.

LFC (1985) *Consumer Protection and Food Legislation*. The London Food Commission.

Linton, M. (1988) 'Think tank urges Mrs Thatcher to abolish four ministries', *Guardian*, 28 March 1988, p. 3.

London Food News (1985) 'We aim to improve London's food' No. 1, Spring 1985, p. 1.

MAFF (1976) *Food Quality and Safety: a century of progress*. London: HMSO.

MAFF (1980) *Proposed Processing Order: Consultation Paper*, 16 April 1980. In C. Barclay (1996) *Bovine Spongiform Encephalopathy and Agriculture*, House of Commons Library Research Paper 96/62, Section II B, p. 13.

MAFF (1989a) Press Release 375/89, Ministry of Agriculture, Fisheries and Food, 25 September 1989.

MAFF (1989b) Press Release 379/89, Ministry of Agriculture, Fisheries and Food, 29 September 1989.

MAFF (1989c) *Food Safety – protecting the consumer.* London: HMSO.

MAFF (1990) *The Food Safety Act 1990 and You: a guide for the food industry.* London: HMSO.

MAFF (1993) Press Release No 350/93, 21 October 1993.

MAFF (1996) *Food Biotechnology must not be over-regulated says Douglas Hogg,* Ministry of Agriculture, Fisheries and Food, Press Release 76/96, 5 March 1996.

Mellanby, E. (1951) 'The chemical manipulation of food', *BMJ,* October 13, 863–86.

Millstone, E. (1984) 'Food additives: A technology out of control?', *New Scientist,* **104** 1426, 20–24.

Nettleton, P. (1989) 'Only science can decide food safety, MPs told', *Guardian,* 30 June 1989, p. 6.

Paulus, I. (1974) *The Search for Pure Food: a sociology of legislation in Britain.* London: Martin Robertson.

Pennington, H. (2003) *When Food Kills: BSE, E. coli, and disaster science.* Oxford: Oxford University Press.

Phillips, Bridgeman J. and Ferguson-Smith, M. (2000) T*he BSE Inquiry: Report: evidence and supporting papers of the Inquiry into the emergence and identification of Bovine Spongiform Encephalopathy (BSE) and variant Creutzfeldt-Jakob Disease (vCJD) and the action taken in response to it up to 20 March 1996.* London: The Stationery Office.

PRO MAF 130/61, Public Records Office, Ministry of Agriculture and Fisheries, file 130/61.

PRO, MH 55/1069, Public Records Office, Ministry of Health, file 55/1069.

Report of the Committee of Inquiry on Food and Mouth Disease – 1968: Part One, 1969, Cmnd. 3999. London: HMSO.

Richmond M. (1990) *The Microbiological Safety of Food,* Report of the Committee on the Microbiological Safety of Food. London: HMSO.

Robbins, C. J. *et al.* (1983) 'Implementing the NACNE Report', *Lancet,* 1351–6.

Roe, N. (1989) 'Swallowed by the market', *Independent,* 19 June 1989, p. 21.

Royal Commission on Environmental Pollution (1979), *Agriculture and Pollution.* London: HMSO.

Sheppard, J. (1987) *The Big Chill: a report on the implications of cook-chill catering for the public services.* Report no 15, London Food Commission.

Smith, M. (1990) *The Politics of Agricultural Support in Britain: the development of the agricultural policy community.* Aldershot: Gower.

Spencer, C. (1991) 'Creaming off the crop', *Guardian,* 1 June 1991, Weekend Section p. 17.

Stigler, G. (1975) *The Citizen and the State.* University of Chicago Press.

Tannahill, R. (1988) *Food in History.* Harmondsworth: Penguin Books.

van Zwanenberg, P. (1996) *Science, Pesticide Policy and Public Health: Ethylene Bisdithiocarbamate regulation in the UK and USA,* Unpublished DPhil, SPRU – Science and Technology Policy Research, University of Sussex.

Walker, C. and Cannon, G. (1984) *The Food Scandal.* London: Century.

Webb, S. and Webb, B. (1904) 'The assize of bread', *Economic Journal,* **14** (54), 196–218.

Webb, T. and Lang, T. (1987) *Food Irradiation: the myth and the reality.* Wellingborough: Thorsons.

Winter, M. (1996) *Rural Politics: policies for agriculture, forestry and the environment.* London: Routledge.

Woodward, L. (1962) *The Age of Reform: 1815–1870.* Oxford: Clarendon Press.

Chapter 4

A new cattle disease

In December 1986, pathologists working at MAFF's Central Veterinary Laboratory (CVL) discovered a new brain disease in cattle. Several dairy cows from farms in the south and south-west of England had died from an unknown neurological disease and brains from some of those animals were eventually sent to the CVL's pathology department for further investigation. Histopathological analysis (i.e. detailed scrutiny of cells taken from the diseased cattle) revealed spongiform changes, or microscopic holes, in the brains.

The discovery of the new disease, later named BSE, gave rise to a very complex and difficult policy challenge. As we explain in this chapter, rising numbers of cases of the new disease were soon diagnosed across the UK, but the paucity of knowledge about the class of diseases to which BSE belonged meant that no one could be sure whether or not humans could be adversely affected. Furthermore, if there was a risk to humans, no one could be sure if that risk was vanishingly slight or potentially catastrophic.

We shall outline what officials and ministers knew, and took the trouble to discover, about the possible risks posed by BSE, and thus the kinds of policy options that they recognised would need to be considered. The overwhelming instincts of both officials and ministers were to avoid perturbing agricultural markets and this was reflected in the absence of any systematic attempt to assess the possible risks, together with efforts to prevent knowledge of the new disease from being disseminated beyond the official veterinary community. This, in turn, necessitated a complete absence of regulatory controls. Amongst other things, those decisions inhibited the detection, diagnosis and reporting of the disease in British herds and impeded learning about the disease and the possible risks.

We describe how agricultural officials eventually responded to an escalating problem, that could no longer be kept secret, by proposing a minimal set of regulatory controls: proposals which were subsequently rejected by ministers. It was in that context that external expert advice was first sought by officials. We argue that the purpose of seeking that advice was not to provide a scientific input to policy deliberations that could not otherwise be obtained from internal scientific resources, but rather to apply political pressure to ministers in order to persuade them to accept a policy proposal – the removal of overtly diseased animals from the human food supply – which they had thus far rejected.

The emergence of BSE

When CVL pathologists first diagnosed spongiform changes in the brains of cattle in late 1986, it was immediately obvious that the pathology closely resembled that of scrapie – a sheep disease that was endemic in British sheep flocks. Scrapie is one of a group of very unusual neurodegenerative diseases, the transmissible spongiform encephalopathies, or TSEs. CVL pathologists were in no doubt that their discovery was significant, and not just because cattle had never previously been diagnosed with what looked like a TSE. When the Head of Pathology, Ray Bradley, informed his departmental colleagues about the initial cases in December 1986, he warned that

> If the disease turned out to be bovine scrapie it would have severe repercussions to the export trade and possibly also for humans if for example it was discovered that humans with spongiform encephalopathies had close association with the cattle. It is for these reasons I have classified this document confidential.
>
> (Phillips *et al.* 2000, vol. 3, para. 1.37)

The Head of Pathology had good reason to be concerned. TSEs were (and at the time of writing still are) untreatable, invariably fatal and very poorly understood. No one had established the identity of the agent responsible for causing the TSEs, but it was clearly quite unlike all other disease agents. TSEs were known to have both infectious *and* inheritable components, incubation periods were measured in years rather than days or weeks and the pathogenic agents are virtually indestructible (Phillips *et al.* 2000, vol. 2, Chapter 2, esp. paras 2.52–2.55). The agent also appeared to be devoid of nucleic acid, which meant that TSEs were inconsistent with dominant assumptions in orthodox molecular biology and especially theories of infections. Viruses and bacteria are living organisms that reproduce using DNA and RNA, but TSE pathogens appeared to be able to reproduce but not by the recognised mechanisms.

A curious characteristic of TSEs is that they do not provoke an immune response in the host (Phillips *et al.* 2000, vol. 2, Chapter 3, pp. 92–94, paras 3.91–3.98). This meant that there was no test available with which to detect infectivity in an animal prior to the onset of clinical symptoms, except an incredibly laborious, expensive and crude approach that involved taking tissues from the suspected host and injecting them into the brains of animals known to be susceptible and then waiting, possibly years, to see whether the recipients subsequently developed a TSE. It was going to be hard to control the disease because asymptomatic animals could not, in practice, be identified nor differentiated from animals that were uninfected. It also meant that TSE research was going to be difficult, slow and expensive.

Prior to 1986, six mammalian species were known to be naturally susceptible to TSEs. Scrapie, by far the most common TSE, afflicts sheep and goats and had been known in Europe since the 1730s (Schwartz 2003, p. 5). The mechanisms by which scrapie was maintained in national flocks were not understood. The disease appeared to transmit vertically, from ewe to lamb, and laterally between unrelated animals. Even unaffected flocks that had grazed in pastures that were previously used by affected flocks developed scrapie, suggesting that there was some environmental vector for the disease (Dickinson 1976). Scrapie had proved extremely difficult to eradicate from countries in which it was endemic and the UK had long given up attempts to do so, despite the fact that many countries refused to accept exports of live UK breeding sheep.

Two much rarer animal TSEs had also been reported. 'Transmissible mink encephalopathy' was first observed in the 1940s in farmed mink (Phillips *et al.* 2000, vol. 2, pp. 23–24, paras 2.16–2.18). Outbreaks of the disease, sometimes killing the majority of animals on a single farm, appeared to be caused by feeding the mink with animal carcasses contaminated with a TSE agent. Another TSE known as 'chronic wasting disease' had also been reported in the late 1960s in wild deer and elk from the western states of the USA (Schwartz 2003, p. 193). It was not known how deer and elk had first contracted the disease nor how it was maintained in the herds.

Humans were the remaining species known to be naturally susceptible to TSEs. One of the human TSEs is known as Kuru, it used to occur within, and was at one time the leading cause of death amongst, the Fore people in New Guinea. Kuru was transmitted by ritual cannibalism during which the brains of deceased relatives were eaten as a mark of respect (Schwartz 2003, pp. 68–72). The best known human TSE is called Creutzfeldt-Jakob Disease (CJD), named after the two doctors who first described the condition in the 1920s. CJD is rare, affecting approximately one in a million of the population worldwide each year, usually in mid to old age. In about 10–15 per cent of cases, CJD appears to have been inherited, but in most of the remaining cases the disease appears sporadically, in other words they have no identifiable cause.

In the late 1980s there were many theories about the nature of the agent responsible for TSEs. Three, in particular, competed for supremacy amongst the small TSE research community: one was that the agent was an unconventional virus (in the sense that it can resist inactivation), a second was that it was an infectious pathogen containing a small piece of nucleic acid, and a third was that it was an abnormal type of protein, known as a prion. By the mid 1990s, several years after the discovery of BSE, the prion hypothesis had become the dominant theory. Prions are normal constituents of healthy tissue but the theory is that prions become pathogenic only once their structural conformations have been transformed. Once aberrant prions have developed, for example if a mutation in the prion gene leads to formation of the abnormal prion, or once they have been introduced into a host by infection, they can somehow trigger similar transformations in the structural conformations of otherwise normal prions, producing a cascade effect, until the aberrant proteins overwhelm the host's brain.

It took only a few weeks for CVL scientists to establish that the new brain disease in cattle was very likely to be a TSE. What are known as 'scrapie-associated-fibrils' – recognised as an identifying feature of TSEs – were discovered in tissue samples from the brains of affected cattle. In the months following the initial identification of the disease, further cattle that had died on farms elsewhere in England were found to have identical spongiform changes in their brains.

By May 1987, five months after the initial discovery of the disease, 6 confirmed cases and 13 suspect cases had been reported (although at that stage no one, not even MAFF's regional veterinary staff, had been told about the new disease and therefore there was almost certainly extensive under-reporting). Three months later there were 10 confirmed and 52 suspected cases of what had then been officially termed bovine spongiform encephalopathy (BSE). By the end of 1987 there were 132 confirmed cases and a further 370 suspect cases. By March 1988 there were 388 confirmed and 600 suspected cases (Phillips et al. vol. 3, Chapter 2).

The majority of the cases were singletons (one per herd) and were occurring simultaneously across the country, but especially in the south of England. Many urgent questions needed to be addressed, including: How had cattle contracted BSE? How was it being transmitted within the national herd? Did the disease pose a hazard to other animals? Crucially, was it transmissible to humans, and if so, how significant were the risks?

Investigations into the possible causes of the disease began in May 1987. Sheep infected with scrapie were recognised as a likely source of infection, but many affected farms did not keep sheep. The CVL's senior epidemiologist, John Wilesmith, eventually discovered that the only factor that was common to all the affected farms was the use of commercial cattle feed. By the end of 1987 Wilesmith was convinced that cattle feed, prepared from rendered slaughterhouse waste contaminated with a TSE agent, was the cause of BSE (Phillips et al. 2000 vol. 3, paras 3.19–3.21) The wastes discharged from abattoirs from sheep, cattle and other animals were routinely rendered into saleable products. The rendering process involved crushing and heating the carcass in order to produce fat, known as tallow, and a solid animal protein residue, known as meat and bone meal (or MBM). Both tallow and meat and bone meal were incorporated into what are termed 'concentrates', in order to provide a protein-rich nutritional supplement to animal feed. The diets of nearly all UK cattle were supplemented with commercial feed, although dairy cows typically received the largest quantities to boost milk yields.

Cattle feed, contaminated with a TSE agent, appeared to be the vector of transmission but CVL scientists did not know the source of that agent. The main suspect, not surprisingly, was scrapie-infected sheep carcasses. There were, however, no precedents for sheep-to-cattle transmission of scrapie, despite the fact that sheep protein had been a constituent of cattle feed for decades. If scrapie was the source of the disease, why had transmission of the disease from sheep to cattle only just been reported, and only in the UK, given that rendered abattoir waste was being used in animal feedstuffs in many countries?

The possible hazard to human health

The most complicated issue for UK regulators was that of establishing the possible consequences of BSE for human health. Familiarity with what was then known about the nature and behaviour of scrapie, and the other known TSEs – which, in principle, was available to anyone willing to consult the existing scientific literature – suggested that there were no easy answers.

As of 1986, all the spongiform encephalopathies were known, on the basis of experimental work, to be transmissible. Transmission of the disease could be demonstrated not only within the host species but also to other mammalian species. In most cases, however, experiments had shown that the infectious dose required to transmit a TSE between species was considerably higher than for transmission between animals of the same species. Furthermore, not all recipient mammalian species appeared to be susceptible to experimental attempts to transmit particular TSEs across species, and not all those species that were susceptible readily succumbed. For any individual TSE, transmission was easier to achieve experimentally with some species and more difficult with others, whilst some species appeared effectively resistant to infection, despite high levels of exposure. Transmission of TSEs between different mammalian species seemed to be limited, by what researchers called a 'species barrier' (Phillips et al. 2000, vol. 2, Chapter 2, pp. 52–54, paras 2.143–2.150).

Although experimental transmission of TSE across species was often possible using appropriate doses and routes of exposure, *spontaneous* cross-species transmission was unusual. Scrapie appeared to transfer under natural conditions from sheep to goats, and farmed mink were believed to have contracted transmissible mink encephalopathy after being fed with the carcasses of other animals infected with an unidentified TSE. As of the late 1980s, however, there were no other known instances of spontaneous cross-species transmission. Importantly, there was no evidence that any of the animal TSEs had transmitted to humans.

In the 1960s, after CJD had been shown to be a transmissible disease, some researchers had suspected that human exposure to scrapie-infected sheep might be the unexplained cause of sporadic CJD. Subsequent epidemiological investigations into the risk factors for sporadic CJD, and of CJD clusters, had, however, failed to identify any association between CJD and exposure to the scrapie agent (Taylor 1989). Epidemiological investigation of very rare diseases is difficult and a link between scrapie exposure and CJD could not be completely ruled out. In the 1970s, US consumer groups had persuaded the US government to ban the sale of sheep meat from scrapie-infected herds on the grounds that a risk to human health could not be entirely discounted (Martin 1998). Nevertheless, by the late 1980s the evidence did not point to any association between the two diseases.

If scrapie did not seem to be pathogenic to humans, it was entirely plausible that the same might be true of BSE. Unfortunately, that was not the only conclusion that could be derived from the evidence. Experiments had indicated that each TSE had its own unique host range and transmission characteristics. The fact that it was not possible, experimentally, to transmit a particular TSE to one animal species did not mean that that species was resistant to all the TSEs. For example, scrapie could be transmitted experimentally to rats but not to guinea pigs, whilst CJD can transmit to guinea pigs but not rats. Such findings, and associated concepts such as a 'species barrier', were empirically determined; they were not based on a clear theoretical understanding of how TSEs were transmitted and why certain species were more or less susceptible to particular strains of TSEs. The fact that scrapie did not seem to be pathogenic to humans did not necessarily mean that other TSEs, such as BSE, would be similarly innocuous.

Scientists at MAFF's CVL suspected, however, that BSE and scrapie might not be different TSEs because a plausible explanation for the emergence of BSE in cattle was that the scrapie agent had crossed the species barrier to cattle, via the consumption of cattle feed containing scrapie-infected sheep protein. BSE might, therefore, simply be 'scrapie in cows' and pose no more risk to human health than scrapie. That was a claim, and a conclusion, that British officials and Ministers were to make publicly on numerous occasions over the next ten years. While both the claim that BSE had derived from scrapie and the conclusion that BSE would therefore behave in the same way as scrapie were by no means implausible, at least until 1988, it was clear to anyone familiar with the scientific literature on the transmission characteristics of TSEs that, even if the scrapie agent had jumped species into cattle, far less optimistic conclusions were also plausible and could not be ruled out.

The experimental evidence, available in 1987, demonstrated that when a species had been infected with a TSE from a different species it could then infect a range of species that the original agent could not infect, and at different doses (Phillips *et al.* 2000, vol. 2, Chapters 2 and 3). Furthermore, if transmission of a TSE between species is successful, subsequent transmission within the recipient species can occur in a shorter time period, dose for dose, as compared to the primary *passage* across species. Experimental precedents for altered host ranges, following passage of a TSE to other species, were well known. For example, human strains of kuru and Creutzfeldt-Jakob disease do not transmit to ferrets or goats unless first *passaged* through primates or cats (Gibbs *et al.* 1979). Once sheep scrapie had been *passaged* through monkeys, the agent no longer produces disease in sheep, goats or mice (Gajdusek 1985). In the absence of a full understanding of the nature and behaviour of TSEs there was no way of predicting, for any given donor species, which recipient species would subsequently be susceptible.

The difficulty in 1987, and for many years thereafter, was that although there was no evidence that animal TSEs could transmit to humans, and in particular no epidemiological evidence that scrapie was a cause of sporadic CJD, one could not conclude that BSE would therefore pose no risk to humans, even if cattle had acquired BSE from sheep scrapie.

The magnitude of any possible hazard

Although no one knew whether or not BSE could, in principle, be transmitted to humans, the significance of any risk, if transmission were possible, would depend on the pattern of human exposure to the BSE agent. It was known experimentally that the ease with which scrapie and other TSEs could be transmitted, both within and between species, varied substantially depending on the route of exposure (Phillips *et al.* 2000, vol. 2, Chapters 2–3). The most efficient way of achieving transmission involved inoculating the TSE agent directly into brain tissue. Inoculation into tissues other than the brain was relatively less efficient. The least efficient way, by about five orders of magnitude compared to intracerebral inoculation, was by ingestion of food containing the agent.

It was also known that the absolute amounts of infected material required successfully to transmit the disease were often extremely small. For example, less than a millionth of gram of sheep brain, from an animal clinically infected with scrapie, contained enough infectivity to transmit the disease to a mouse if it were injected directly into its brain. Thus, for any particular recipient species, successful transmission of a TSE, even via a relatively inefficient route of exposure, might still involve quite small amounts of infected material (Phillips *et al.* 2000, vol. 2, Chapter 3).

The significance of any possible risk from BSE was also going to depend on the level, as well as the route, of human exposure to the BSE agent. Estimating that would require, amongst other things, data on the numbers of animals infected with BSE (and the point in time at which they became infected), the distribution of infectivity over time in different cattle tissues, and the end uses of the various tissues once cattle had been slaughtered. Only the latter information was, in principle, available in the late 1980s.

No one knew, or would be able to find out for some time, how many cattle might have been exposed to, or infected by, the BSE agent because animal feed could not be tested for the presence of a TSE agent and because there was no test to detect asymptomatic but infected animals. The best way of estimating the numbers of subclinically affected animals would have been to have taken brain tissues from a large enough sample of apparently healthy cattle and inoculate them into the brains of other cattle sourced from outside the UK, and see how many subsequently developed the disease. Such experiments would, however, have taken many years to complete.

Knowledge about how the BSE agent spreads and is distributed in different cattle tissues was also going to take many years to acquire. With no test available to detect the presence of a TSE agent in the tissues of a host, what are known as pathogenesis studies are required. They involved lengthy experiments in which various tissues were taken from experimentally infected host animals, at different time periods following initial infection, and then diluted in tenfold steps. Attempts were then made to transmit various dilutions of the tissues to animals known to be vulnerable to infection. The level of infectivity per gram of a particular tissue can be calculated from the lowest dilution sufficient to induce disease in 50 per cent or more of the test recipients.

In the absence of pathogenesis data from BSE-infected cattle, all that could be done was to draw on analogies with pathogenesis studies using other TSEs and animals. Those data indicated that the TSE agent initially spreads and replicates in lymphatic tissues (for example, the spleen, tonsils, thymus and lymph nodes) (Hadlow *et al.* 1982; Phillips *et al.* 2000, vol. 2, para 3.198). It would then spread to the central nervous system, via nerve fibres, where it replicated to high concentrations, or titres, in the brain. Over time the levels of the agent would drop in lymphatic tissue and rise to such high levels in the brain that it caused severe physical damage. Symptoms would appear and the host would invariably die.

Pathogenesis experiments with scrapie and other TSEs had shown that the infectious agent was sometimes present in non-lymphatic and non-neural tissues too, but at much lower levels and less frequently. A study published in 1982 had shown that sheep scrapie could be transmitted to mice, not only by injecting neural and lymphatic tissues into the brains of mice, but also using mucosa, pancreas, liver and bone marrow suspensions (Hadlow *et al.* 1982). The study found the highest level of infectivity in neural tissues where certain types of brain tissue contained 15 million infective units of the agent per gram of tissue. In other words, a 15,000,000th of a gram of infected brain material was sufficient to induce disease in mice via intracerebal exposure. Next highest was lymphatic tissue (including intestines which contain lymph nodes) which contained between 18 and 24,000 infective units per gram, depending on the tissue selected and the time since initial infection. A gram of mucosa contained between 60 and 270 infective units, a gram of pancreas contained 30 infective units, a gram of liver 27 infective units and a gram of bone marrow contained 18 infective units (Hadlow *et al.* 1982). No infectivity had been detected in muscle i.e. in what would normally count as 'meat'.

Most pathogenesis experiments had been performed using mice as the recipient species because they showed signs of disease in a few months, rather than the years typical of larger mammals, and because they are comparatively cheap to use. One problem, however, was that to cause infection in mice the TSE agent had to cross a species barrier. This meant that, when compared to sheep-to-sheep transmission for example, the data on levels of infectivity in sheep-to-mice transmission would be an underestimate. The absence of disease in the recipient mouse meant only that there was no infectivity in the innoculum at or above the limits of detection. It did not mean that infectivity was absent, or indeed that infectivity was not present in sufficient quantities to cause a TSE in a species more sensitive than the mouse.

Some pathogenesis studies had been conducted using the same species as both host and recipient and these had also indicated that infectivity was present in peripheral tissues, including, in some cases, muscle tissue. For example, studies conducted in the late 1950s and early 1960s by researchers working for the UK Agricultural Research Council found that intracerebral transmission of scrapie from goat-to-goat was routinely successful using 1 gram of neural and lymphatic tissues, and that it was also intermittently successful using 1 gram of pancreas, liver and muscle tissues (Pattison and Millson 1962). Another

1969 study using mink as both host and recipient managed to transmit mink spongiform encephalopathy by intramuscular inoculation with liver, kidney, lung, bladder, muscle and faeces, as well as neural and lymphatic tissues (Marsh *et al.* 1969). The highest level of infectivity was in brain tissue which contained 100,000 infective units per gram. By comparison, a gram of liver was found to contain 1000 infective units of the TSE agent, a gram of kidney or bladder or faeces contained 100 infective units and a gram of muscle contained 10 infective units (Marsh *et al.* 1969).

Risk scenarios and policy options

Given what was already known about scrapie and other TSEs, a range of different possible risk scenarios could be identified. On the most optimistic scenario, BSE would not be transmissible to humans. The 'species barrier' would be so large that even high exposure to the agent would fail to induce a TSE in humans. That scenario appeared quite plausible to some but not all scientists, given what was known about natural transmission of TSEs. Epidemiologists had not found any association between scrapie exposure and CJD and even amongst subpopulations that routinely consumed sheep brains, or that were occupationally exposed to sheep, no elevated levels of CJD had been discovered.

The worst case scenario was extremely alarming. A very large number of UK cattle might be incubating BSE, there might be a very low species barrier such that transmission readily occurred via oral exposure and the agent might be present in tissues such as muscle and kidney. Even if the agent was only present in significant quantities in neural and lymphatic tissues, there would still be widespread exposure to the agent, given that tissues such as brain and spinal cord entered the human food chain and because nervous and lymphatic tissue such as lymph nodes and nerves are present in all cuts of meat. In these worst case scenarios a large proportion of the UK population might succumb to CJD. Unfortunately there was a precedent for that scenario: where there had been outbreaks of mink spongiform encephalopathy, presumably through feeding farmed mink with TSE-infected farm animal carcasses, the death rate in the mink colonies were sometimes in the order of 60 per cent or more (US Department of Agriculture 1999; Phillips *et al.* 2000, vol. 11, para. 5.169).

In 1987, and until early 1996, there was no way of knowing where, on the spectrum between the best and worst case scenarios, the risks posed by BSE might be located. Research over the medium term could diminish some of the uncertainties about the ways in which the BSE agent behaved but it would not be able to answer all the policy-relevant questions. Transmission experiments might have helped to characterise the host range of BSE, but even if the host range was found to differ from that of scrapie, one would still not know whether humans were more or less likely to be susceptible to BSE as compared to scrapie. Pathogenesis experiments would have helped identify which cattle tissues might contain infectivity, and at what levels, and which tissues might even be pathogen-free. In the absence of knowledge about the existence or magnitude of a species barrier between cattle and humans, however, no one could know the significance of those data as far as the risk to humans was concerned. Whether or not BSE could cross the species barrier to humans was unknown and untestable. It was nevertheless enormously important for public health, for public policy and for the meat trade. When Alvin Weinberg in 1972 had coined the term 'trans-science' as a policy-relevant question that could be posed using scientific vocabulary but which was unanswerable by science, he was referring to just such an issue (Weinberg 1972).

Given the spectrum of possible risks to human health, a wide range of possible policy responses was available. The only way to prevent any further human exposure to the BSE agent would have been to exclude from the food chain all animals which were known or suspected of harbouring the disease. As there were no ways of knowing which animals were contaminated, that would have entailed excluding almost the entire national herd from both the human food chain and other products manufactured using bovine ingredients, such as certain pharmaceutics. Once contaminated feed was recognised as the vector of the disease, in late 1987, rapid elimination of the BSE pathogen from food and agriculture would have entailed decontaminating the entire feed chain and slaughtering and restocking the national herd. We estimate that that option would have cost in the order of £20 billion at 2000 prices (cf. National Audit Office 1998). It is difficult to imagine any government, then or now, having been keen, or even willing, to devote such a huge sum to an entirely unknown and speculative risk.

Very many other policy options were available, however, to diminish human exposure to the disease agent but at far lower cost. These ranged, for example, from a ban on human consumption of nervous system and perhaps lymphatic tissues from clinically diseased animals, to a ban on human consumption of the entire carcass of animals exhibiting conspicuous clinical symptoms of BSE, to a ban on the use of all animals from affected herds as human food. More precautionary, but more expensive measures, included a ban on the use of bovine tissues that were suspected of harbouring significant levels of the transmissible agent from each and every animal that entered the human food chain.

In deciding how to respond to BSE, scientific considerations were certainly a crucial component of decision-making but they did not and could never provide a sufficient basis for reaching a decision. Non-scientific judgements had to be made, first about how significant the risks might be as a result of consumption of, and exposure to, bovine tissues, and second about how those risks should be juxtaposed against the costs and difficulties of removing bovine material, and of other actions to reduce or eradicate the disease in the cattle herd. Policy-makers had to make political judgements about which level of protection was worth paying for (which would be borne by public finances and by many commercial activities in the food chain), and how the costs should be distributed as between public and private sources, to avoid or diminish the uncertain risks which BSE might be posing.

The early policy responses

Given the emergence of a novel disease, the implications of which were entirely unknown, one might have expected some effort to have been expended on characterising the possible risks, identifying the kinds of policy responses that might be appropriate, deciding which responses to introduce, and initiating a research programme to diminish some of the policy-relevant uncertainties. Yet, during the first 12 months following the discovery of BSE, possible human health risks appear to have been neither a primary nor even a subordinate concern amongst MAFF's senior veterinary and policy officials. There is no evidence that anything remotely resembling a proper risk assessment concerning the nature and possible extent of any threat to human health from BSE was conducted within MAFF, or indeed anywhere else, during that period. A risk assessment of that sort could have drawn on the literature that then was available on the transmissibility and pathogenicity of TSEs. There is also no evidence that policy-makers gave any serious consideration to whether policy measures to protect human health were appropriate or might be required.

Responsibility for co-ordinating policy on diseases such as BSE fell, in the late 1980s, to an administrative branch of MAFF called the Animal Health Group. Many other branches within MAFF contributed to policy-making on BSE, in particular the State Veterinary Service which was run by a Chief Veterinary Officer (CVO) and consisted of a field service, a regional network of veterinary investigation centres, and a research arm, the Central Veterinary Laboratory. The State Veterinary Service provided a subordinate input to policy, as compared to the co-ordinating role of Animal Health Group, but in practice final responsibility for policy advice on BSE rested with the CVO, rather than with one of his administrative colleagues.

In 1987, the overriding issue for MAFF's senior veterinary and policy officials was that domestic and overseas consumers might become aware of a new TSE in British cattle and that this could have disastrous consequences for the UK meat industry. In particular, there was a concern that trading partners would ban imports of live cattle and beef from the UK, once they learnt of the disease. Consequently, in the six month period following the initial discovery of BSE, senior veterinary and administrative officials refused to allow any details of the disease to be disseminated beyond a small circle of CVL scientists and senior staff in MAFF's Animal Health Group and the State Veterinary Service.

MAFF had been jointly funding (with the Agriculture Research Council) a specialist scrapie research institute known as the Neuropathogenesis Unit (NPU) which employed the UK's leading experts in transmissible spongiform encephalopathies, but MAFF officials did not even inform the head of the NPU about BSE until June 1987. The State Veterinary Service's regional veterinary investigation centres were also not notified about BSE, or even of the need to inform CVL of suspected cases, until June 1987, for fear of information leaking out of official circles (Phillips *et al.* vol. 1, para. 176). Even after June 1987, staff at the investigation centres were instructed not to publish accounts of the disease in veterinary newsletters or discuss BSE with universities or other research institutes; a move that prompted one of MAFF's senior veterinary investigation officers to complain of a 'total suppression of all information on the subject' (Gallagher 1987). Most significantly, no information about BSE was then given to the Department of Health (DoH) or to the government's Chief Medical Officer who was located in the DoH.

Ministers in MAFF first learnt about BSE in the summer of 1987 in a submission written by the Chief Veterinary Officer. The submission explained that '[t]he Secretary [of State] will wish to be aware of this development since the disorder could have potentially serious implications, not only domestically but for UK exports' (Rees 1987). As far as risks to humans were concerned the submission stated only that '[t]here is no evidence that the bovine disorder is transmissible to humans' (ibid.). It then went on to add that

In the absence of such evidence [of transmissibility to humans], and in the absence also of the epidemiological knowledge or of a definitive test to establish the disorder's presence in a live host, it does not seem appropriate to impose restrictions on affected farms or on the sale of produce from cattle in affected herds. Irresponsible or ill-informed publicity is likely to be unhelpful since it might lead to hysterical demands for immediate, draconian Government measures and might also lead other countries to reject UK exports of live cattle and bovine embryos and semen.

(Rees 1987)

Thus, from the point of view of MAFF's senior veterinary officials, a regulatory response to BSE would serve as an admission that consuming meat, milk or dairy products from British cattle might be harmful and this would have undermined domestic and international confidence in the safety of British beef. Senior officials even advised later that year against the option of making the disease notifiable, an essential tool for disease surveillance on the grounds that such action:

> Might interfere with trade in animals, cattle products, embryos and semen to the detriment of the industry and the country's balance of payments [and because it] might imply to the general public we know something they don't like the meat or milk is a source of danger for humans.

(Phillips *et al.* 2000, vol. 3, para. 2.130)

Throughout 1987 and the first half of 1988, no regulatory measures whatsoever were introduced in response to the emergence of BSE. It even remained entirely lawful in the UK to sell meat from animals known to have died from BSE.

With an increasing rate of reported cases, information about BSE could not be kept secret indefinitely. By mid-1987, CVL staff were anxious to claim scientific credit for discovering a new disease and veterinarians in private practice were threatening to accuse MAFF of a cover-up. CVL scientists were subsequently given permission to release details of the new disease at specialist meetings with selected members of the veterinary profession and the cattle trade, and to prepare short written communications about BSE for the specialist veterinary press. They were told, however, that authorisation from the CVO would be required and that if any comparisons were made with scrapie, or if scrapie was even mentioned in planned oral presentations or in publications, approval would be withheld (Wells 1998, para. 53). In October 1987 a short paper written by CVL staff which provided details of the initial cases of BSE was published in the *Veterinary Record*, the journal of the British Veterinary Association (Wells *et al.* 1987). The submission process had been delayed by several months because all of the scientists employed at CVL considered it scientifically indefensible to delete references to scrapie. The paper was only submitted after the CVO agreed to drop his objection to making references to scrapie (Phillips *et al.* 2000, vol. 3, Chapter 2, Dissemination of Information).

It is difficult to establish what MAFF's own scientists and officials actually knew, and took the trouble to discover, about the possible nature and magnitude of the potential risks to humans during the first year of the BSE epidemic. One senior CVL official has claimed that his department, and MAFF more generally, did not have any medically trained staff and were in no position to make a detailed assessment of the possible risks to humans from BSE

(Phillips *et al.* 2000, vol. 3, para 5.145). There is no evidence of any proper or even outline risk assessment having been performed internally or commissioned from elsewhere in government. Most of MAFF's senior veterinary and policy officials have claimed that they merely assumed that BSE was unlikely to pose a risk to humans, on the grounds that none of the other veterinary spongiform encephalopathies had been linked to human disease (Phillips *et al.* 2000, vol. 3, paras 5.8–5.12 and 5.16).

Nevertheless, we have already noted that senior CVL officials were told, as soon as the first cases of BSE had been diagnosed, that the new cattle disease might have severe repercussions for humans. MAFF's senior veterinary and policy officials were clearly aware of such concerns. As the Head of MAFF's Animal Health Group later recalled, during the period between December 1986 and June 1987

> We [the Chief Veterinary Officer and I] discussed whether the new disease might affect humans. This was felt to be unlikely, given that scrapie had been present in the country for several hundred years and did not affect humans but it was clear that the possibility could not be ruled out. The similarity with kuru and CJD was worrying.
>
> (Cruickshank 1998, para. 2.2)

The extent of any informal discussions within MAFF, in 1987, on issues such as the possible routes and levels of exposure to the BSE agent, the possible magnitude of any risks to human health, or the kinds of policy measures that might be available to reduce possible risks, were not recorded in official documents, at least not in those gathered by the staff of the Phillips Inquiry. It is, however, difficult to imagine that such issues were not raised informally amongst MAFF's veterinarians. The extent to which they might have been subsequently discussed with Ministers, however, also remains unknown.

Agriculture Ministers do not appear to have learnt much from their officials in 1987 about the possible risks to human consumers, only about the risks to the cattle and beef industry. In July of that year Ministers requested a written paper from their officials with more information on the possible risks to the livestock industry and, in particular, the risks of transmission to humans and the research that would be required to assess those risks (Bowles 1987). On possible risks to humans Ministers were told only that scrapie was not believed to present a risk to humans and that a disease of this nature in cattle 'could give rise to concern about any human health risks, although there is no reason at all to believe that such risks exist' (Watson 1987). On research, they were just told that '[a]ny possible relationship between BSE and similar diseases in humans could only be demonstrated by analysis of clusters of cases in the respective populations. Experimental work to prove animal to human transmission is impossible' (ibid.). No further documented information was provided on that occasion.

A proposed slaughter scheme

In December 1987 many of MAFF's senior veterinary and animal health policy officials changed their minds about there being no need for regulatory controls. Several events seem to have contributed to that shift of opinion. Numbers of reported cases were rising rapidly, the CVL's epidemiologist had become convinced that cattle had acquired BSE from animal feed infected with the sheep scrapie agent, and the media were also beginning to take an interest in the new disease (Phillips *et al.* 2000, vol. 3, paras 2.116 and 2.127).

At a meeting of senior officials in mid December it was decided that various policy options should be identified, such as making BSE a notifiable disease (i.e. making it a legal requirement to inform MAFF of cases of the disease). As then deputy Chief Veterinary Officer recalled '[i]t was also decided that the human health aspects which had been raised by the media should be addressed' (Meldrum 1998, para. 39). A curious feature of that remark is that it suggests that if the media had not posed the question, human health considerations would not have been addressed.

Animal health officials decided to recommend that Ministers make BSE a notifiable disease and to introduce a slaughter and compensation scheme for clinically affected cattle. Consideration had been given, at that mid-December meeting, to whether more stringent options might need to be taken in respect of meat from subclinically infected animals, but they were rejected. The CVO at the time later recalled that 'it would be impossible to identify these [subclinical cases]. We had no live test for animals' (Rees 1998).

In January 1988, in a minute to senior colleagues, the head of MAFF's Animal Health Group explained that the Government could not be sure there was no risk to human health and that without notification and slaughter of clinically diseased animals, Ministers would be criticised for allowing meat from diseased animals to be sold for human consumption (Cruickshank 1988). He argued that:

> If we believed the risk to human health was so remote as to be negligible we might advise Ministers to ride out the criticism. I would however be reluctant to say the risk is negligible. One theory is that BSE may have originated from sheep affected with scrapie . . . If this theory is correct – and I emphasise that it is only one of a number of possible explanations – we have to face up to the possibility that the disease could cross another species gap.

> (Cruickshank 1988, p. 1)

MAFF scientists and officials were never as emphatic in public. One month earlier, in an article for a group of cattle breeders known as the British Holstein Society, CVL's senior pathologist Ray Bradley had written:

> Just making the suggestion that BSE is a transmissible disease leads to the inevitable question 'Is there a danger to humans?' No there is not. There is no evidence yet for the spread of BSE between herds or individual cattle let alone to humans. There are well known but rare transmissible spongiform encephalopathies of humans but there is no known connection between them and BSE. There is no evidence either of any similar human disease developing as a result of contact with affected cattle or their products.

> (Bradley 1987)

Bradley's published remarks contrast markedly with his private comments to colleagues six months later in which he acknowledged that '[w]e cannot answer the question is BSE transmissible to humans. That natural experiment is underway in the human population' (Bradley 1988).

Although most of MAFF's senior officials had decided, by January 1988, that a slaughter and compensation policy was necessary the Agriculture Minister, John MacGregor, was, as his private secretary put it, 'very cautious' (Haine 1988). In a submission to MacGregor, officials had explicitly stated that the main reason why they were recommending a policy of slaughter with compensation was to safeguard public health in the absence of knowledge about possible transmissibility to humans (Cruickshank 1988). MAFF's Permanent Secretary (i.e. the Department's senior official) also told MacGregor that

> I do not see how you could defend taking no action now unless you had the support of the Chief Medical Officer [and that] on the face of it, it seems unlikely that he would feel able to endorse a wholly reassuring statement of the likely risks of transmission of this disease to man.

> (Andrews 1988)

Officials also told the Minister that a slaughter and compensation policy would help control the disease, that the costs were estimated to be in the order to £250,000 in the first year (i.e. relatively cheap) and that, although there were likely to be short term difficulties with exports, in the longer term a slaughter policy was likely to be more acceptable to importing countries.

MacGregor's private secretary outlined the Minister's response:

> He does not see how we could proceed without being clear where the offsetting savings are coming from [i.e. reductions in other parts of MAFF's overall budget] . . . More importantly, there is a read across to such things as rhizomania [a disease of sugar beet which was not subject to compensatory funding]. The Minister has commented that although he knows the analogy is not completely exact, he feels that this is not the way it will be seen. The argument that slaughter compensation

policy would help to stem the spread of the disease (advocated in these papers) is precisely the one sugar beet growers have been making, and which we have strongly and publicly been rejecting. He also thinks that action along the lines recommended now would make the export position much worse, not better.

(Haine 1988)

MacGregor later claimed that more positive evidence of a risk would have been required before government expenditure would have been warranted (Phillips *et al.* 2000, vol. 3, para. 5.186), but his remarks at the time appear to suggest that he was primarily concerned about safeguarding exports and avoiding anything that was inconsistent with the government's more general strategy of insisting that industry pay the costs of eradicating animal and plant diseases (Rees 1987). Given that senior officials had clearly informed Ministers that the primary purpose of a slaughter policy would be to safeguard public health in the absence of knowledge about possible transmissibility to humans, the government's policy on BSE was the antithesis of precaution. Its primary objective appeared to be rather one of trying to diminish, as far as possible, the short-term adverse impact of BSE on the profitability of the food industry and on the level of public expenditure.

Seeking expert advice

MAFF officials had told MacGregor that the only credible option available to him if he rejected his officials' advice was to obtain the support of the Department of Health's Chief Medical Officer (CMO). On 3 March 1988, the CMO, Donald Acheson, was formally notified about BSE – a full 17 months after MAFF were first alerted. Acheson was not however asked whether he would endorse a reassuring statement about the risks of BSE. Instead he was asked for advice 'on the view [MAFF] should take of the possible human health implications' (Phillips *et al.* 2000, vol. 3, para. 5.196).

On the same day several Department of Health (DoH) officials attended a meeting with MAFF's CVO and the Director of the CVL. The DoH officials reported to Acheson that MAFF officials' proposals to slaughter diseased animals and to provide compensation to farmers had been rejected because the Treasury had refused to meet the public expenditure costs, and because of knock-on effects on exports and meat and milk consumption (Dawson 1988). The minutes of that meeting note that '[t]he question is, do infected animals entering the human food chain present a risk to the general public' (ibid.).

Acheson subsequently organised a meeting with the Head of MAFF's Animal Health Group, the Director of the CVL and his own senior officials from the DoH, the Public Health Laboratory Service and the Communicable

Diseases Surveillance Centre. Those present at the meeting acknowledged that '[t]here was evidence that these infectious agents could change their host range' (Anon 1988) and that there were very few answers to some very long-standing questions on the transmission of TSEs. MAFF's minutes of the meeting noted that 'all those present found it very difficult to give any clear advice on the subject' (Phillips *et al.* 2000, vol. 3, para. 5.66). The meeting concluded by agreeing to recommend the setting up of an expert advisory group, specifically to provide urgent advice on biological products and the disposal of sick animals (ibid.). Acheson told his colleagues at the meeting that he thought it highly probable that the advice would be that carcasses of affected animals should not go for human consumption (ibid.).

The immediate, and irredeemably political, problem at that juncture was how to respond to the uncertainty about the risks posed by BSE. It is therefore appropriate to ask why Acheson agreed to establish an expert committee to advise on specific policy measures when what was required was a scientific opinion about the possible risks posed by BSE, and a separate policy recommendation as to whether the direct and indirect costs associated with a slaughter and compensation policy were worth enduring in return for a reduction in the levels of BSE contaminated material, of uncertain risk, entering the human food chain.

Acheson could have decided to advise that the human health implications of BSE were unknown, and that in those circumstances a slaughter and compensation policy was a sensible response. Yet, it appears he either wanted to avoid taking responsibility for that type of decision, or he didn't consider that he had sufficient power or authority to make a judgement that was at odds with Ministerial wishes. It is possible that he didn't think the risks were such that a slaughter policy needed to be adopted, but that he wanted external justification to support advising that no action was necessary. The latter seems unlikely given that Acheson had initially acknowledged that it was very likely that the expert group would recommend that diseased animals should be destroyed.

In retrospect Acheson has argued that the unanimous opinion at the meeting on 7 March 1988 was to appoint an advisory committee and that

> Had I attempted to overrule the unanimous advice of the scientists at the meeting on this point, [by recommending a slaughter policy] I regard it as highly unlikely that my personal advice, unsupported by experts, would have been accepted by the Treasury.

(Acheson 1999, paras 27–28)

Acheson noted that he had been told by MAFF officials at the meeting that a formal risk appraisal was a prerequisite for the introduction of a slaughter and compensation policy in order to justify the costs to the Treasury (Phillips *et al.* 2000, vol. 3, para. 5.209).

The Phillips Inquiry did not find Acheson's account of these events entirely convincing, in particular his claim that MAFF officials had told him that a more formal risk assessment was required prior to considering regulatory intervention. The Inquiry concluded that Acheson must have been confused about events at that time because his claims were at odds with the testimony of MAFF officials who argued that they were slightly disappointed that Acheson had failed to back an immediate slaughter policy (Phillips *et al.* 2000, vol. 3, paras 5.209 and 5.213). The contemporaneous minutes of the meeting do note, however, that: 'Mr Cruickshank [a senior MAFF official] thought it necessary to assess the risk in humans in order to justify the cost of any control measures taken by MAFF' (Anon 1988). Whether MAFF officials did in fact argue that such appraisal need to be conducted *in advance* of any control measures is disputed, but it is clear that Ministers had already rejected official advice in part because they wanted more positive evidence of a risk to humans before the expense of government compensation could be recommended (Phillips *et al.* 2000, vol. 3, para. 5.193).

Our interpretation of events is that since evidential support could not be provided, Acheson and other officials chose to seek what has been termed 'eminential' support for the policy that Ministers had thus far rejected (cf. Isaacs and Fitzgerald 1999). Acheson therefore recommended that Ministers appoint an expert committee of eminent scientists (none of whom were experts on TSEs) in order to provide urgent policy advice. In making that recommendation Acheson explained to the Health Minister that MAFF had not felt able to make BSE notifiable or face the costs of compensation to farmers for destroyed livestock without advice on the potential human health hazard.

Just to be sure, in April 1988, Acheson wrote to the chair of the new committee, Professor Richard Southwood, suggesting that 'it may be desirable for your group to have an early meeting to decide whether any urgent action is prudent' (Acheson 1988). Acheson also enclosed a list of questions for the committee, one of which asked: 'what steps if any is prudent to take . . . in clinically affected animals covering . . . meat, offal and meat products for human consumption' (ibid.). At a meeting with the committee chair and senior MAFF officials held in the following month, Acheson again asked that Southwood and his colleagues provide advice as soon as possible on whether there were immediate steps which should be taken to safeguard human health. Finally, prior to the committee's first meeting on 20 June 1988, a DoH colleague of Acheson also provided a draft answer for the committee to Acheson's question concerning the steps, if any, that were prudent to take as regards clinically affected animals. That answer stated that meat, offal and meat products from clinically affected animals were 'not acceptable' for human consumption. When the committee did immediately recommend taking clinically affected carcasses out of the human food chain, Acheson wrote to the Health Minister arguing that 'such action is indeed essential' (Phillips *et al.* 2000, vol. 3, para. 5.109).

Our interpretation of the evidence is that what became known as the 'Southwood Working Party' was established primarily to provide officials in MAFF and the Department of Health with a political resource with which to push for the introduction of regulations which they believed Agricultural Ministers and the Treasury would not otherwise accept, rather than by a perceived need for scientific advice per se. The fact that none of the committee members were experts on TSEs was thus relatively unimportant to that objective. The one required quality was the eminence that the members possessed in abundance.

Summary

In the absence of a test to identify animals that were subclinically infected with BSE, the destruction of overtly diseased cattle was not going to be sufficient to remove all infectivity from the food chain and thus reassure consumers that beef was safe. Senior civil servants' political judgement, until early 1988 at least, was that any such intermediate response would have alerted domestic consumers and potential importers of UK cattle and meat to the presence of a new potentially fatal zoonotic disease and would have inevitably forced policy-makers to adopt far more stringent precautionary measures to maintain demand. Thus, from the perspective of MAFF civil servants, any regulatory response – indeed any admission that consuming meat, milk or dairy products from British cattle might not be entirely safe – would have undermined domestic and international confidence in the safety of British beef. The only credible options, given the objectives of maintaining stable markets and control over public expenditure, were to pretend that the disease did not exist and, once that position became untenable, to claim that BSE did not pose a risk to human health, as evidenced by a total lack of regulations (and information).

The policy of secrecy and denial was not based on scientific evidence or advice, but rather on a decision to avoid consulting or involving external scientific advisors and researchers. Scientists internal to the policy regime, on the other hand, had little choice but to conform to the wishes of senior management, but they were clearly unhappy at the restrictions placed on dissemination of information about the new disease. Those restrictions had obvious ramifications for learning about the new disease. Gathering knowledge about the extent of the epidemic was difficult because, as the chair of the British Cattle Veterinary Association recalled, '[t]hroughout most of 1986 and 1987 most veterinary surgeons . . . were ignorant of the presence of this disease, and were not informed of its clinical signs or its significance as a potential national disease problem' (Phillips *et al.* 2000, vol. 3, para. 2.171).

The concern to promulgate a superficially reassuring vision of BSE also contributed to delays in addressing and resolving crucial questions about the risks posed by BSE. No attempt to conduct a proper risk assessment was attempted, and collaborative research between the staff at CVL and the Neuropathogenesis Unit in Edinburgh was seriously delayed (Phillips *et al.* 2000, vol. 3, para. 2.141).

Despite the inflexibility inherent in taking the stance that there were no risks whatsoever to human health from BSE, officials eventually decided that to take no action would have been worse than introducing a policy of requiring the slaughter of overtly diseased cattle. Southwood and his colleagues were used by senior officials in MAFF and the DoH to pressurise ministers into agreeing to remove clinically diseased cattle from the food chain. The Southwood Working Party therefore had a distinct policy role, but not an autonomous role. The danger, from MAFF's point of view, was that the working party might go too far by recommending a more stringent set of measures. The way in which that tension played out is the subject of the next chapter.

Bibliography

Acheson, D. (1988) Letter dated 20 March 1988 to Sir Richard Southwood, *BSE Inquiry Year Book* Reference No. 88/4.20/1.1–1.2. In Phillips *et al.* 2000, op. cit.

Acheson, D. (1999) *Witness Statement No. 251a*, in Phillips *et al.* 2000, op. cit.

Andrews, D. (1988) *Bovine Spongiform Encephalopathy (BSE)*, Memo dated 24 February 1988, *BSE Inquiry Year Book* Reference No. 88/2.24/2.2. In Phillips *et al.* 2000, op. cit.

Anon (1988) Note of a meeting on bovine spongiform encephalopathy 17 March 1988 Venue, DHSS, Richmond Terrace, Whitehall. *BSE Inquiry Year Book* Reference No. 88/03.17/8.1–8.3. In Phillips *et al.* 2000, op. cit.

Bowles, C. (1987) Minute from C. Bowles dated 23 July 1987, 'Bat Rabies and Bovine Spongiform Encephalopathy (BSE)' *BSE Inquiry Year Book* Reference No. 87/7/23/2.1.

Bradley, R. (1987) BSE Article, *BSE Inquiry Year Book* Reference No. 87/12.10/5.1–5.6. In Phillips *et al.* 2000, op. cit.

Bradley, R. (1988) BSE Research Projects, Minute dated 19 July 1988 to WA Watson. *BSE Inquiry Year Book* Reference No. 88/07.19/2.1–2.2. In Phillips *et al.* 2000, op. cit.

Cruickshank, A. R. (1988) Bovine spongiform encephalopathy, Memo, *BSE Inquiry Year Book* Reference No. YB88/2.16/1.1. In Phillips *et al.* 2000, op. cit.

Cruickshank, A. R. (1998) Witness Statement No 75 to the BSE Inquiry.

Dawson, A. (1988) Minute from Dr Ann Dawson, dated 7 March 1988 'Bovine spongiform encephalopathy (BSE)'. *BSE Inquiry Year Book* 88/3.7/6.1–6.2.

Dickinson, A. G. (1976) Scrapie in sheep and goats. In R. H/ Kimberlin (ed.) *Slow Virus Diseases of Animals and Man*, Chapter 10. Amsterdam, Oxford & New York: North Holland & Elsevier.

Gallagher, J. (1987) 'Bovine spongiform encephalopathy – confidentiality'. Letter to Richard Cawthorne, MAFF, dated 19 June 1987, YB 87/06.19/6.1. In Phillips *et al.* 2000, op. cit.

Gajdusek, D. C. (1985) Unconventional viruses causing subacute spongiform encephalopathies. In B. N. Fields *et al.* (eds) *Virology.* New York: Raven Press.

Gibbs, C. J., Gajdusek, D. C. and Amyx, H. (1979) Strain variation in the viruses of Creutzfeldt-Jakob disease and kuru. In S. B. Prusiner and W. J. Hadlow (eds) *Slow Transmissible Diseases of the Nervous System,* vol. 2, pp. 87–110. New York: Academic Press.

Hadlow, W. J., Kennedy, R. C. and Race, R. E. (1982) 'Natural infection of Suffolk sheep with scrapie virus', *The Journal of Infectious Diseases,* **146** (5), 657–64.

Haine, D. B. (1988) Minute to the Private Secretary of Mr Thompson, dated 29 February 1988, BSE Inquiry Document No. YB 88/2.29/4.1. In Phillips *et al.* 2000, op. cit.

Isaacs, D. and Fitzgerald, D. (1999) 'Seven alternatives to evidence-based medicine', *BMJ,* **319,** 1618.

Marsh, R. F., Burger, D. and Hanson, R. P. (1969) 'Transmissible mink encephalopathy: behavior of the disease agent in mink', *American Journal of Veterinary Research,* **30,** 1637–43.

Martin, W. B. (1998) Involvement with scrapie as Scientific Director of the Moredun Research Institute. The BSE Inquiry/Statement No. 5. In Phillips *et al.* 2000, op. cit.

Meldrum, K. (1998) Statement No 184 to BSE Inquiry.

National Audit Office (1998) *MAFF and the Intervention Board: BSE: The Cost of a Crisis,* Report by the Comptroller and Auditor General, HC 853 1997/98, 8 July 1998. The Stationery Office, London.

Pattison, I. H. and Millson, G. C. (1960) 'Further observations on the experimental production of scrapie in goats and sheep,' *Journal of Comparative Pathology,* **70,** 182–93.

Pattison, I. H. and Millson, G. C. (1962) 'Distribution of the scrapie agent in the tissues of experimentally inoculated goats', *Journal of Comparative Pathology,* **72,** 233–44.

Phillips, Bridgeman J. and Ferguson-Smith, M. (2000) *The BSE Inquiry: Report: evidence and supporting papers of the Inquiry into the emergence and identification of Bovine Spongiform Encephalopathy (BSE) and variant Creutzfeldt-Jakob Disease (vCJD) and the action taken in response to it up to 20 March 1996.* London: The Stationery Office.

Rees, H. (1987) Minute dated 5 June 1987 to Parliamentary Secretary and others. 'Newly identified bovine neurological disorder – Bovine Spongiform Encephalopathy. *BSE Inquiry Year Book* 87/06.05/2.1–2.2. In Phillips *et al.* 2000, op. cit.

Rees, H. (1998) BSE Inquiry transcript of oral hearings, Day 54, 10/9/1998, p. 106. In Phillips *et al.* 2000, op. cit.

Schwartz, M. (2003) *How the Cows Turned Mad,* trans. E. Schneider. Berkeley, CA: University of California Press.

Taylor, D. M. (1989) Bovine spongiform encephalopathy and human health, *The Veterinary Record,* **125,** 413–15.

US Department of Agriculture (1999) *Transmissible Mink Encephalopathy,* Fact Sheet, Veterinary Services, Animal and Plant health Inspection Services, September 1999. Available at: *http://www.idfa.org/reg/bse/fstme.pdf*

Watson, W. (1987) Minute dated 30 July 1987 'Bovine Spongiform Encephalopathy (BSE)'. *BSE Inquiry Year Book* 87/7.30/1.1–1.4. In Phillips *et al.* 2000, op. cit.

Weinberg, A. (1972) 'Science and trans-science', *Minerva,* **10,** 209–22.

Wells, G., Scott, A., Johnson, C., Gunning, R., Jeffrey, M. and Bradley, R. (1987) 'A novel progressive spongiform encephalopathy in cattle', *Veterinary Record,* **121,** 419–20.

Wells, G. (1998) Statement No. 65 to the BSE Inquiry. In Phillips *et al.* 2000, op. cit.

Chapter 5

The Southwood Working Party

This chapter explores in detail the operation and impact on policy of the first expert committee on BSE, known as the Southwood Working Party, after its chair, Sir Richard Southwood. The working party was established in the spring of 1988, a few weeks after MAFF told the government's Chief Medical Officer about the existence of BSE. Although it existed for only nine months its role in and impact on policy-making is key to understanding the dynamics of the entire BSE saga.

The working party was invariably portrayed by Ministers and government officials as a wholly independent, and entirely scientific body. Its advice in relation to BSE was also represented as the most authoritative and definitive available, not only at the time at which it was provided but for many years afterwards. Ministers always insisted, too, that they had no option but to rely entirely on that independent and authoritative advice in formulating policy. As the Agricultural Minister, John Gummer, later told the House of Commons in a debate on BSE: 'the first question the House must address is whether the government have any alternative but to accept the advice of the experts' (Gummer 1990). The then Prime Minister, Margaret Thatcher has also recalled that 'we were almost completely dependent on the scientists . . . It would have been irresponsible and perhaps even counterproductive to second guess the experts' (Thatcher 1999). There was nothing unusual about the ways in which MAFF was characterising the Southwood Working Party. Virtually all of the Department's expert committees and regulatory policy processes were portrayed in a similar technocratic fashion.

As this chapter explains, however, most of the important policy developments in the late 1980s emerged unilaterally from MAFF rather than in response to the advice of the Southwood Working Party. Much of what was portrayed as independent advice had, in any case, been strongly influenced by, and in some cases was merely a recycling of, the concerns and perspectives of officials in both the DoH and especially in MAFF. Even the nominally scientific aspects of the working party's advice – its assessment of the possible risks posed by BSE – reflected and embodied officials' policy commitments and objectives.

The key analytical aim in this chapter is to show how, in practice, scientific and non-scientific considerations interacted and were coupled together in the process of providing expert advice to policy-makers. The chapter will explore both the extent to which expert advice on BSE was influenced by the social and political context in which it was produced and the ways in which those influences operated. We shall also explain what those patterns of interaction indicate about the range of social and political roles that the working party played in BSE policy-making.

Chapter 4 argued that some officials wanted an expert committee so as to provide a political resource to persuade Ministers to accept a slaughter policy for diseased animals. The committee did indeed fulfil that intended political function, but the Southwood Working Party played a variety of additional social and political roles too. We believe that the evidence in this chapter demonstrates that the advice from the working party already incorporated or anticipated officials' prior policy objectives and preferences. As a result we argue that the same officials were able to use the working party as a source of apolitical authority to sanction, and deflect challenges away from, a series of potentially contestable policy decisions – many of which had been adopted prior to the solicitation of expert advice, and which government officials believed Ministers, other government departments, the meat industry and the general public might not otherwise accept. Officials were also able to invoke the scientific authority of the working party for policy decisions that had been taken on entirely different grounds and for policies for which scientific evidence and knowledge was no longer reliable.

Although we will argue the Southwood Working Party (and science more generally) served strategically as a legitimatory resource – as a means of taking the politics out of policy-making – that does not necessarily exclude other rationales. In part, the working party was an autonomous producer of 'policy' and it did provide some scientific information for policy-makers about what was, and was not, known about BSE. Yet neither of those roles was especially significant. In particular, much of the expertise and scientific knowledge required already existed within government, and within affiliated institutions, such as the Neuropathogenesis Unit. The working party's assessment of what was and was not known about BSE had largely been written by its secretariat and by other MAFF officials. Furthermore, although there always was (and continues to be) a need for rigorous scientific and technical advice on BSE, the immediate problem for UK policy-makers in the late 1980s was not so much that that they were unaware of the possible risks posed by BSE but rather that they urgently needed to respond to the profound uncertainty about the nature of those possible risks. This was primarily a political rather than a scientific dilemma.

Composition and remit

Sir Richard Southwood, Professor of Zoology at Oxford, and formerly chair of the Royal Commission on Environmental Pollution, was selected, on the basis of a recommendation from the Chief Medical Officer (CMO), as a suitable chair for the new working party. The preference of MAFF's Permanent Secretary had been for Southwood to provide advice alone, on the basis of help from civil servants, and without any terms of reference (Andrews 1988a). As the Permanent Secretary told his Minister: 'Departments need to be in the position to say that they are seeking appropriate expert advice. But we do not want to over dramatise things at this stage by announcing the appointment of an expert group' (ibid.). The CMO had insisted, however, that external experts join the committee (Andrews 1988a).

The 'Southwood Working Party' consisted of Richard Southwood and three additional members. They were Anthony Epstein, emeritus Professor of Pathology at Bristol University and joint discoverer of the Epstein–Barr virus, Professor Bill Martin, a veterinarian and former director of the Moredun Research Institute in Edinburgh, and Sir John Walton, former Professor of Neurology at Newcastle upon Tyne. All members of the working party were eminent senior scientists who had previously served on numerous government committees (Inquiry Secretariat 1999, para. 1). None of them, however, were experts on TSEs. Southwood had insisted that no active TSE researchers should be included on the committee as he believed that they would inevitably have entrenched views about the nature of the transmissible agent.

In common with most UK advisory committees, the working party had no staff, no budget, the members were unpaid and they were expected to carry on with their existing professional duties. An official secretariat, which in this case comprised one official from MAFF and one from DoH, was therefore crucial to the operation of the committee. Although the Members could and did spend time working on their report outside of the formal meetings they were inevitably dependent on the resources and knowledge of their secretariat and other MAFF and DoH officials. Prior to the working party's first meeting, officials from MAFF and DoH had helped Richard Southwood to draw up a list of 28 questions for the working party to address. Those officials then subsequently drafted the answers to all of those questions, supplied most of the relevant data and evidence to the committee, drafted much of the committee's final report, and entered into discussions and negotiations with the committee over the practicality of its recommendations. As we shall show, this asymmetry between the committee and the two government departments entailed that several aspects of the committee's output were effectively a recycling of departmental views, albeit sanctioned with a veneer of independent scientific credibility.

The Southwood Working Party was formally appointed to 'advise on the implications of Bovine Spongiform Encephalopathy and matters relating thereto' (MAFF/DoH, 1989). That phrase was crucially ambiguous as between providing scientific advice or policy advice or both. There was also consider-able ambiguity about precisely what issues and topics fell within and outside the committee's remit. Such ambiguities were a source of confusion amongst protagonists but also a strategic opportunity for both officials and committee members to shift what the working party was responsible for, and what it was represented as responsible for, on different kinds of issues. Furthermore, as we shall show, the actual alignment reached between the respective roles of gov-ernment and advisors, and on what specific issues fell within and outside the working party's remit, was often never made explicit, even to those within the agricultural and health policy communities. This subsequently caused substantial problems for the nature and dynamics of BSE policy.

From the outset, however, it was clear that most officials were expecting the working party to provide advice on both the risks posed by BSE and the meas-ures that should be taken to counter those risks. That is what the CMO told his Minister and that understanding is evident from official discussions about the precise wording for the Southwood Working Party's terms of reference (Phillips *et al.* 2000, vol. 4, paras. 1.5–1.8). The CMO had also written to Southwood explaining that '[a] very brief note with recommendations is all that is expected' (Phillips *et al.* 2000, vol. 4, para. 1.10).

In making recommendations, instead of only indicating what the scientific evidence implied about the possible risks from BSE, the working party inevitably exercised judgements about how the highly uncertain benefits of different types of regulatory interventions should be juxtaposed against the anticipated costs. A key question then is how were such policy judgements formed? We believe the evidence shows that in practice public officials were actively involved in attempting to manage the advice which they had requested. It also shows how committee members pre-empted the government's political objectives by tacitly structuring them into their advice, and indeed even into their scientific assessment of risk.

The advice from the Southwood Working Party

The Southwood Working Party met on four occasions between June 1988 and the publication of its report in February 1989 (MAFF/DoH, 1989). Some interim recommendations were made after each meeting but the bulk of the working party's advice, and its analysis of the possible risks, appeared in its 35 page report. That report contained a discussion of the history and possible causes of BSE, predictions about the future course of the epidemic, an assessment of the possible risks, and recommendations in regard to the protection of human and animal health and future research needs. The key points contained in the report are summarised below.

The assessment of risk

With a phrase that was to be subsequently repeated on numerous occasions by UK policy-makers, the Southwood Working Party report's General Conclusions articulated perhaps the most optimistic conclusion that could have been drawn from what was known about BSE and other TSEs, stating that '[f]rom the present evidence, it is . . . most unlikely that BSE will have any implications for human health' (MAFF/DoH 1989, para. 9.2).

The working party also implied that its general conclusion was valid regardless of the kinds of tissue to which humans were exposed or the route by which they were exposed. In a subsection of the report entitled 'Possible Transmission to Man', the working party explained that different routes and sources of exposure presented varying levels of theoretical risk with the highest theoretical risk arising from inoculation of infected neural and lymphoid tissues (MAFF/DoH 1989, para. 5.3.2). It provided examples of such theoretically high risk exposure scenarios, including inoculation of pharmaceutical products derived from bovine tissue and accidental inoculation of slaughterhouse workers and veterinarians. The working party argued, however, that '[i]n these, as in other circumstances [i.e. oral routes of exposure such as eating contaminated food], the risk of transmission of BSE appears remote' (MAFF/DoH 1989, para. 5.3.5).

The working party's optimistic conclusions were, nevertheless, qualified with caveats. Thus, the phrase that it was 'most unlikely that BSE will have implications for human health' was followed by the warning that '[n]evertheless, if our assessments of these likelihoods are incorrect, the implications would be extremely serious' (MAFF/DoH 1989). Elsewhere the report noted that given the long incubation period it would be a decade or more before 'complete reassurance can be given' (MAFF/DoH 1989, para. 5.3.1) and it pointed out that transmission, even by the relatively less efficient oral route of exposure, 'cannot be entirely ruled out' (MAFF/DoH 1989, para. 5.3.5).

Anyone expecting a structured description of the working party's risk assessment, or even an explanation of their analysis, was going to be disappointed. Most significantly, the rationale for the working party's general conclusions about the risks of transmission to humans was not explained. Neither was there any explanation as to why the working party regarded the risks of inoculation with neural or lymphatic tissue to present no less 'remote' a risk than the risks of oral exposure to non-neural and non-lymphoid tissues. The report provided no substantive discussion about which cattle tissues might contain infectivity; it only noted that the agent would be most likely to be present in spleen and lymphatic tissues in the early stages of infection and, as the disease progressed, in the brain and neural tissue (MAFF/DoH 1989) The only acknowledgement that non-neural and non-lymphatic cattle tissues might carry the agent was the comment that 'the risk is far less with other tissues' (MAFF/DoH 1989, para. 5.3.2) Finally, the report neglected to discuss the possible magnitude of the 'remote' risks, although the phrase 'if our assessments of these likelihoods are incorrect, the implications would be extremely serious' implied that they could be quite high.

In retrospect, it is worth noting that the absence of a proper explanation of the reasoning behind the working party's assessment of the possible risks of BSE to human health was the focus of the principal criticism of the Southwood Working Party from the Phillips' Inquiry report. Phillips and his team argued that the Southwood report was worded in a way that failed to alert the British government to the need to review the committee's judgements and advice as and when new evidence emerged that might undermine the committee's conclusions. On the other hand, the working party's approach was consistent with traditional practices amongst British expert committees.

Risks of BSE transmission were also discussed briefly in relation to animals by the working party. The report argued that ruminants other than cattle and sheep (i.e. deer and antelope) 'would clearly be at considerable risk' (MAFF/DoH 1989, para. 5.2.4). It also suggested that 'domestic pets could well be susceptible to BSE were the agent to reach them in an adequate dose by an appropriate route' (MAFF/DoH 1989). Non-mammalian species, on the other hand, such as poultry, were considered 'unlikely to be susceptible to BSE' (MAFF/DoH 1989). The possible risks to mammals, other than domestic pets and ruminants, were not mentioned at all, aside from a general comment in the conclusions of the report that the recycling of ruminant material in animal feed exposed herbivores to 'infective risks against which they have not evolved any defences' (MAFF/DoH 1989, para. 9.4). No reasons were provided as to why domestic pets might be more susceptible to BSE than humans, or indeed any other mammals.

The working party agreed with MAFF that there was convincing evidence that feed was the vector of transmission by which cattle acquired BSE but it implied that there would be no other transmission vectors because it concluded that '[f]rom present evidence, it is likely that cattle will prove to be a 'dead-end host' for the disease agent' (MAFF/DoH 1989, para. 9.2) – a phrase which the report had earlier noted meant that there would no direct animal to animal transmission of the disease (MAFF/DoH 1989, 5.1.2). The working party appeared, however, to contradict that statement because it had stated that '[a]t the present state of knowledge it is impossible to predict whether cattle to cattle transmission of BSE will occur' (MAFF/DoH 1989).

Policy recommendations

As expected, the working party moved swiftly to recommend the slaughter and destruction of clinically diseased animals. That advice had been given 'as a matter of urgency' (Inquiry Secretariat 1999, para. 4.1) on 21 June 1988, the day after the working party's initial meeting. Aside from recommending that milk from suspected BSE cases should not enter the human food chain, a piece of advice that MAFF had invited the working party to endorse in November 1988, no other policy measures in relation to the protection of human health appeared during the course of the working party's deliberations.

One additional piece of human-health related advice was issued, but it was not a policy recommendation but rather advice to the food industry. In its final report the working party stated that '[w]e consider that manufacturers of baby food should avoid the use of ruminant offal and thymus' (MAFF/DoH 1989, para. 5.3.5). That recommendation applied to the offal and thymus of all cattle and was intended to capture those animals that were infected with BSE but not yet displaying clinical symptoms. No such advice was made in regards to the composition of food for non-infants; indeed the report noted that

> It has been suggested . . . that consideration should be given to products containing brain and spleen being so labelled, to enable the consumer to make an informed choice. The working party believes that risks as at present perceived would not justify this measure.
>
> (MAFF/DoH 1989)

No explanation was provided as to why offal and thymus might pose an unacceptable risk to infants but not to children or adults. Neither was there an explanation as to why lymphatic and nervous tissue other than offal and thymus could be included in baby food.

As for non-food borne routes of exposure to the BSE agent, the report only suggested that the attention of the human and veterinary medicine licensing authorities 'be drawn to the emergence of BSE so that they can take appropriate action' (MAFF/DoH 1989, para. 8.2) and that the potential problems caused by BSE should be brought to the attention of the Health and Safety Executive 'who can consider whether further guidance should be given' (MAFF/DoH 1989, para. 8.3).

As far as the protection of animal health was concerned, immediately prior to the first meeting of the working party, MAFF had itself decided to ban, for a period of six months, the use of ruminant protein (i.e. slaughterhouse waste from cattle and sheep) in the feed of ruminants. The working party endorsed MAFF's feed ban, although it advised that it should continue indefinitely, but no further measures to protect animal health, such as extending the feed ban to cover domestic pets or other farm animals, were issued. The report's conclusions did, however, make a very general recommendation to Ministers, urging them to 'address' the problem of recycling 'inadequately sterilised' animal products as animal feed 'as part of the adjustment of the framework of the agricultural policy of the EC in the coming years' (MAFF/DoH 1989, para. 9.4).

Four recommendations regarding research were considered by the working party to be sufficiently urgent that they were issued the day after the working party's initial meeting in June 1988. One of these was to set up an experiment to determine whether maternal transmission of BSE occurred by monitoring a sample of the offspring of cows with the disease. MAFF had not done this by the time the working party had completed its work and the working party therefore repeated that particular recommendation in its final report, 'urg[ing] that all necessary resources are made available' to ensure that the offspring of cows with BSE were monitored (MAFF/DoH 1989, para. 8.1).

A second recommendation was to test whether scrapie was transmissible via milk or muscle. The working party believed such an experiment would provide a rapid analogy for assessing the possible transmissibility of BSE from milk and muscle (Phillips et al. 2000, vol. 4, para. 2.4). Again, MAFF had not acted on that recommendation by the time the working party had completed its work and in its final report the working party again repeated that particular piece of advice.

A third recommendation was to test the hypothesis that scrapie-infected feedstuffs were the origin of BSE (Phillips et al. 2000, vol. 4, para. 2.4). Once again MAFF had not acted on that recommendation by the time the working party had completed its work. In fact MAFF never acted on that recommendation and such an experiment has never been performed in the UK, despite the fact that the hypothesis that BSE was caused by a conventional scrapie agent was the key reason for believing that the disease would not present a risk to humans.

The final recommendation, issued immediately following the working party's first meeting, did not concern a specific experiment but was rather advice to establish an entirely new expert committee to advise on existing and further research in to BSE and other TSEs (Phillips et al. 2000, vol. 4, para. 2.4).

Several additional recommendations regarding research appeared in the working party's final report. One was for epidemiologists to monitor cases of

Creutzfeldt-Jakob Disease (CJD) for atypical cases or changing patterns of incidence on the grounds that any human cases of BSE would probably present as CJD. Others concerned various areas of research which the working party wanted the new research advisory committee to pursue; these included epidemiological studies, transmission studies to a variety of possible host species, formal monitoring of pigs and domestic pets and studies to compare the molecular structure of the BSE and scrapie agents.

The Southwood report was completed and published in February 1989. Despite the inconsistencies, unanswered questions and caveats that were apparent on close inspection of the report, the overall impression it provided was largely sedative. After all, the working party had endorsed the optimistic hypothesis that BSE would behave just like scrapie and present no risk to humans. The optimism was boosted by the fact that the working party's warning that 'if our assessments . . . are incorrect the implications could be extremely serious' (MAFF/DoH, 1989, para 9.2) was usually deleted from government pronouncements on the report's findings. Instead, policy-makers insisted that BSE was an innocuous version of scrapie and therefore that the presence of BSE in British dairy and beef herds posed no threat to human health. MAFF claimed, for example, that '[t]here is no reason to believe BSE will be any different from scrapie and independent experts have concluded that BSE is most unlikely to have any implications for human health' (MAFF 1990a). That was a message that was widely accepted, not only by those outside of government but also by most of those within MAFF and the Department of Health (Phillips *et al.* 2000, vol. 4, paras 11.6–11.10).

The production of advice in relation to human health

The Southwood report had endorsed the most optimistic available conclusions about the potential risks of BSE to human health. It had also failed to make any substantive recommendations aside from that of removing overtly diseased animals from the food chain. We now examine in more detail the working party's deliberations and advice in relation to the protection of human health. The discussion below focuses on three topics: the assessment of risk to humans, the recommendation to slaughter and destroy clinically affected cattle, and the anomalous absence of policy recommendations to restrict the sale and/or consumption of tissues from infected but asymptomatic cattle.

Risk to humans

Chapter 4 argued that during the late 1980s the potential for BSE to transmit to humans was simply unknowable. In 1988, MAFF's own scientists and administrators had acknowledged that fact. For example a senior veterinary pathologist, who was amongst the best informed of MAFF scientists on TSEs, had written to the Director of the CVL in July 1988 pointing out that '[w]e cannot answer the question is BSE transmissible to humans. That natural experiment is underway in the human population and it remains for epidemio-logists to collect data and produce a hypothesis based on it' (Bradley 1988). Yet, on the basis of much the same evidence, the Southwood Working Party had concluded that it was 'most unlikely' that BSE would have any implica-tions for human health. Why had working party reached what was in effect the most optimistic conclusion possible?

The Southwood Working Party were certainly aware that the BSE agent *might* be different from, and/or have different transmission characteristics to, the scrapie agent. Prior to the working party's first meeting, one of the 28 questions to which MAFF and DoH officials had provided answers had asked: 'what are the risks of a species jump?' MAFF's answer had stated that even if BSE had originated from scrapie, 'the effects of *passage* of the agent in cattle, in terms of altered risks for other species, will be difficult to ascertain' (Phillips *et al.* 2000, vol. 4, annex, p. 78). Richard Kimberlin, the former Director of the Neuropathogenesis Unit, had been invited to the working party's second meeting in November 1988 and had also told the members that, even if the BSE agent originated as a particular scrapie strain in sheep, it had to be assumed to be a hazard because no one could predict what was going to happen to a given strain of agent when it entered another species (BSE Inquiry Transcript, 1 July 1998, p. 141). Furthermore, the working party recognised that BSE might not even have derived from scrapie since they had recom-mended an experiment to test whether scrapie was responsible for BSE.

Nevertheless, the working party eventually reported that it was highly likely that the BSE agent was simply 'scrapie in cattle', and moreover a version of scrapie that had not altered on *passage* to cattle. Section 4 of the working party's report entitled 'The cause of Bovine Spongiform Encephalopathy: the epidemiological evidence' provided an explanation for that conclusion. It argued, first, that the consumption of meat and bone meal containing mater-ial from scrapie-infected sheep was the most likely cause of BSE. It suggested that scrapie may always have been capable of infecting cattle, but that during the 1980s there may have been higher exposure to scrapie-infected tissue as a result of a possible increase in both the prevalence of scrapie in the UK sheep flocks, and in the numbers of sheep heads and diseased sheep included in material used for rendering; although no evidence was provided to support those claims. At the same time it noted that rendering technologies had begun to treat material at lower temperatures and/or for shorter time periods than had previously been the case, thus perhaps allowing greater amounts of infectivity to survive; once again, no evidence was provided to support those claims. The report suggested, therefore, that an increased level of exposure to the scrapie agent may itself have resulted in transfer of the scrapie agent to cattle (MAFF/DoH 1989, para. 4.2.8).

Section 4 of the report then discussed one 'further hypothesis', namely that BSE had derived from a mutant strain of the scrapie agent pathogenic for cattle. It argued that such a hypothesis was unlikely because the pattern of the epidemic (single or dual cases per herd across a wide geographical area) would mean that a mutant scrapie strain would have had to emerge simultaneously in a large number of sheep flocks, or cattle, throughout the country. In the words of the report:

> If [BSE] had resulted from a localised chance transmission of the scrapie strain from sheep to cattle giving rise to a mutant, a different pattern of disease would have been expected: its range would have increased with time.

> (MAFF/DoH 1989, para. 4.2.9)

As was later confirmed by the working party (Inquiry Secretariat 1999) the arguments presented in Section 4 of the report provided the basis for the working party's optimistic conclusions about the risks of BSE transmission to humans. Section 6 of the report, entitled 'The Future Course of the Disease', had in fact indicated just that line of reasoning:

> It cannot be automatically assumed that animals and man will react to BSE agent exposure as they have done to scrapie, which in the human case has not led to any clear association with disease. BSE agent may for example be an adapted or particularly virulent form of scrapie although the results of the epidemiological study indicate otherwise.

> (MAFF/DoH 1989, para. 6.3)

A number of points are worth making about this line of reasoning. First, Sections 4 and 6 of the report had not been written by the members of the working party but rather by MAFF's senior veterinary epidemiologist, John Wilesmith (Pickles 1998, para. 41.3). Section 4 bears remarkably close resemblance to the text of an article published by Wilesmith and MAFF colleagues in the previous year (Wilesmith *et al.* 1988).

The members of the working party simply assumed the validity of Wilesmith's evidence and arguments. They did not critically review the arguments and they did not see the underlying data. In fact, even if they had wanted to review the underlying data they would not have been able to because they were told by Wilesmith that the data were confidential (Inquiry Secretariat 1999, para 113). Thus, the rationale underpinning the working party's important conclusions that it was 'most unlikely that BSE will have any implications for human health', was not its own, but rather belonged to the very Department that was supposedly seeking its advice. This may not have been a deliberate attempt by the secretariat or Department to steer the beliefs and judgements of the Southwood Working Party. Rather it seems that departmental views were recycled through, and sanctioned by, a nominally independent committee because of the structural asymmetries of knowledge that characterised the relationship between that committee and government, and because the working party had acquiesced to those structural limitations.

The second point to make about the working party's rationale for concluding that BSE was probably just like scrapie, and therefore of no significant risk to humans, was that whilst it was plausible, it was based on a set of hypotheses some of which were very poorly supported by the available evidence. Thus, whilst the evidence strongly supported a feed-borne vector of transmission for the agent, the argument that scrapie was the source of the agent was entirely speculative. Additional hypotheses about the origin of BSE, such as that the disease originated in cattle or some other non-scrapie source, were not even mentioned in the report.

The epidemiological evidence was at least consistent with the theory that there was a common source for BSE (rather than a single point source of origin) because cases had occurred simultaneously in geographically separate regions. This in turn was consistent with the hypothesis that transmission of scrapie to cattle had occurred only as a result of higher exposure to the scrapie agent and not a localised transmission of a modified strain of the scrapie agent, pathogenic to cattle. Wilesmith was assuming, however, that he had described the epidemic at an early stage, and that every case was an index case resulting from a cross-species transfer from scrapie-infected sheep material to cattle. In fact, it subsequently emerged that the epidemic had been underway for some considerable time and had already spread geographically, and through several cohorts of cattle, but had often not been noticed (Phillips *et al.* 2000, vol. 2, Chapter 3). Thus by the time MAFF began reporting BSE cases, those animals had probably contracted the disease from the recycled remains of previous cohorts of BSE-infected cattle. Whether, in fact, the epidemic had a common source or a single point source remains unknown, as does the origin of the disease.

The Southwood Working Party had recognised that Wilesmith's epidemiological work might be incorrect. Dr Hilary Pickles (the DoH Secretary) and Richard Southwood both appear to have had doubts about Wilesmith's estimate of the future course of the BSE epidemic; although those doubts were not set out in the working party's report and members of the working party subsequently indicated that that was something they regretted. Subsequent statements from both Pickles and Southwood, indicating that the working party was concerned that if they were to have specified a higher figure for the number of diseased animals that they anticipated, it might have implied unacceptably high rates of compensation, were never challenged (Southwood 1998, 1999; Pickles 1998). Wilesmith's predictions were nevertheless reproduced in the working party's report. Those predictions were based on the assumption that scrapie-infected material was the only vector of disease, and not BSE-infected material from subclinically infected animals; precisely the same reasoning that led to the conclusion that there must be a common scrapie source for BSE. Southwood later claimed that the members of the working party self-censored their doubts about the quality of Wilesmith's work in anticipation of an otherwise unfavourable Ministerial response to other aspects of their advice. He recalled that

> It is tempting to speculate that if we had given a higher estimate [of the eventual incidence of BSE], the costs of compensation [for clinically diseased animals] would then have been seen as so considerable that only partial compensation would have been offered and the risks consequently increased.

> (Southwood 1998, para. 23, pp. 5–6)

There was an additional problem with the working party's reasoning, regardless of the validity of Wilesmith's hypotheses that scrapie was the source of BSE, that there was a common source to the epidemic and that therefore greater exposure to the scrapie agent had allowed transmission to cattle, as opposed to the presence of a modified strain of scrapie pathogenic for cattle. The working party appeared to be assuming, as indeed they later confirmed, that if BSE was caused by an unmodified version of scrapie this would mean that the host range of that agent, once present in cattle, ought to be identical to that of the agent in its sheep host (Phillips *et al.* 2000, vol. 4, para. 10.27; Inquiry Secretariat 1999, para. 10). Yet crucially, the fact that the transmission characteristics of a TSE agent sometimes change in unpredictable ways after that agent *passages* to a new host species does not require that the agent must be an altered or mutant form prior to transmission to the new host.

That point was made clear in one of the written answers provided by Wilesmith to the 28 questions posed prior to the working party's first meeting. The question had asked 'what are the risks of a species jump?' Wilesmith's answer was as follows:

> If BSE is a result of cattle becoming infected with the scrapie agent, it will be some time, if ever, [before it is known] whether only a particular strain, and possibly a new one, is involved. Similarly the effects of *passage* of the agent in cattle, in terms of altered risks for other species, will be difficult to ascertain.

> (Phillips *et al.* 2000, vol. 4, annex, p. 78)

In other words, the selection of new strains of scrapie pathogenic to cattle, and changes in the transmission characteristics of the scrapie agent following *passage* to cattle are two separate issues. Thus even if BSE was caused by a conventional scrapie agent that was irrelevant to the question of whether or not BSE would subsequently have the same transmission characteristics as sheep scrapie. Yet the working party appeared to have assumed that the two points were one and the same issue. As one of the members, Bill Martin, recalled: 'we were talking, in these days, about the possibility of a mutant strain having made the leap across the species barrier, and therefore could it continue to cross the species?' (BSE Inquiry Transcript, 11 March 1998, p. 113).

During the course of the working party's deliberations evidence also began to emerge that challenged the validity of the assumption that BSE would have the same host range and transmission characteristics as scrapie. For example, in 1987 and 1988 attempts by the CVL to transmit BSE to hamsters were unsuccessful, even though hamsters are a species readily susceptible to scrapie (Phillips *et al.* 2000, vol. 2, para. 3.51). In September 1988, moreover, researchers at the NPU found that following transmission of BSE to mice, the incubation period was shorter than the incubation period for known scrapie strains (Phillips *et al.* 2000, vol. 2, para. 3.54). None of that evidence was mentioned in the working party's report. In fact, as we shall discuss in Chapter 6, in the months and years after the working party reported, evidence continued to accumulate demonstrating that BSE behaved quite differently from scrapie. We shall describe, in due course, some of the ways in which MAFF responded to that evidence, but it is striking that many aspects of government policy on BSE were for years subsequently made (and defended) on the premise that BSE was simply 'scrapie in cows', and hence the working party's optimistic judgement about human risk was entirely and unproblematically reliable.

To recapitulate briefly, the working party's conclusions about the likely absence of a risk to humans were based on the hypothesis that BSE was an unmodified form of scrapie that would behave in the same way in cows as it did in sheep. That hypothesis was problematic in several respects; it had little or no supporting evidence, and it faced some contrary evidence. The members of the Southwood Working Party seem to have recognised the fragility of the analysis, partly because they had privately acknowledged that they were sceptical of Wilesmith's epidemiological work. Moreover, Southwood had written a private letter in August 1988 stating that 'my colleagues and I have made various recommendations based, I have to admit, largely on guesswork' (Phillips *et al.* 2000, vol. 4, para. 10.33). Yet, the fact that the working party's members knew they were guessing was not made clear in their report; nor did those concerns translate into a more cautious overall conclusion.

There was one crucial reason why the most optimistic risk scenario available was sanctioned by the working party and why doubts about the validity of that scenario were not made more explicit. In written evidence to the Phillips Inquiry, the working party members had described what they considered to be their role, stating that '[w]e were fully aware that the consequences of an alarmist report from the Southwood Working Party would be disastrous' (Inquiry Secretariat 1999, para. 2). By 'disastrous' the working party explained that they were referring in part to the possibility that the childhood vaccination programme would have been put in jeopardy if they had given the impression that the existing stock of vaccines were unsafe.

Southwood has recalled that because of the use of bovine materials in the manufacture of pharmaceutical products such as vaccines '[w]e really thought the medical problem was severe' (BSE Inquiry Transcript 21 July 1999, p. 73). In other words, the members were far from convinced that BSE would be harmless to humans. Southwood and his colleagues were especially concerned about the use of bovine products in the production of pharmaceutical products. Early drafts of the working party's report had drawn attention to those concerns but the members were persuaded by the Department of Health secretariat to modify the relevant passage of the committee's report on the grounds that public confidence in the vaccination programme might have been put in jeopardy (Phillips et al. 2000, vol. 4, para. 8.14). Thus, the working party adopted verbatim the DoH officials' suggested wording for the relevant section of their report (Phillips et al. 2000, vol. 7, para. 5.21). It stated that the risks of transmission via medicinal products appeared 'remote' (MAFF/DoH 1989, para. 5.3.5). Earlier drafts of the report. had only used the term 'remote' to refer to the risks from food-borne sources of exposure (Pickles 1988a). As one of the members of the Southwood Working Party later recalled:

> [the] use of the word 'remote' was done on purpose, because the consequences for the vaccination programme, for the use of medicines, could have been really quite disastrous if the public at large had been alarmed by this.
>
> (BSE Inquiry Transcript 21 July 1999, p. 65)

The working party had also been privately worried about the possible risks to those occupationally exposed to BSE; they had drawn attention to the risks in earlier drafts of its report (Phillips et al. 2000, vol. 4, para. 6.11). Yet in its published report the working party again publicly played down its concerns by describing such risks as 'remote'. As Richard Southwood explained: 'causing alarm – which may be totally unnecessary – is not something a responsible body does' (BSE Inquiry Transcript, 21 July 1999, p. 96). When asked by counsel to the

Phillips Inquiry why the working party had been concerned about being alarmist in relation to occupational risks when there was no likelihood of adverse consequences arising from the reactions of those working in farming or the slaughtering industry, as there were in relation to non use of vaccines, one of the working party members, Bill Martin, explained:

> I think there is more to it than that . . . One could see slaughtermen downing tools and going on strike because of the possible risks of handling cattle. There were all sorts of possibilities there. I could not see veterinarians doing that, but they would take precautions by wearing long plastic sleeves and so on in any calving they were doing. But slaughtermen and abattoir workers were a different category. They could down tools and refuse to handle cattle.

(BSE Inquiry Transcript, 21 July 1999, p. 97)

At the Phillips Inquiry members of the working party defended their decision deliberately to play down their concerns, in print, about non-food-borne risks from BSE by claiming that they had privately alerted the Medicines Control Agency and the Health and Safety Executive to their real beliefs about the potential risks of transmission. The working party argued that since those bodies were 'responsible' they would act on that private advice, and thus the phrase 'remote' to describe non-food-borne risks was accurate in the sense that it would refer to the situation once the appropriate steps had been taken by the relevant statutory bodies (Phillips *et al.* 2000, vol. 4, para. 10.87).

That strategy, if it was not a post hoc justification, ultimately turned out to be naive because the relevant agencies were persuaded by the working party's published advice that the risks were already remote (Phillips *et al.* 2000, vol. 4, paras 10.83–10.109). For example, in September 1989 a Working Group of the Committee of Safety of Medicines referred to 'the findings of the Southwood Report in which it was stated that 'the risk to man of infection via medicinal products was remote" (BSE Inquiry Transcript 21 July 1999, p. 81). Existing stocks of vaccines continued to be used until 1993, for example, and it took the Health and Safety Executive three years to issue advice to high-risk trades (Phillips *et al.* 2000, vol. 1, p. xxvii).

Although the working party acknowledged that they self-censored their concerns about both occupational and pharmaceutical exposure to the BSE agent, they maintained that their published assessment of the risks from oral, food-borne exposure to the BSE agent had not been similarly modified; indeed early drafts of the report had always referred to the risks from oral exposure to the BSE agent as 'remote'. There are, however, several reasons for suggesting that a concern to avoid public alarm did in fact have some influence on the presentation of the working party's assessment of the risks of oral routes of exposure to the BSE agent.

For example, following its initial meeting, when the working party decided to recommend the slaughter of clinically affected animals, Southwood wrote to the MAFF Permanent Secretary justifying that piece of advice by noting that 'my colleagues would wish to join me in emphasising to you the magnitude of the potential risks involved' (Phillips *et al.* 2000, vol. 4, para. 2.4). There was, however, a marked discrepancy between that private correspondence and the language adopted in the first draft of the working party's report that had been written on the basis of deliberations at the initial meeting. That draft, referring to the risks from oral exposure to the BSE agent, contained the phrase 'the risk of transmission of BSE to humans appears remote', but that phrase had been written by the DoH secretariat and not the Members.

One possible explanation for this discrepancy is that the same rationale for the reassuring public representation of the risks was assumed as in relation to pharmaceutical and occupational exposures to BSE; namely, that the public language referred to the dangers that existed after regulatory intervention (in this case the slaughter and destruction of clinically affected animals) and not in its absence. Indeed, in evidence to the European Parliament in 1996, Southwood explained that the principles that should guide a scientific committee advising a government include 'a duty not to cause unwarranted public anxiety, more particularly if the "damage", if any, has already been incurred' (Southwood Working Party 1999, para. 81.5). Yet in this case, even with a slaughter policy in place for clinically diseased cattle, there would still have been substantial oral exposure to the BSE pathogen from subclinically infected animals.

The members of Southwood Working Party have recalled that they had been very worried about allowing consumption of some types of bovine offals (BSE Inquiry Transcript, 11 March 1998, p. 142). Nonetheless, their final report gave the impression that there were no risks associated with such animals; not only because the term 'remote' was used to describe the risks of transmission of BSE to humans but also because subclinical animals were barely mentioned. In 1989, in response to a letter from a retired neurologist who had criticised what she believed to be the implication in the working party's report that food from subclinically infected cattle was safe, Southwood hinted that the working party had decided to underplay their concerns about the risks from a-symptomatic animals. He explained:

> As you can imagine it was extremely difficult to steer the proper course between causing excessive alarm and undue complacency. The evidence to date seems to indicate that the BSE agent is very similar to scrapie . . . It was this line of argument that finally convinced us not to press the point, that you have made in your letter, any more strongly.

> (Phillips *et al.* 2000, vol. 4, para. 10.66)

A lawyer representing the members of the working party at the Phillips Inquiry acknowledged that Southwood and his colleagues were concerned to avoid alarming the meat-eating public. He explained that in wishing to avoid alarm the working party didn't just mean a possible lack of uptake of childhood vaccinations but also the possible economic consequences for farmers and those involved in the livestock industry (BSE Inquiry Transcript, 21 July 1999, p. 7) which presumably meant the consequences of members of the public ceasing to purchase British beef.

Officials had also made clear to the working party that any new regulations, *let al*one a risk assessment that drew attention to the uncertainties, would undermine confidence in beef markets. For example, in November 1988, three months before the working party's report had been completed, Southwood told ministers and officials that current Health and Safety Executive regulations were inadequate. The response from the Chief Veterinary Officer, Keith Meldrum was that 'new precautions would escalate the issue unnecessarily when we were saying there was no hazard to man from BSE' (Phillips *et al.* 2000, vol. 4, para. 6.11). We think that the working party acquiesced, at least in part, with those types of concerns.

The remarks in the discussion above suggest that both MAFF and the members of the working party were concerned to avoid saying anything publicly to indicate the existence of possible risks, and consequently a narrative was constructed suggesting that there were negligible risks, and implying that their reassurances were scientifically legitimated, even though that played down both the possible risks and their underlying reasoning. The portrayal of hybrid judgements as if they were purely scientific and robust caused numerous subsequent problems, and could be said to have made a difficult problem considerably more difficult than might otherwise have been the case. The representations of the risks from BSE were based on a set of epidemiological hypotheses that were developed by Wilesmith and his colleagues at CVL, endorsed by MAFF officials, and then *passaged* through the Southwood Working Party. Those hypotheses were useful to MAFF because, by providing a reassuring narrative, they could contribute to stabilising the market for British beef. That account is consistent with what in Chapter 2 we referred to as a co-evolutionary model; it indicates how a seemingly scientific account was in practice constructed out of some fragments of evidence and several non-scientific considerations that framed MAFF's approach and that of the working party.

Other factors may also have contributed to the reasons why the members of the working party under-emphasised the uncertainties in relation to their assessment of risk. For example, some of the comments made by members of the working party to the Phillips Inquiry suggest that they had been unwilling to question the analogy with scrapie. Members of the working party have stated that

> There was no, or virtually no scientific knowledge concerning BSE available at this time. We worked on the basis that scrapie was the most likely cause of the BSE epidemic; we had to base our advice on the science relating to scrapie at that time.

> (Inquiry Secretariat 1999, para. 42)

Similarly, the working party collectively indicated that

> Whilst our Report drew attention to the uncertainties that existed, we did not and do not consider that the highlighting of numerous 'potential' risks was then or is now desirable especially when such potential risks are based on speculation rather than scientific knowledge.

> (Southwood Working Party 1999, para. 9)

Those comments invite two interpretations. One is that the members of the working party adopted the orthodox scientistic practice of preferring to focus just on what was known – i.e. about scrapie – even if it did not directly apply to BSE. An alternative explanation would be that the members of the working party were providing a post hoc justification for judgements that were initially based on different, but unacknowledged, considerations.

The failure of the scientific advisors fully to acknowledge the uncertainties that characterised their understanding of, for example, the risks to human health from asymptomatic but infected animals can not, we suggest, simply be explained by reference to their adherence to the social conventions of academic research. If they had been willing only to endorse well-supported claims, their representation of the risks would have been far more tentative. Our analysis of the evidence suggests that the Southwood Working Party acquiesced in MAFF's desire to provide reassurance to consumers to ensure market stability.

In the long run, we argue, the willingness of the Southwood Working Party to endorse a very optimistic narrative, and to provide a seeming scientific secure defence of that narrative, served to insulate MAFF's policy from many contemporaneous challenges and (as we will explain in later chapters) from subsequent reviews as new and troubling evidence emerged. The rigidity that came to characterise MAFF's policy regime, and the representation of the science, was not (as Phillips et al. suggested) a consequence of the fact that the working party failed to make its reasoning explicit, but because it was never MAFF's intention to ensure that policy-making was informed by a proper science-based analysis of the possible risks.

Slaughter of clinically affected animals

As we explained in Chapter 4, in late 1987 MAFF officials had decided to recommend that Ministers introduce a slaughter and compensation scheme for cattle clinically affected with BSE. The Minister had refused to follow that advice and this led to the decision to inform the government's Chief Medical Officer, Donald Acheson, about BSE. That in turn led to a subsequent decision by Acheson to recommend that an expert committee be established to provide urgent advice on the risks of biological products and the disposal of sick animals. We argued that Acheson's decision to establish the committee was motivated primarily by his desire to gather additional political support – in the guise of an advisory committee – for a policy that Ministers had been resisting.

Even after MacGregor learnt that the proposed expert committee would be very likely to recommend that carcasses of overtly diseased animals should not enter the human food chain, he was adamant that there would be no government funding for a slaughter scheme (Phillips *et al.* 2000, vol. 3, para. 5.80). MAFF officials therefore initiated discussions with the cattle industry to see if they would fund a slaughter scheme, but the industry was clearly reluctant to do so. MAFF's Permanent Secretary subsequently tried to persuade Southwood that the new Working Party, yet to begin meeting, should avoid recommending a slaughter policy. According to Southwood, the Permanent Secretary 'expressed the hope to me that any recommendations we would make "would not lead to an increase in public expenditure"' (Southwood 1998, para. 25). The Permanent Secretary maintained, however, that as the minutes of the encounter noted, he only told Southwood that the government wanted to examine a range of alternatives to compulsory slaughter and that the Working Group's deliberations should be restricted to the scientific evidence and not make policy recommendations (Strang 1988). The minutes suggest that Southwood responded by stating the 'Group would not specify what administrative mechanisms would be appropriate. That would be a matter for the Government' (ibid.).

Despite the promise, and the pressure from the Permanent Secretary, the working party did recommend that arrangements should be made to ensure that clinically diseased animals were slaughtered and destroyed. As we noted in Chapter 4, guidance in that direction had been provided by officials at the Department of Health. The CMO had written to Southwood in April 1988 asking his working party to address the question: 'what steps if any is prudent to take . . . in clinically affected animals covering . . . meat, offal and meat products for human consumption' (Acheson 1988). A draft answer to that question, written by DoH officials for the Southwood Working Party, had commented that 'meat, offal and meat products for human consumption – not acceptable' (Phillips *et al.* 2000, vol. 4, annex, p. 78). MAFF officials responsible for animal health also provided a draft answer and, despite the Agriculture Minister's concerns, the answer was also that 'it may be prudent to condemn, for any use, the whole carcass of affected animals' (Phillips *et al.* 2000, vol. 4, annex, p. 78).

Ministers reluctantly agreed to the Working Party's recommendation but were only prepared to provide farmers with 50 per cent of the value their animals would have fetched in the marketplace if they had been healthy. That decision was not supported by the head of MAFF's Animal Health Division, the CMO or the members of the Southwood Working Party because they recognised that it gave farmers a strong disincentive to report that their cattle had BSE (Cruickshank 1988, para 4.25; Acheson 1998, para. 54). MAFF officials told Southwood that the decision to provide compensation at 50 per cent of the average market value would, however, be reviewed when they received the Working Party's final recommendations (Andrews 1988b).

On 10 November 1988, the working party held its second meeting and was told by MAFF officials that there was no evidence of any evasion of the law requiring the reporting of suspected BSE cases. The DoH secretariat later stated that

> My recollection is that this was mostly verbal reassurances from MAFF officials, backed up with the changes in reporting rates said to have followed the introduction of the scheme. I cannot recollect having even anecdotal evidence of evasion presented to the working party at that time.
>
> (Pickles 1998a, para 40.6)

Nevertheless, the minutes of the meeting note that 'It was agreed that this reassuring position should be referred to in the Report and that precise figures should be sought' (Anon 1988).

The final report of the Southwood Working Party, published three months later, included the following text, which had been written by the DoH secretariat:

> It has been suggested that because compensation is set at 50% some farmers are evading the law and that as a result the carcasses of affected animals are reaching the human food chain. However the evidence does not support this view.
>
> (MAFF/DoH 1989, para. 7.2.3)

The report then goes on to cite some supporting evidence: however, it was unconvincing. It noted that:

> The number of suspect cases being reported has gone up since the compulsory slaughter programme was introduced. It also seems likely that should a farmer try to sell an animal for slaughter, rather than report suspected BSE, the transportation to a market and abattoir will exacerbate the clinical signs of the disease. . . . BSE was confirmed in only 40 out of a total of 63 suspect cases reported from markets and slaughterhouses. None of these cases was from herds in which BSE had previously been recognised: so there was no evidence that early signs had been suspected and that evasion was deliberate.
>
> (MAFF/DoH 1989, para. 7.2.3)

However, the fact that the number of suspects cases being reported had increased since the slaughter programme was introduced merely reflected the fact that the epidemic was increasing (and even if the epidemic was stable, an increase in reporting rates would tell you only that there was more reporting compared to when there was no compensation). Furthermore, given that almost all early cases of BSE were singletons (i.e. one per herd) one could not take comfort from the fact that cases picked up in markets were also singletons. Southwood later recalled that in their report they had 'cited evidence, that we had been given by MAFF, suggesting that [the level of compensation at 50%] was effective; however privately we remained concerned' (Southwood 1998, para. 25).

That evidence was, however, subsequently represented as factual and authoritative by policy-makers because it had appeared in the Working Party's report. For example, the Agricultural Minister, John MacGregor, recalled that in the Spring of 1989 he had resisted increasing the compensation payable to farmers in the absence of firm evidence given that

> The Southwood Report had advised that there was no evidence to support the view that because compensation was set at 50% some farmers were evading the law and carcasses of affected animals were reaching the human food chain.

> (MacGregor 1998, para. 91)

Similarly, Donald Thompson, MAFF's junior Minister in the late 1980s, has recalled that:

> *I could only rely on expert scientific and legal advice.* For example, the Southwood Report stated that it had been suggested that because compensation is set at 50 per cent, some farmers are evading the law and that as a result, carcasses of affected animals are reaching the human food chain. However, the Southwood report said: 'Evidence does not support this view'.

> (BSE Inquiry Transcript, 8 July 1999, pp. 16–17; emphasis added)

Thus an empirically weak claim was written into the Working Party's report by government officials, without complaint, by members of the Working Party. Importantly, it was subsequently cited in support of the policy in question as if it were a reliable, evidence-based scientific fact that had been sanctioned by a committee of experts.

The lack of controls on asymptomatic animals

One of the most problematic discrepancies in the advice provided by the Southwood Working Party was that clinically affected animals were deemed sufficiently risky to be removed entirely from the human food chain whilst subclinically infected animals that were not yet showing symptoms of BSE – potentially almost as hazardous as clinically infected animals – were considered acceptably safe. It was not even thought necessary to label food products containing bovine brain and spleen. That discrepancy was further compounded by the Working Party's advice to baby food manufacturers to avoid the use of ruminant offal and thymus. If offal and thymus were not considered acceptably safe for infants then why were they considered acceptable for children and adults? This section explores the rationale for the Working Party's advice in relation to subclinically infected animals.

First, however, it is interesting to note that in early June 1988, before the working party began to meet, sections of the food industry appear to have considered ceasing to use bovine brain in their food products but were dissuaded from doing so by MAFF officials. An article published on 4 June in the *British Medical Journal* had criticised the 'alarming indifference' on the part of the medical profession and the general public to press reports about the emergence of BSE (Holt and Phillips 1988). It argued that the view that slaughter of animals with clinical symptoms of the disease would be sufficient to remove any risk to consumers was 'naive, uniformed, and potentially disastrous' because asymptomatic cattle might be just as infective as those with overt symptoms, and it concluded that the use of cattle brain in food should be abolished (Holt and Phillips 1988). In response to the article, the food industry asked MAFF's Food Standards Division whether they should stop using brains in meat products. The Head of MAFF's Animal Health Division 'advised strongly', however, that Food Standards Division should not suggest to the food industry that it should voluntarily cease to use bovine brains in meat products on the grounds that there was no evidence to justify such a move (BSE Inquiry Transcript 20 July 1999, pp. 39–42).

It is also interesting to note that in 1988 the rendering industry had asked MAFF to stop permitting the use of brain spinal cord and other potentially infected tissues as a contributory source for meat and bone meal (Phillips *et al.* 2000, vol. 6, para. 3.223). Similarly, the pet food industry decided in July 1988 that it would stop using certain cattle offals as ingredients in its products. (Phillips *et al.* 2000, vol. 6, para. 3.192). If the rendering and pet food industries could see the benefits of excluding bovine offals from their products, MAFF's approach seems distinctly anomalous.

Although the working party did not recommend any restrictions on the consumption of subclinically infected animals – save the advice to baby food manufacturers – the working party members have recalled that they were very worried about allowing consumption of some types of bovine offals (BSE Inquiry Transcript, 11 March 1998, p. 142). In fact the first draft of the Working Party's report, written by the DoH Secretariat on the basis of deliberations from the first meeting of the working party had suggested that: '[b]rain and lymphoid tissue could be omitted from meat pies without any important consequences for the industry and certainly without any culinary loss' (Phillips *et al.* 2000, vol. 4, para. 10.53).

The working party subsequently decided, however, to omit that recommendation. The minutes of its second meeting on 10 November 1988 note that 'it was inappropriate to recommend banning all ox-brain for human consumption' (Phillips *et al.* 2000, vol. 4, para. 5.11). The rationale for that decision was not, however, recorded. In written evidence to the Phillips Inquiry, the members of the working party claimed that at the time they did not consider the costs and practicalities of banning bovine brain tissue to be proportionate to their beliefs about the possible risks (Southwood Working Party 1999, para. 28). The question, is how were judgements about what was, and what was not, a proportionate response reached?

In evidence to the Phillips Inquiry, Southwood argued that

> A general ban on bovine materials of certain sorts ... [would imply] immediately moving into a more alarmist phase. The Prime Minister after all thought our report was very alarmist as it was. Once you moved to the whole British herd, you are moving to an alarmist phase, and that has implications for life not just through the vaccination programme but for the farming industry, for people's lives there. So we were very conscious that that was a pressure. We had to be totally persuaded that there was some real significant risk to adults and we were not.

> (BSE Inquiry Transcript, 21 July 1999, p. 121)

In 1996, however, Southwood provided a more illuminating answer. He told a journalist from the *New Scientist* that a recommendation to ban the use of all cattle brains in food would have stood little chance politically: 'We felt it was a no-goer. [MAFF] already thought our proposals were pretty revolutionary' (Pearce 1996). In other words, Southwood implied that his committee believed it could not issue advice restricting the consumption of cattle brains, and perhaps lymphatic tissues too, because it knew that advice would be politically disagreeable to Ministers. Direct pressure from officials was not required; in this case, mere anxiety seems to have been sufficient.

Although the working party had decided in November 1988 not to recommend a ban on the human consumption of cattle brains, they did, at that time, suggest alternatively that processed food which contained cattle brain should be labelled (Phillips *et al.* 2000, vol. 4, para. 5.12). The working party recognised that in practice this would mean that the food industry would stop using brains rather than include them with labelling (Pickles 1988b). Thus a draft of the Working Party's report, dated 22 December 1988, included the following in parenthesis: 'we also recommend that use of ox brain and ? lymphoid tissue in meat products [? for young children and/or any cooked food] be limited and or indicated by labelling' (MAFF/DoH, 1988, para. 9.4).

The working party was, however, already having second thoughts about its labelling recommendation. MAFF officials had told Southwood that a labelling requirement could not be introduced unilaterally under European Community rules and might be viewed as a disguised barrier to trade (Southwood Working Party 1999, para. 33.3). MAFF officials were also concerned about other ramifications of a labelling recommendation. In a note written in early January 1989, entitled *Sensitive Issues in the Animal Health Sector*, the CVO noted that labelling meat products as containing bovine brain, spinal cord and spleen:

> Would create considerable presentational difficulties since the consumer would be invited to make up his own mind on whether or not they believe there to be a risk from BSE through the consumption of such products and would hedge the issue as to whether such products carry a risk to the consumer.

(Meldrum 1989)

The Working Party's labelling suggestion was omitted from its published report. Southwood later claimed that his Group had been advised that a labelling requirement would be difficult to enforce and that the UK was having problems with EEC proposals on food labelling (Southwood 1998, para. 28i). Despite deciding to omit the recommendation to ban or label the use of brain and lymphatic tissues in human foodstuffs, Southwood and his colleagues did decide, at their final meeting, that they would advise manufacturers of baby food to avoid the use of ruminant offal and thymus. The working party were concerned that young people might be more vulnerable to infection than adults.

Several senior MAFF officials were dismayed by the baby food recommendation, in part because offals such as liver and kidney were widely used in baby food and because their suitability for adults might be questioned as a result of the recommendation. After the Working Party's report had been completed, but before it had been published, Elizabeth Attridge, who was head of the of the Emergencies, Food Quality and Pest Control Group at MAFF, sent a memo to colleagues noting the difficulties with preventing the use of liver and kidney in baby food. She argued that MAFF should assess more fully what the actual risks were and not create problems 'simply on the basis of poorly substantiated speculation' (Phillips *et al.* 2000, vol. 6, para. 3.32). She pointed out that '[m]y understanding is that the evidence is not clear-cut and does need further consideration' (ibid.). She therefore suggested that the press notice accompanying the Southwood report should include the following passage:

> I understand the Committee did not have the opportunity to examine thoroughly all the scientific evidence relating to offal, particularly liver and kidney in human and baby food and I am therefore proposing to refer [I have therefore referred] the matter to the CMO to seek his advice before taking any further action.

(Phillips *et al.* 2000, vol. 6, para. 3.32)

Before the Southwood report was published the CMO checked the definition of offal with Southwood who agreed that the term 'offal' did not in this case refer to liver and kidney but only to only to spleen, brain, spinal cord and intestine (ibid., para. 3.51) The government were thus able to claim, at the time the Southwood report was published, that no bovine offal, in the sense used by the Working Party, was currently used in baby food.

The debate over what to say and do about liver and kidneys appears to reveal that senior officials were willing to assert and accept that some of the underlying evidence was not critically examined by the working party (when the conclusions drawn from that evidence were apparently deemed unacceptable). At the same time officials were apparently prepared to accept that all the remaining evidence had been robustly examined because the rest of the report was not reviewed and was uncritically accepted. This implies that senior officials saw the working party tactically as a scientific-seeming resource to serve political purposes and to provide legitimation for the prevailing policy regime rather than as a vital resource to help protect public health.

Several aspects of the evolution of the Working Party's advice concerning the possible risks from subclinically infected animals are worth highlighting. First, the decision to omit recommendations to ban some tissues and to label others appears to have been a result of direct political pressure, and in anticipation of a negative response from officials and Ministers. It is not that the Southwood Working Party chose only to make scientific judgements; it made, as we argue above, numerous policy judgements. Its report, however, was represented as purely scientific. The final report of the working party did not explain the basis for any of the decisions that had been taken in regard to subclinically infected animals. Instead the working party represented the risks from consuming asymptomatic cattle as negligible, as again apparently a purely scientific decision. For example, the report had noted that 'the Working Party believes that risks as at present perceived would not justify [labelling bovine brain and spleen]' (MAFF/DoH 1989, para. 5.3.5).

We believe the interactions between the scientific advisors comprising the Southwood Working Party and policy-makers in MAFF and the DoH show how risk management considerations shaped not just the representations of the risks but their assessments too. Nonetheless, both the Southwood Working Party and policy-makers chose to represent the advice of the working party as if it were purely, and robustly, scientific. By doing so, we argue that the central role of political judgements about what was and was not acceptable was disguised. The representations of the risks were adjusted to correspond with policy advice. The report of the Southwood Working Party we believe failed to draw attention to those risks that were not covered in the policy advice it provided. That failure was crucially important, because the report was subsequently interpreted by Ministers as having implied that the only necessary controls were those recommended in that report, and that all the residual uncertainties could be discounted. For example, Ministers and several senior officials believed that there was no need seriously to consider imposing controls on asymptomatic animals. As the then Agricultural Minister, John MacGregor, later recalled: 'some people were concerned about subclinical animals . . . others were not, because Sir Richard Southwood had made clear that was not a real problem' (Phillips *et al.* 2000, vol. 6, para. 3.262). The struggle over the introduction of controls on so-called 'specified bovine offals' will be discussed at length in the next chapter.

Animal health risks

Almost no policy measures to protect animal health were recommended by the Southwood Working Party. The only exceptions were its insistence that MAFF's ruminant-to-ruminant feed ban should be extended indefinitely, and a general recommendation to 'address' the problem of recycling 'inadequately sterilised' animal products as animal feed as part of the adjustment of the EC's agricultural policy framework (MAFF/DoH 1989, para. 9.4). There was little doubt that the available evidence supported MAFF's theory that contaminated animal feed was the main vector of transmission of BSE, and therefore that the ruminant-to-ruminant feed ban, introduced by MAFF and endorsed by the Working Party, would help limit infection spreading from animal to animal. There were, however, several outstanding issues in relation to animal health. In particular, was the scope and nature of the ruminant feed ban sufficient to protect cattle and other animals from food-borne transmission of the agent, given what was known and not know about BSE? Analysis of MAFF's deliberations and decisions in relation to that issue, and its subsequent interaction with the Southwood Working Party, is especially revealing.

The scope of MAFF's ruminant feed ban

Once it had been established that cattle were almost certainly becoming infected with BSE through the consumption of contaminated animal protein (i.e. meat and bone meal), there were several means of preventing further feed-borne transmission. One option was a complete ban on the use of animal protein in animal feed, but initial discussions within MAFF highlighted the fact that just over 10 per cent of commercial meat and bone meal was fed to cattle and sheep. Most of the remainder ended up in pig and poultry feed, although some was consumed by animals in zoos. As MAFF officials noted, a complete ban on the use of animal protein in animal feed would deprive the rendering industry of its principal market but a ban limited to the use of animal protein for cattle and sheep feed would have relatively little effect on the industry (Cowen 1988). Officials also recognised that a partial ban would enable exports of meat and bone meal to continue (Rees 1988).

Animal health officials consequently decided that the diets of pigs and poultry were not going to be affected by the proposed feed ban; the measure would only ban the use of animal protein in the feed for ruminants. MAFF's Chief Veterinary Officer, Howard Rees, justified that decision to Ministers by asserting that 'there was no evidence that these species [pigs and poultry] were susceptible to such diseases' and that 'even if [they were susceptible], their life cycle is such that clinical disease is unlikely to occur' (Rees 1988).

That decision was potentially problematic for two reasons. First, it merely assumed that non-ruminants, such as pigs, poultry and domestic pets would not be susceptible to BSE. Evidence either to indicate susceptibility or lack of susceptibility did not exist. Indeed, in June 1988, the new CVO, Keith Meldrum, admitted privately to a colleague that '[t]he most we could say is that any ruminant protein fed to [pigs] might contain the agent of BSE or scrapie. Whether or not infection would be established in the pig and whether it might replicate is unknown' (BSE Inquiry Transcript, 16 June 1998, p. 99). Second, unless those countries that imported UK animal feed were to introduce a ban on use of animal protein in ruminant feed there was nothing in the proposed feed ban to prevent exported ruminant protein ending up in the feed of cattle herds in other jurisdictions. Officials were aware of that possibility but in practice, exported feed containing ruminant proteins was not labelled; in fact, importing countries were not told that they might be receiving contaminated animal feed.

In early June 1988, MAFF announced that the feeding of rations containing animal protein to ruminants was to be banned until 31 December 1988. A few days later, however, following representations from the animal foodstuffs industry, the scope of the feed ban was narrowed (Phillips *et al.* 2000, vol. 3, para. 4.21). The definitions were revised to limit 'animal protein' to proteins derived from a *ruminating* animals. Thus cattle feed would still be able to contain recycled animal proteins derived from pigs, poultry and other non-ruminant animals. That further narrowing of the ban was potentially problematic. The reason why MAFF officials had initially decided that *all* animal protein, rather than just ruminant protein, should be banned from ruminant feed was because existing analytical techniques were not sufficiently advanced to distinguish between ruminant protein and those from other mammals (Evans 1988). Indeed, once the animal foodstuffs industry had managed to persuade animal health officials to exempt non-ruminant protein from the proposed ban, an official from MAFF's Food Standards Division, in a memo to the head of the Animal Health Division, noted that 'I appreciate there is a case for minimising the damage to the rendering industry. Nonetheless there are clearly problems in drafting legislation in which we know the essential point to be unenforceable' (Owen 1988).

In order to protect the viability of the rendering industry, MAFF had therefore limited the feed ban to such an extent that it was effectively gambling that pigs and poultry were not susceptible to BSE, and that the animal feed industry would police itself by ensuring that its members did not, either deliberately or accidentally, use ruminant proteins in ruminant feeds. Officials also effectively decided that maintaining the domestic animal feed industry's export markets, in the very short term, was worth the risks to veterinary and public health in the UK's trading partners. It was inevitable that many overseas countries would discover that the UK was exporting feed that posed a risk to their domestic herds and take protective measures; MAFF's actions were just delaying the inevitable.

As we shall note in later chapters, the potential problems with the scope of MAFF's ruminant feed ban – anticipated by officials – all materialised. Domestic pets and a number of other species went on to develop TSEs from exposure to contaminated ruminant proteins and pigs were found to be susceptible, experimentally at least, to the disease. BSE was also exported to, and became a severe problem for, many other countries that imported UK animal feed. Furthermore, it transpired that there had been widespread disregard of the ruminant feed ban and extensive cross-contamination between animal protein destined for non-ruminants and animal protein destined for cattle. In 1988 and early 1989, however, MAFF managed to ensure that what were then only potential problems with the scope of the ruminant feed ban were not raised overtly by the Southwood Working Party. That was sometimes relatively straightforward. For example, officials simply did not tell the working party that ruminant protein could not be distinguished from other mammalian protein, and that officials were concerned that the Department's legislation would be unenforceable. Not surprisingly, the committee members did not raise that particular issue. The remaining potential problems required more careful management.

Exports

When Southwood was first told by MAFF officials, in May 1988, that the Government were intending to ban the use of meat and bonemeal in feed for ruminants he 'expressed concern about exports of feed' (Strang 1988). Those concerns were subsequently ignored. The Minister, John McGregor, on learning of Southwood's comments had told his officials that 'it is particularly important that the trade implications for feed . . . be handed very carefully' (Haine 1988).

Southwood and his colleagues returned to the issue of exports of ruminant protein-based feeds at their final meeting in February 1989. They had wanted to recommend that some restrictions should be placed on such exports but as a minute written by the MAFF secretary pointed out:

> A number of other changes [to the committee's report] were made, most of which were helpful. In addition, there had been some suggestion that a recommendation should be made in relation to exports of meat and bone meal. However, *the Working Party was persuaded not to include such a recommendation* because importing countries were well aware of our health status and it was therefore up to them to decide whether or not to import and under what conditions.
>
> (Lawrence 1989a, emphasis added)

Southwood told the European Parliament in 1997 that his committee was not in fact asked about the consequences of exporting UK ruminant protein. He stated that:

> If you ask me whether in 1988 the working party would have considered there was a risk to herds in other countries if UK-produced meal (with meat and bone meal) was exported I am totally confident that we would have answered in the affirmative. Knowing that the meal was almost certainly the cause of the outbreak in the UK it is clear that it was irresponsible (whatever the law) to make it available as cattle food elsewhere.
>
> (European Parliament 1997a, p. 8)

In the absence of inconvenient comments on feed exports from the Working Party, the diversion of contaminated ruminant protein overseas continued in the full knowledge of officials and Ministers. For example, in January 1989 a representative of the United Kingdom Renderers Association told MAFF's junior agricultural minister that members were experiencing difficulty in selling animal protein but were exporting as much as possible (Thompson 1989). As one senior MAFF official told a colleague later that year, '[t]he rendering industry has survived the July 1988 prohibition, in part because they have been able to fill the gap in the market through exports' (Lawrence 1989b).

Although the Southwood Working Party had been persuaded not to comment on the export of MBM in its report, the issue was taken up by the Chief Medical

Officer who attempted on several occasions during 1989 to persuade MAFF to ban exports of MBM or at least label the feed as unfit for ruminants (Acheson 1998, para. 64). Senior veterinary officials refused to follow the CMO's advice, believing that if they informed third countries that ruminant feed was not permitted to be fed to ruminants in the UK, the countries concerned would just cease to import the feed (Phillips *et al.* 2000, vol. 3, para. 6.54).

Eventually, in January 1990, John Gummer, by then Secretary of State at MAFF, told the CVO Keith Meldrum that there was a moral obligation to ensure that importing countries were aware that the UK did not permit the feeding of these products to ruminants. The CVO then warned his opposite number in each recipient country (ibid., Strang). As a DoH official subsequently put it, however: 'the action taken so far overseas suggest the message has not got through . . . I fail to understand why this cannot be tackled from the British end which seems to be the only sure way of doing it, preferably by banning exports' (ibid., para. 6.57). Exports of animal feeds were not banned, however, until after March 1996.

From the point of view of the UK's trading partners, the failure to control exports of ruminant protein was one of the more problematic aspects of the BSE saga. In 2001, the WHO/FAO warned that more than 100 countries which had imported meat and bone meal or live cattle from western Europe during the 1980s were at risk from BSE (FAO 2001). Contaminated UK ruminant protein continued to be exported right up until March 1996 when the EU imposed a worldwide export ban on all exports of cattle and cattle products from the UK. Directive 94/38, issued in June 1994, banned the use of proteins derived from mammals for feeding to ruminants, and Directive 96/239, issued in March 1996, banned, amongst other things, the export from the UK of mammalian-derived meat and bonemeal. MAFF's policy of continuing with exports of ruminant meal for as long as possible was easier to sustain politically than it would have been if the Southwood Working Party had alerted stakeholders to the risks posed by exports and had argued publicly for controls.

Risks to non-ruminant animals

The minutes of the Southwood Working Party's first meeting, prepared by the MAFF secretariat, noted that 'although there was no certainty that the agent could not jump the species barrier into pigs and poultry, action in relation to these species would not be recommended' (Lawrence 1998, para. 85). It is not entirely clear whether that was a decision that originated with the committee or a decision that MAFF officials had persuaded the committee to adopt.

It would have been curious, however, if the working party had decided a priori not to make recommendations in relation to pigs and poultry. More significantly, there is evidence that the working party was concerned, at that meeting, about the risks of transmission of BSE to non-ruminant animals. A note of that meeting, prepared by the DoH secretariat, pointed out that the proposed ruminant feed ban still allowed 'affected cattle (minus heads) to enter the human food chain and allow affected sheep/cattle to be rendered for feed (with existing low-temperature processes) for pigs and poultry. This caused concern' (Pickles 1988c).

There is also evidence that MAFF officials did not want the working party to even mention the possible risks to pigs in its report. In January 1989 the DoH secretariat wrote to Southwood stating that: 'The surplus production [of ruminant meat and bone meal] is now going into pigs and poultry, I believe. I suppose we cannot make any comments about that' (Pickles 1989). Furthermore, the Working Party's final report had noted that 'domestic pets could well be susceptible to BSE' (MAFF/DoH 1989, para. 5.2.4) but had neglected to mention the possible risks to pigs or indeed any other other mammalian species. The impression was conveyed that there were no reasons to be concerned about farm animals that received the bulk of UK-produced meat and bone meal.

The implications of extending the ruminant feed ban to other mammals went substantially and problematically further than the immediate loss of markets to the rendering industry. If, for example, ruminant protein was banned from pig feed it would be an obvious step to ask why it was still considered safe to feed the same material to humans. Even mentioning the fact that other animals might be at risk of catching BSE from the same kind of food that was entering human food chains would be problematic, let alone introducing regulations.

Southwood had in fact attempted, indirectly, to recommend that the ruminant feed ban should be extended to cover pigs. In December 1988, Southwood drafted the conclusions to his Working Party's report. They included the following paragraph:

> This problem [BSE] has arisen as a result of the practice of feeding animal materials to herbivores which are thus exposed to infection/infective risks against which they have not evolved any defences. . . . we believe the inevitable risks are such that it would be prudent to change agricultural practice so as to eliminate these novel pathways for pathogens. We urge the Minister to address this general problem.
>
> (Phillips *et al.* 2000, vol. 4, para. 9.21)

Once the Secretariat saw that draft conclusions the DoH secretary wrote to the Chief Medical Officer pointing out that 'alarm bells will be ringing already in MAFF and they may attempt to steer Sir Richard away from a general statement of this sort' (ibid., para. 9.22). She added that

> Perhaps it's just as well that we have now arranged for DH to take over from MAFF the final stages in preparing the report. The official excuse was that I had better secretarial support than my colleague in MAFF.
>
> (Phillips *et al.* 2000, vol. 4, para. 9.22)

As predicted by the DoH secretary, the draft conclusions 'caused great anxiety' when MAFF officials first saw the text (Cruickshank 1998, para 7.1). A MAFF official noted that although:

> It may be difficult, and perhaps even inappropriate, for MAFF to intervene at this stage. . . . I would suggest that, at the very least, the members of the Working Party should be made aware of what the rendering industry does and its scale of activity so that they can reflect on the implications of the draft recommendation. . . . If a MAFF paper is provided this might perhaps offer a more flexible form of words which would at least leave room for the Government to examine a number of options besides a prohibition on the recycling of animal waste for feed rations.
>
> (Suich 1989)

The junior agriculture minister Donald Thompson comment was unambiguous: 'I cannot say how strongly I regard this matter. Of course we must take all due care but the environmental, economic and competition consequences would be dire if Prof S was to go forward' (Phillips *et al.* 2000, vol. 4, para. 9.25).

Prior to the Southwood Working Party's final meeting in early February MAFF officials spoke to two of the members of the Working Party, John Walton and Bill Martin, about the implications of effectively shutting down the UK's rendering industry (ibid., para. 9.28). Bill Martin subsequently wrote to Sir Richard Southwood and although he acknowledged that all the committee members were unhappy about the recycling of animal wastes, he argued that

> Disposal of the vast amount of animal waste does present a difficulty . . . Rendering and recycling, despite its limitations would seem to be the most acceptable method at present. . . . I think we have to be restrained in the view we express in the report, on this subject.
>
> (Martin 1989)

At the Working Party's final meeting on 3 February, where the report was signed, alterations to the final paragraph were agreed. Whilst the draft section had stated that:

> This problem has arisen as a result of the practice of feeding *animal* materials to herbivores . . . we believe *the inevitable risks* are such that *it would be prudent to change agricultural practice* so as to eliminate these novel pathways for pathogens.
>
> (Phillips *et al.* 2000, vol. 4, para. 9.21; emphasis added)

The final published version stated that:

> This problem has arisen as a result of the practice of feeding *ruminant* materials to herbivores . . . we believe that *the risks* from *inadequately sterilised animal products* are such that *this method of disposing animal waste should be changed* so as to eliminate these novel pathways for pathogens.
>
> (MAFF/DoH 1989, para 9.4; emphasis added)

As Southwood later noted, '[r]ecognising the practical problem of extensive quantities of [meat and bone meal], we did not recommend extending the ban to pigs and poultry' (Inquiry Secretariat 1999, para. 124).

As we noted earlier, however, the absence of a recommendation to extend the feed ban to pigs and poultry was represented in the Working Party's report as if had been based solely on scientific grounds concerning the absence of risk, rather than as a decision to acquiesce to MAFF's concerns about the consequences of preventing the recycling of animal waste. It would of course have been very difficult presentationally to raise concerns about the risks of feeding ruminant protein to pigs and poultry, while at the same time suggesting that there was no need for regulatory restrictions on the ingredients of those animals' feed, without making explicit the fact that the committee were not making purely scientific judgements. Officials were consequently able to represent the decision not to extend the feed ban to pigs and other non-ruminant animals by claiming that the working party had objectively examined the evidence and concluded that there was no scientific basis for making that particular recommendation.

In the next chapter we will describe some of the pressures on MAFF officials to extend the feed ban to non-ruminants. At this stage, however, we note that in January 1990 MAFF issued a Press Release which stated that:

> There is no scientific justification to extend the ruminant feed ban to pigs and poultry. The Southwood report acknowledged the importance of the feed ban for ruminants, but did not recommend that it be extended to pigs and poultry.

> (MAFF 1990b, emphasis added)

Officials made a similar private response to the animal feed industry and to their Ministers. (Phillips *et al.* 2000, vol. 5, paras 3.102 and 3.125). In a briefing paper for the Prime Minister for example, officials noted that: 'It is argued that if the scrapie agent can cause BSE in cattle, it could do the same in pigs and poultry. Professor Southwood has advised that there are no grounds for such an action' (Lowson 1990).

We believe that the above demonstrates that the Southwood Working Party's conclusions about the adequacy of the ruminant feed ban were subordinated to the prior policy judgements of MAFF officials and Ministers. Furthermore, as we have argued, those prior decisions, taken on political and commercial grounds, tacitly shaped the ostensibly scientific assessment of risk provided by an ostensibly independent committee. Officials then drew on the scientific veneer of authority provided by the working party to justify officials' policy preferences to the public, the animal feed industry and even their own Ministers; a tactic that the members of the working party did not overtly challenge.

Bibliography

Acheson, D. (1998) Letter dated 1988 to Sir Richard Southwood, *BSE Inquiry Year Book* Reference No. 88/4.20/1.1–1.2, in Phillips *et al.* 2000, op. cit.

Acheson, D. (1999) Witness Statement No. 251a. In Phillips *et al.* 2000, op cit.

Andrews, D. (1988a) Confidential – Bovine Spongiform Encephalopathy (BSE), Memo dated 31 March 1988, *BSE Inquiry Year Book* Reference No. 88/3.31/5.1–5.2, in Phillips *et al.* 2000, op. cit.

Andrews, D. (1988b) Letter to Sir Richard Southwood dated 12 July 1988, *BSE Inquiry Year Book* Reference No. 88/7.12/2.1, in Phillips *et al.* 2000, op.cit.

Anon (1988) Working Party on Bovine Spongiform Encephalopathy (BSE) Note of a Meeting Held on 10 November in Room 37D at the Department of Zoology, South Parks Road, Oxford. *BSE Inquiry Year Book* Reference No. 88/11.10/2.1–2.6, in Phillips *et al.* 2000, op. cit.

Bradley, R. (1988) *BSE Research Projects*, Minute dated 19 July 1988 to WA Watson, see *BSE Inquiry Year Book* Reference No. 88\07.19\2.1–2.2, in Phillips *et al.* 2000, op. cit.

BSE Inquiry Transcripts, in Phillips *et al.* op. cit.

Cowen, J. R. (1988) Bovine Spongiform Encephalopathy, Minute dated 26 February 1988, *BSE Inquiry Year Book* Reference No. 88/2.26/3.1–3.3, in Phillips *et al.* 2000, op. cit.

Cruickshank, A. (1998) Statement to the BSE Inquiry No 75, in Phillips *et al.* 2000, op. cit.

European Parliament (1997a) *Report on Alleged Contravention or Maladministration in the Implementation of Community Law in Relation to BSE.* Part A, PE220.544/fin./A, 7 February 1997. European Parliament, Brussels.

Evans, D. (1988) Parliamentary Secretary (Commons)'s meeting on BSE-Friday 27 May 1988, Minute dated 2 June 1988. *BSE Inquiry Year Book* Reference No. 88/6.2/3.1–3.3, in Phillips *et al.* 2000, op. cit.

FAO (2001) Press Release 01/41, 21 June 2001, 'FAO: More Than 30 Countries Have Taken Action On BSE, But More Needs To Be Done.', available at: http://www.fao.org/livestock/AGAP/FRG/Feedsafety/ffsp2.htm (1 March, 2002)

Gummer, J. (1990) *Hansard* 21 May 1990, vol. 173, No. 110, column 82. The Stationery Office, London.

Haine, D. B. (1988) Bovine Spongiform Encephalopathy: Secretary's Meeting with Sir R Southwood and the CMO, Minute dated 24 May 1988. *BSE Inquiry Year Book* Reference No. 88/5.24/2.1, in Phillips *et al.* 2000, op. cit.

Holt, T. A. and Phillips, J. (1988) 'Bovine spongiform encephalopathy', *BMJ*, **296**, 1581–2.

Inquiry Secretariat (1999) Information provided by Sir Richard Southwood, Sir Anthony Epstein, Dr William Martin and Lord Walton. Statement of Information No. 483, in Phillips *et al.* 2000, op. cit.

Lawrence, A. (1989a) BSE: The Southwood Report, Minute dated 7 February 1989, *BSE Inquiry Year Book* Reference No. 89/2.7/1.1, in Phillips *et al.* 2000, op. cit.

Lawrence, A. (1989b) BSE: Exports of Meat and Bonemeal to other Member States, Minute dated 3 July 1989, *BSE Inquiry Year Book* Reference Number 89/7.03/5.1–5.2, in Phillips *et al.* 2000, op. cit.

Lawrence, A. (1998) Statement No. 76 to the BSE Inquiry, in Phillips *et al.* 2000, op. cit.

Lowson, R. (1990) BSE: Note for the Prime Minister, dated 26 January 1990. *BSE Inquiry Year Book* Reference No. 90/01.26/13.1–13.6, in Phillips *et al.* 2000, op. cit.

MacGregor, J. (1998) Statement to the BSE Inquiry No 302, in Phillips *et al.* 2000, op. cit.

MAFF/DoH (1988) *Draft Report of the Expert Working Party on Bovine Spongiform Encephalopathy. BSE Inquiry Year Book* Reference No. 88/12.22/3.1–3.58, in Phillips *et al.* 2000, op. cit.

MAFF/DoH (1989) *Report of the Working Party on Bovine Spongiform Encephalopathy.* London: Ministry of Agriculture Fisheries and Food/Department of Health.

MAFF (1990a) *Government Action on BSE,* News Release FF 1/90, 9 January 1990. London: Ministry of Agriculture Fisheries and Food.

MAFF (1990b) *News Release 184/90,* 15 May 1990. London: Ministry of Agriculture Fisheries and Food.

MAFF (1990c) *British Beef Is Safe, Gummer,* News Release 185/90, 15 May 1990. London: Ministry of Agriculture Fisheries and Food.

Martin, W. B. (1989) Letter to Sir Richard Southwood, dated 16 January 1989, *BSE Inquiry Year Book* Reference No. 89/1.16/1.1, in Phillips *et al.* 2000, op. cit.

Meldrum, K. (1989) Confidential – Sensitive Issues in the Animal Health Sector. *BSE Inquiry Year Book* Reference No. 89/1.10/7.1–7.4, in Phillips *et al.* op. cit.

Owen, E. (1988) Bovine Spongiform Encephalopathy (BSE) – Emergency Order, Minute dated 10 June 1988. *BSE Inquiry Year Book* Reference No. 88/6.10/8.1, in Phillips *et al.* op. cit.

Pearce, F. (1996) 'Ministers Hostile to advice on BSE', *New Scientist,* 30 March 1996, 4.

Pickles, H. (1988a) The Transmission of Bovine Spongiform Encephalopathy. *BSE Inquiry Year Book* Reference No. 88\11.07\1.2–1.5, in Phillips *et al.* op. cit.

Pickles, H. (1988b) Bovine Spongiform Encephalopathy, Minute dated 11 November 1988. *BSE Inquiry Year Book* Reference No. 88/11.11/1.1/1.2, in Phillips *et al.* op. cit.

Pickles, H. (1988c) Bovine Spongiform Encephalopathy: first Meeting of Working Party Minutes dated 20 June 1988. *BSE Inquiry Year Book* Reference No. 88/6.20/3.1, in Phillips *et al.* op. cit.

Pickles, H. (1989) Letter to Sir Richard Southwood, dated 17 January 1989, *BSE Inquiry Year Book* Reference No. 89/1/17/1.1–1.2, in Phillips *et al.* op. cit.

Pickles, H. (1998), Statement to the BSE Inquiry No 115. Available at *http://www.bseinquiry.gov.uk/files/ws/s115.pdf* in Phillips *et al.* 2000, op. cit.

Rees, W. H.G. (1988) Bovine Spongiform Encephalopathy, Submission dated 6 May 1988. *BSE Inquiry Year Book* Reference No. 88/5.6/3.1–3.22, in Phillips *et al.* op. cit.

Southwood, R. (1998) Statement No 1 to BSE Inquiry, in Phillips *et al.* 2000, op. cit.

Southwood, R. (1999) BSE Inquiry Witness Statement No. 1, para. 23 (BSE Inquiry Transcript, Day **106**, 21 July 1999, pp.127–8. Available at *http://www.bseinquiry.gov.uk/files/ws/s001.pdf*

Southwood Working Party (1999) Witness Statement No. 1D, in Phillips *et al.* 2000, op. cit.

Strang, F. (1988) Bovine Spongiform Encephalopathy: Secretary's Meeting with Sir Richard Southwood and the CHO. *BSE Inquiry Year Book* Reference No. 88/05.19/4.1–4.3, in Phillips *et al.* op. cit.

Suich, J. C. (1989) BSE – Southwood Working Party, Minute dated 10 January 1989. *BSE Inquiry Year Book* Reference No. 89\1.10\3.1–3.2, in Phillips *et al.* op. cit.

Thatcher, M. (1999) Statement No 401 to the BSE Inquiry, in Phillips *et al.* 2000, op. cit.

Thompson, D. (1989) BSE – Southwood Working Party. Minute dated 19 January 1989, *BSE Inquiry Year Book* Reference No. 89/1.19/4.1, in Phillips *et al.* 2000, op. cit.

Wilesmith, J. W. *et al.* (1988) 'Bovine spongiform encephalopathy: epidemiological studies', *Veterinary Record,* **123**, 638–44.

Chapter 6

Regulatory rigor mortis

Introduction

With the publication of the Southwood Report in February 1989 the UK government might have been forgiven for thinking that BSE would not cause any further significant scientific or political difficulties. After all, Southwood and his colleagues had endorsed the hypothesis that BSE would probably behave just like scrapie and, on that basis, had concluded that the risks to human health were 'remote'. Regulations were also in place to remove clinically diseased animals from the food chain, and supposedly to halt the epidemic amongst cattle.

Nevertheless, BSE was about to become a far more complex and politically fraught issue. The rate at which new cases of BSE were diagnosed was rising much faster than many had expected. More importantly, the Southwood Working Party's conclusion, enthusiastically endorsed by the UK government, that the risks of BSE to humans were 'remote' was provisional, and had provided just about the most optimistic interpretation that could have been put on the available evidence. In the months and years that followed the publication of the Southwood Report, a wide range of new evidence emerged indicating that BSE was not like scrapie and that the assumptions about the possible risks posed by BSE (and the policy implications that flowed from those assumptions) might need to be changed. Just as importantly, Southwood's recommendations, and the set of regulations that had been established by the UK government by February 1989, were beset by anomalies, not least because there were no scientific grounds for the contrasting comments and actions in relation to the risks from clinically diseased animals on the one hand and subclinical cases on the other.

This chapter explores some of the key determinants and dynamics of regulatory change in BSE policy during the seven year period following the publication of the Southwood Report in February 1989. That period came to an abrupt end in March 1996 when Ministers acknowledged that atypical cases of CJD in unusually young people were most likely to have been caused by exposure to beef products contaminated with the BSE agent. The analytical focus, once again, is on the interactions between science and policy, but this will not be an exhaustive account. We focus on examples chosen to illustrate the most important types of interactions that occurred, and the most important consequences of those patterns of interaction for the dynamics of policy.

We will describe how UK policy-makers desperately attempted to maintain the regulatory status quo that had been established by the beginning of 1989, despite the anomalies and the changing evidence. The paramount policy objective was to maintain market stability and the confidence of domestic and overseas consumers, and neither of these was compatible with introducing new regulations. Our argument is that officials were reluctant to make incremental changes to policy, not, or rather not only, because of the direct commercial consequences of introducing further regulatory controls, but because such changes would undermine the technocratic rhetoric that knowledge about BSE was reliable, and that the existing regulations were sufficient to ensure that there were no risks from the consumption of British beef. Changes to policy would have made it evident that knowledge was more fragile than previously claimed, and that consumers had already been exposed to risks of a non-negligible type. Having embarked on a representation of policy along technocratic lines, market stability required the initially chosen representation – and the credibility of those who provided it – to be maintained. This was why, as we argue, it became (perversely) logical for officials to strenuously resist introducing what were known to be risk-reducing, practical and cheap controls.

The discussion will, we believe, illustrate how policy-makers continued to try to use science to endorse their prior policy preferences. We say, they did this in time-honoured fashion by representing their decisions and preferences as resulting in complete safety and as emerging directly and unproblematically from the scientific evidence. Our analysis, as set out below, is that in order to maintain that fiction, however, policy-makers deployed a variety of tactics. First, they disguised some of the uncertainties and their judgements about acceptability of risk. Second, they papered over regulatory anomalies by deploying ambiguous or empirically empty scientific-seeming claims. Third, they played down the implications of new evidence, rather than reacting to it in candid and prudent ways. Finally, they deployed their expert advisors tactically, seeking advice only when useful to shore up authority (rather than as providing an input to policy), and as with the Southwood Working Party in 1988, seeking to steer the committee into endorsing the department's preferred policies. We show how one effect of adopting what we say was a misleading, technocratic and antiscientific deployment of seemingly scientific argument was further policy ossification. That occurred partly because

Ministers were not always fully informed and were therefore not always aware of the scope for, and necessity of, incremental shifts in policy, but also we say because policy changes that were inconsistent with misleading scientific claims were officially deemed unacceptable.

This chapter is organised around a chronological discussion of some of the most important aspects of policy decision-making, over the period 1989–1996, concerned with the protection of human health. As will become apparent, despite our arguments about a tendency towards policy inertia verging at times on rigor mortis, the scientific evidence, the government's expert committees, and the broader scientific community did not always conform to the wishes of policy officials. Science and scientists were not, and could not be, entirely subordinated to politics. In response to some of the emerging evidence, the efforts of scientists, and associated political reactions, both domestic and international, regulatory controls were tightened, but in ways that were primarily reactive, often many months or years after action had first been proposed, and then only when there were no alternatives available to policy-makers. Every time policy shifted, however, the regime's credibility was undermined, just as officials had anticipated, but the longer officials tried to resist policy changes, the more difficult it became to reiterate unscientific and antiscientific claims to support the status quo. For these reasons the government's technocratic defence of BSE policy-making was always fragile and it finally imploded in March 1996.

New expert committees

One of the earliest recommendations of the Southwood Working Party had been to establish a new expert committee to advise on TSE research. The Consultative Committee on Research, chaired by the virologist David Tyrell, and known commonly as the 'Tyrell Committee' began meeting in the Spring of 1989 after the Southwood Working Party had been disbanded. In addition to Tyrrell there were four other members, three of whom had been nominated by MAFF and one by the DoH. The MAFF appointees were: William Watson, the director of MAFF's Central Veterinary Laboratory, John Bourne, the director of the Institute for Animal Health, and Richard Kimberlin, a scrapie expert who had recently left the Neuropathogenesis Unit in Edinburgh and was then an independent TSE consultant. Robert Will, a consultant neurologist, was the DoH appointee.

The Tyrell Committee had a remit to advise MAFF and the DoH on TSE research then in progress and on future priorities for research. In practice, that meant the production of a report outlining priorities for a future research programme that was finalised in June 1989 (MAFF/DoH 1990). In late 1989, MAFF and DoH officials decided that a successor to the Tyrell Committee would be required in order to maintain the research oversight function but that would also respond to specific questions from government and provide policy advice (Phillips *et al.* 2000, vol. 11, paras 4.6 and 4.7). Consequently, in February 1990 the remit of the Tyrell Committee was widened to that of advising MAFF and the DoH on 'matters relating to spongiform encephalopathies'. It was also renamed the Spongiform Encephalopathy Advisory Committee, or SEAC.

All of the Tyrell Committee members were invited to join SEAC, with the exception of John Bourne who was replaced by Fred Brown, a veterinary virologist. Later in 1990 the CMO, Donald Acheson, suggested that two medical experts should be appointed to strengthen the human health expertise on SEAC. He proposed a neuropathologist and Professor Joseph Smith, a microbiologist, who was then Director of the Public Health Laboratory Service. MAFF officials successfully resisted the idea of appointing Joseph Smith but agreed to the appointment of Professor Ingrid Allen, a neuropathologist. One of MAFF's Deputy Secretary's commented that

> [Allen's] appointment, which pleased us, was to inject her particular specialism and indicate to the Royal College of Pathologist that their interests will be covered so forestalling them from setting up their own BSE committee.

> (Capstick 1990)

MAFF officials argued that to counterbalance the appointment of Ingrid Allen, an extra veterinarian should also be appointed. In practice two veterinarians joined SEAC later in 1990: Professor Richard Barlow, a veterinary pathologist, and David Pepper, a practising veterinary surgeon. The overall balance of SEAC membership was thus skewed towards veterinary expertise.

The membership of SEAC did not change again until 1994. William Heuston, a veterinary epidemiologist joined in January 1994 as a replacement for Richard Barlow. It was not until January 1996, however, that the bias towards veterinary expertise was reversed. As we describe later in this chapter, in 1994 the CMO had wanted to strengthen the clinical membership of SEAC, in the wake of increased anxiety about the possibility of CJD transmission to humans. This resulted, initially, in the appointment of Professor John Pattison, a medical microbiologist, in February 1995. Once Pattison became chair of SEAC, in November 1995, he was anxious to redress the balance within the Committee and he appointed five new members, most of whom had a medical or public health background. By that point, however, it was becoming increasingly apparent that BSE might be transmissible to humans.

From the time SEAC was first established its official role, in addition to maintaining the Tyrell committee's function of providing oversight on the government TSE research programme, was to respond to specific questions about policy (Phillips *et al.* 2000, vol. 11, paras 4.6 and 4.65). The provision of ad hoc policy advice was a role with which, initially at least, the members were uncomfortable. In July 1990, for example, in the context of being asked to advise on whether farmers should be allowed to breed from the offspring of BSE-infected animals, SEAC pointed out that its role was 'to produce "opinions" which set out clearly what was implied by scientific knowledge. It was for others to decide what policy decision should flow from this' (Phillips *et al.* 2000, vol. 11, para. 4.85). The previous month it had also stressed that 'what action might be appropriate depended not just on what the science indicated but also on what the policy objective was' (Phillips *et al.* 2000, vol. 11, para. 4.83). In practice, however, SEAC frequently provided policy recommendations, covering a very wide range of issues.

As with the Southwood Working party, SEAC had no staff or budget and thus relied heavily on its joint secretariat (one official from the DoH and one from MAFF) and on other officials. The secretaries again played a key role, both in providing information and background papers for the committee and, once again, in helping to draft the advice that SEAC provided to government (Phillips *et al.* 2000, vol. 11, para. 4.31 and 4.36).

The Specified Bovine Offal ban

By far the most important policy development to occur after February 1989 was the introduction of a ban on the use in the human food chain of bovine brain, spinal cord, tonsils, spleen, thymus, and intestines from all adult cattle, also known as the Specified Bovine Offal or SBO regulations. The ban was announced by Ministers on 13 June 1989, only four months after the Southwood Report had been published. In making that announcement, Ministers effectively overturned Southwood's advice that the risks from subclinical animals did not warrant regulatory restrictions.

Ministers had been willing to consider further regulatory restrictions as soon as the Southwood Report had been published, but were repeatedly advised not to do so by their officials. The day before the Southwood Working Party report was published, for example, the Secretary of State, John MacGregor, told his officials that the press were already claiming that subclinically infected animals were entering the food chain, and he asked: 'Should we not be taking further action on offal in new product preparations? Why not ban? Seems likely a ban will come anyway' (Stagg 1989a). Once the report had been published, several articulate independent scientists continued to point out, publicly, the inconsistency between Southwood's advice on clinically diseased animals and that on subclinically infected cattle, and they argued that it was vital to prevent cattle brain and other nervous tissues from entering the human food chain (Phillips *et al.* 2000, vol. 6, paras 3.60 and 3.61). On 21 March, a few weeks after the publication of the Southwood Working Party report, MAFF's junior Minister, Donald Thompson, asked the Animal Health Division to consider a policy of excluding cull cows (i.e. dairy cattle that had reached the end of their milking life) from human consumption (Phillips *et al.* 2000, vol. 6, para. 3.149).

Animal health officials were very reluctant to support Thompson's idea on the grounds that it would involve significant economic and practical problems and claimed it was not necessary (Lawrence 1989). The CVO, Keith Meldrum, also pointed out that '[t]o remove all cull ruminants would . . . run counter to the line that we have taken previously, e.g. there is no known hazard from either scrapie or BSE to human health' (Phillips *et al.* 2000, vol. 6, para. 3.154). In the following seven years, concerns that any tightening of policy might undermine the credibility of the Department were to reappear time and time again as an important consideration in BSE decision-making.

Meldrum thought that the Minister might respond to the government's critics by seeking a voluntary restraint on the use of brain and spinal cord from the meat industry (Phillips *et al.* 2000, vol. 6, para. 3.155). He suggested, therefore, that animal health officials might want to 'leave the door open fractionally on the end use of brains and spinal cords originating from adult cattle and sheep' (Phillips *et al.* 2000, vol. 6, para. 3.155). He later asked Alan Lawrence in the Animal Health Division to prepare an options paper on the use of brain and spinal cord, in consultation with Ray Bradley, the Head of Pathology and BSE research co-ordinator at MAFF's Central Veterinary Laboratory (Phillips *et al.* 2000, vol. 6, para. 3.158).

Bradley recognised that, so long as one assumed there was a non-zero risk of transmission, there was a clear rationale for restrictions on the consumption of brain, spinal cord and certain other ruminant tissues. In a background note he argued that central nervous and lymphatic tissues, endocrines and gut in pre-clinical animals are 'highly likely to be infected to a high titre of significance to humans if the agent is transmissible to them' (Phillips *et al.* 2000, vol. 6, para. 3.164). He also pointed out that sheep offal should also be considered a problem because sheep had been fed with meat and bone meal and BSE could have been transferred (back) to sheep. Some unknown proportion of sheep infected with scrapie might therefore actually have BSE (Phillips *et al.* 2000, vol. 6).

As for regulatory options, Bradley noted that:

> *It would be relatively simple to reduce risks considerably* by sending for rendering or incinerating specified easily identified organs . . . Spleen, uteri . . . all endocrines, heads . . . and spinal cord from sheep over 1 year and cattle over 2.5 years could be designated unsaleable for human consumption.

> (Phillips *et al.* 2000, vol. 6)

Bradley added that vertebral column 'is highly likely to be seriously contaminated in an infected animal. You might consider not permitting recovery of meat scraps from vertebral column' (Phillips *et al.* 2000, vol. 6, para. 3.165). That comment referred to the production of what is known as mechanically recovered meat.

The options paper for the junior Minister, which had been written by Alan Lawrence, did not mention Bradley's point that vertebral columns in cattle were likely to be contaminated, or his argument that sheep might also have contracted BSE. Lawrence argued that the only tissues at risk were bovine brain, spinal cord, spleen, lymph nodes, thymus and intestines. He also noted that a prohibition on those tissues would not cause any problems to the meat trade, principally because they were not widely used as food ingredients. Nevertheless, Lawrence argued strongly against a ban, for reasons that in retrospect are very revealing:

> There would not appear to be any reason to take any further action at this stage, particularly since Southwood did not recommend it. In fact he concluded that even the labelling of products would not be justified in the present state of knowledge. . . . To take action would probably invite criticism as to why it was not taken earlier. It is also possible that it will arouse public concern, even if we make the point that it is very much a precautionary measure. Indeed the public may conclude that there is some reason to be concerned and that MAFF are being unduly secretive. This would do nothing to improve consumer confidence.

> (Lawrence 1989)

As argued in Chapter 5, the reason why Southwood had not recommended an offal ban is that his Working Party did not think that such advice would have been politically welcome to Ministers. The circularity of a policy judgement being recycled through a scientific committee, in the guise of a purely scientific claim, in order to dissuade Ministers from moving away from that very same pre-existing policy judgement is clear. Although Lawrence had been the MAFF secretary to the Working Party, he might not have been aware of the reasons why the Working Party decided not to recommend a ban on bovine offal. Lawrence must have realised, however, that the Working Party had wanted to recommend that offal should be labelled because it had been

Lawrence who had persuaded the committee to drop that piece of advice (Southwood Working Party 1999, paras 33.2 and 33.3). Lawrence was thus reinforcing the Working Party's misrepresentation of its decision not to recommend labelling, though to his Minister rather than to the public, even though he was best placed to know that that judgement had never been made on purely scientific grounds.

Lawrence's arguments also indicate that officials were concerned that, having failed to eradicate or substantially diminish possible risks, any tightening of the existing regulations threatened to reveal that those risks were not, and had never been, negligible, and were not, and had never been, fully characterised or eradicated. As far as officials were concerned, the only way to maintain stable markets was to pretend that risks were known and that the measures being taken were sufficient to ensure those risks remained negligible; even if this implied that additional, relatively cheap, risk reduction measures had to be avoided to sustain that fictional narrative. Indeed, it is worth stressing that officials' reluctance to support an offal ban was not because the department's own scientists failed to recognise the scientific case or because officials acquiesced with, or were captured by, part of an industry reluctant to bear increased costs. Rather, regulatory measures that officials knew to be unproblematic to the meat industry, and which would have considerably reduced possible risks, were being opposed to maintain the credibility of the Department's antecedent policy and its technocratic narrative of legitimation.

The tactic of preventing Ministers from pursuing the introduction of controls on subclinically infected animals was soon undermined. By May 1989, Ministers and officials had learnt that two major pet food manufacturers had decided, independently of MAFF, to exclude certain high-risk cattle tissues from commercial pet food products (Phillips *et al.* 2000, vol. 6, para. 3.203). One of the pet food companies had taken that decision after commissioning a risk assessment from Richard Kimberlin in July 1988. Kimberlin had recently left the Neuropathogenesis Unit in Edinburgh and had become a self-employed consultant. By the spring of 1989, Kimberlin was also a member of the Tyrell Committee.

Kimberlin's risk assessment was commercially confidential and he had not told MAFF officials about it, or even the Southwood Working Party, one of whose meetings Kimberlin had attended in late 1988. In mid-May 1989, however, the Pet Food Manufacturers Association asked Kimberlin to share his information with MAFF on the grounds that it might be more widely applicable (Phillips *et al.* 2000, vol. 6, para. 3.197). Kimberlin had conducted his assessment by dividing bovine tissues into four categories of risk, based on analogies with the scrapie infectivity levels that had been found experimentally in various sheep tissues. For each category Kimberlin attempted to provide quantitative estimates of the levels of infectivity in the relevant tissues. Category IV, the lowest risk, included tissues that were widely consumed such as bone marrow, kidney, lung, heart, thymus, and muscle.

Having learnt of Kimberlin's risk assessment, an official from MAFF's Food Standards Division suggested that it might be prudent for his colleagues to conduct a similar risk assessment exercise, focusing on meat and meat products for human food (Phillips *et al.* 2000, vol. 6, para. 3.199). In a remarkably revealing document, Dr Mark Woolfe, the Head of MAFF's Food Science Division, responded to that suggestion by telling colleagues that he had decided such an exercise would be inappropriate. Woolfe explained:

> The reason for my reluctance is that I would have to use the same data as Dr Kimberlin . . . Dr Kimberlin has had to make intelligent guesses at the fact that even though the assay, which has an interspecies barrier, has not detected the agent [in Category IV tissues], it might still be present in Category IV organs [because the assay underestimates absolute levels of infectivity]. In fact when all the effects are built in to figures, the infectivity levels are not insignificant in this Category.

> (Phillips *et al.* 2000, vol. 6, para. 3.202)

Woolfe also noted that since consumption of Category IV tissues would determine human exposure to the BSE agent

> *There would be no way of reducing such a calculated exposure of BSE agent to the public without recommending certain restrictions to Ministers.* However, if challenged, the basis of our conclusions would still be intelligent guesswork rather than hard facts and would be difficult to substantiate.

> (Phillips *et al.* 2000, vol. 6, para. 3.202, emphasis added)

We believe the above means that, because a proper risk assessment would have indicated that there were potential significant risks, which might in turn necessitate restrictions that were inconsistent with the government's policy objectives, Woolfe thought it best not even to conduct such an assessment. This suggests that, in effect, science was being treated as little more than a tactical tool. If it could not be deployed in circumstances that could be used to support a pre-existing policy commitment, then it was better not to deploy it at all. We note that, until March 1996, no efforts were made by the UK government or its expert advisors to quantify the possible levels of human exposure to the BSE agent.

Although MAFF officials continued to tell Ministers that there was no scientific justification for an offal ban (Phillips *et al.* 2000, vol. 6, paras 3.206 and 3.214) they decided in early June to go ahead anyway. Ministers had discovered not only that the pet food industry had unilaterally banned offal from its products (one company had been doing so for over a year), but also that the Bacon and Meat Manufacturers Association, whose members produced approximately 80 per cent of the meat products consumed in the UK, was advising its members to exclude bovine brain, spinal cord, pancreas, thymus, spleen and intestine from their products. As a DoH minute revealed:

> From the outset it was clear Mr MacGregor believed there was an overriding political case for action even if the science had not changed. He was under increasing pressure from the public and the industry to ban bovine offal from the human food chain. There was talk of the food industry taking its own measures and he could not allow MAFF to be upstaged by the industry.

> (Metters 1989)

The SBO ban was to be one of the most important public health measures that diminished the risks from BSE, but it seems the motivation for its introduction had little to do with public health, and a great deal to do with the political credibility of the Minister and the desire for market stability. Indeed, the Department of Health only learnt about the decision to introduce an offal ban after officials read about the decision in a newspaper report (Pickles 1990a). Furthermore, given the conclusions of the Southwood Working Party several (although not all) policy-makers appeared to believe that an offal ban could not be scientifically justified. Consequently the importance of the SBO regulations as a risk reducing measure was not always conveyed to the meat and farming industries or to the veterinary profession. As John MacGregor later recalled:

> Some people were concerned about subclinical animals . . . others were not, because Sir Richard Southwood had made clear that was not a real problem . . . So others were more concerned about the thing I was bothered about, public presentation.

> (Phillips et al. 2000, vol. 6, para. 3.262)

As we argued in the previous chapter, the Southwood Working Party underplayed its concerns about the risks posed by subclinically infected animals so as not to undermine Ministers' and officials' overriding commitment to maintaining stability in the beef market. Yet seemingly that tacit framing assumption was not recognised even by those from whom it had first originated. One consequence was that it became increasingly difficult for Ministers and other policy actors to appreciate the possible risks and the extent of the uncertainties, and so they failed to appreciate the scope for, or the strength of the case for, exercising precaution.

This fundamental problem was further compounded when Ministers and officials agreed that they should represent the SBO ban, not as a means to reduce possible risks to human health, but rather as the easiest way to implement Southwood's advice to manufacturers of baby food not to use bovine offal and thymus. That rhetorical strategy was adopted to provide a narrative so that 'the Minister would thereby not be appearing to contradict the scientific evidence in the Southwood Report by taking more comprehensive action than recommended' (Phillips *et al.* 2000 vol. 6, para. 3.248). In other words, the government could maintain, not so much the integrity of Southwood and his colleagues, but rather the impression that all the advice that it had received was reliable and complete and, by implication, that the policy measures it had thus far imposed were scientifically sound.

The message that the SBO ban was only a measure of 'administrative convenience' to implement Southwood's recommendation on baby food was not only conveyed to the meat industry, and to those responsible for enforcing slaughter house regulations (Phillips *et al.* vol. 6, para. 3.305, 3.309); it was maintained internally too. Inevitably, the primary justification for misrepresenting the reasons for the ban was soon forgotten. For example, after a cabinet reshuffle in July 1989, MAFF officials prepared a briefing for the new Ministerial team which did not mention any public health reasons for the proposed offals ban. Instead it stated that:

> The Southwood Working Party did not identify any general need to prohibit the use of offal in meat products. It did, however, suggest that manufacturers of baby foods should avoid the use of ruminant offal and thymus. . . . In working out the details, it was concluded that a better way of dealing with this would be to ensure that the relevant types of bovine offals . . . were rejected at abattoirs as unfit for all human consumption.
>
> (Lowson 1989)

A regulation which Ministers, numerous officials and in due course veterinary inspectors and the farming and meat industry believed was not strictly necessary, was never going to be rigorously implemented and enforced. Before being implemented, however, it had to be designed.

The scope of the SBO ban

In early June 1989, MAFF officials had prepared a submission for Ministers discussing the possible scope of an SBO ban (Cockburn 1989). Using the same logic that Kimberlin had used for the pet food industry, the submission divided different bovine tissues into four risk categories, listed below, albeit omitting any quantification of the levels of infectivity in the four categories.

Category i   brain and spinal cord

Category ii   spleen, lymph nodes, tonsils, intestines, nerves and thymus

Category iii   all remaining organs, except for milk, serum and faeces

Category iv   milk, serum and faeces

The submission stated that if an SBO ban was to be introduced 'it might include brain and spinal cord (category i) and spleen (category ii), *possibly with other organs which are not used in preparation of cooked meat products*' (Phillips *et al.* 2000, vol. 6, para. 3.237, emphasis added). The assumption that the SBO ban was primarily a measure to reassure an irrational and ill-informed public must have contributed to policy-makers' decision that the ban should not cover tissues that were of commercial value.

John MacGregor subsequently met with the Chief Veterinary Officer (CVO), the deputy Chief Medical Officer, two senior officials from MAFF's Animal Health Group, MAFF's Head of Information and MAFF's Special Advisor to decide, provisionally, on the scope of the SBO ban. Those present decided that, in addition to brain, spinal cord and spleen, as proposed in the submission, tonsils and thymus would be included in the ban. Three of the category ii tissues were thus excluded from the proposed ban, i.e. lymph nodes and nerves because they were 'everywhere in the carcass' and it was considered impracticable to take action on these, and intestines on the grounds that they were scraped and cleaned of lymphatic material before being used for sausage casings (Phillips *et al.* 2000, vol. 6, para. 3.245).

All category iii tissues were excluded although many of them, such as lung, liver, kidney, bone marrow, oxtail, pancreas and adrenal and pituitary glands could be expected, by analogy with experiments on scrapie, to have contained the infective agent. Sheep were not included in the proposed ban because the CVO argued that there was much less of a concern about scrapie as compared to BSE and because sheep are not usually split after slaughter and the removal of their spinal cords would have raised abattoir costs (Stagg 1989b). As we have already noted, Ray Bradley, BSE research co-ordinator at CVL, had previously suggested that the problem was not so much scrapie, but rather that sheep that might have been infected with BSE from exposure to animal feed. Bradley's advice had not, however, been included in the options paper later circulated by Alan Lawrence to Ministers and senior officials; neither Bradley nor any of his CVL colleagues (or indeed any of MAFF's expert advisors) were present at that crucial meeting.

The CVO, Keith Meldrum, told those present the proposed ban would enable MAFF to provide 'complete reassurance to the general public since the rest of the carcass would not contain the BSE agent in any significant quantities' (Phillips *et al.* 2000, vol. 6, para. 3.245). In the absence of the relevant experimental data, or even a crude indication of estimated levels of infectivity in the various tissues (as provided by Kimberlin for the pet food industry), we believe Meldrum's claim was misleading and unscientific.

Exclusion of calves

Although the government's intention to legislate on cattle offal was announced in June 1989, the SBO ban itself did not come into force for another five months. In the meantime there was extensive internal deliberation about the scope of the ban although in the end only a few changes were made to the initial proposals. One important change was that cattle aged six months or less were completely excluded from the ban.

That decision is worth highlighting for several reasons, not least because, we argue, it illustrates how potentially infectious tissues were exempted from the regulations, not because their inclusion would have increased direct costs, but in order to disguise the fact that, even with the SBO ban, exposure to the BSE agent was never going to be zero.

Initially, MAFF's veterinary and animal health officials had wanted to exclude only the spinal cord of calves because, like sheep, the carcasses were not normally split in abattoirs and the removal of their spinal cords would have raised abattoir costs (Phillips et al. 2000, vol. 6, para. 3.519). The public justification for that exemption was to be that there would be no risk from consuming calves because they would have been born after the ban on recycling ruminant protein in cattle feed. This of course ignored the possibility that BSE might transmit vertically from cow to calf, a mechanism that was known to occur in sheep scrapie (Phillips et al. 2000, vol. 6, para. 3.523). MAFF officials realised, however, that if the justification for excluding spinal cord was that there was no risk at all that calves could have become infected with BSE, it would be difficult to explain why calf offal other than spinal cord remained prohibited. Rather than suggest altering the justification, for example by explaining the real basis for excluding calf spinal cord, officials recommended instead that all calf offal be excluded from the SBO controls in order to appear consistent (Phillips et al. 2000, vol. 6, para. 3.523 and 3.524). Officials also realised if MAFF could portray calves as posing no risk to human health, this would deflect any potential pressure from continental European countries to restrict the important export trade in live calves (Phillips et al. 2000, vol. 6, para. 3.532).

If calves had become infected from their mothers then, at the time of slaughter (i.e. at six months), the BSE agent would be expected to be present in the gut and lymphatic system but not in the brain and spinal cord, given that infectivity does not reach nervous tissues at detectable levels until relatively late in the incubation period. Thus by suggesting that all calf offal, rather than just spinal cord, be exempted from the ban, officials were effectively proposing to increase human exposure to the BSE agent. The increased risk was primarily to maintain the credibility of the government's antecedent technocratic portrayal of risk regulation. The available scientific evidence, however, pointed in the opposite direction.

MAFF's veterinary and animal health officials were initially unable to persuade all of their departmental colleagues or the CMO to support the proposed exemption for calves. MAFF therefore sought the support of Richard Southwood and two members of the Tyrell research committee, David Tyrell and Richard Kimberlin, but they too objected on the grounds that vertical (and horizontal) transmission to calves could not be ruled out. Kimberlin told the Chief Veterinary Officer, Keith Meldrum, on 4 October that whilst he could accept exempting nervous tissues 'I cannot find a way of exempting the major LRS [lymphoreticular system] tissues at any age . . . I appreciate the implications of banning LRS tissues but I see no choice' (Phillips *et al.* 2000, vol. 6, para. 3.544, 3.545 and 3.549). Meldrum subsequently told Kimberlin that he had discovered that, in the UK, spleen and thymus were not used for human consumption and that it was therefore totally reasonable to exempt calves from the ban. Kimberlin was persuaded by that argument bearing in mind, according to Meldrum, 'the importance of the issue and the need to protect the UK's export markets' (Phillips *et al.* 2000, vol. 6, para. 3.553). Southwood and Tyrell also agreed with Meldrum's proposal (Phillips *et al.* 2000, vol. 6, para. 3.563).

It appears, however, that Meldrum was wrong when he said to Kimberlin, Southwood and Tyrell that spleen and thymus were not used in human food, because on 20 October the Meat Industry Liaison Group (MILG), which represented all the major meat trade associations, told senior MAFF officials that 'there was a small specialist trade in thymuses, but they could not say what tonnage was involved' (Phillips *et al.* 2000, vol. 6, para. 3.558). (MAFF's minutes of that meeting were not retrieved by the Phillips Inquiry.) Furthermore, whatever the level of consumption of thymus in the UK, the vast majority of UK-born calves were not consumed in the UK but were exported live for slaughter and consumption in continental Europe; some 250,000 calves were exported live each year compared to about 25,000 that were slaughtered in the UK. In countries such as France the thymus is considered a delicacy and relatively large amounts, from UK cattle aged under six months, were therefore almost certainly entering human food chains. MAFF officials failed to draw their independent scientific advisors' attention to that possibility when obtaining support for the exemption.

Department of Health officials were, however, aware of that fact because the Deputy Chief Medical Officer wrote to Meldrum on 19 October pointing out that

> You put forward strong arguments for total exemption of young cattle and tell me Dr Kimberlin is content. You mention the importance of this issue for exports and yet you do not comment on human consumption of thymus outside the UK.

> (Phillips *et al.* 2000, vol. 6, para. 3.564)

Nevertheless, the Deputy Chief Medical Officer went on to say that 'we are content for all organs of young calves to be exempt. After all, the Southwood report concludes vertical transmission is unlikely' (Phillips *et al.* 2000, vol. 6, para. 3.564).

As noted in Chapter 5, the Southwood report had concluded that cattle were likely to be a dead-end host for the disease, despite that fact that scrapie was known to transmit vertically. The Working Party had provided no supporting evidence, no explanation of their reasoning, and had contradicted itself because an earlier section of the report had acknowledged that 'it is impossible to predict whether cattle to cattle transmission of BSE will occur' (MAFF/DoH 1989, para. 5.1.2). Yet Department of Health officials were treating the Working Party's conclusion as scientifically validated and therefore as providing grounds for allowing MAFF to exempt a high risk tissue from the SBO ban.

Having persuaded Southwood, Tyrell, Kimberlin and DoH officials, it was relatively straightforward to get Agriculture Ministers to agree. The submission from officials seeking Ministerial agreement did not, however, refer to the export trade in calves or the possible risks to continental European consumers (Phillips *et al.* 2000, vol. 6, para. 3.568).

Mechanically recovered meat

One additional aspect of the government's deliberations over the scope of the SBO ban is worth scrutinising. It concerns the exemption of mechanically recovered meat (also known as MRM), obtained from the vertebral column of cattle. Vertebral column provided the main source of MRM. As we have already noted, Ray Bradley, BSE research co-ordinator at CVL, had written a note to colleagues in April 1989 stating that bovine vertebral column 'is highly likely to be seriously contaminated in an infected animal . . . ' and he had suggested that 'You might consider not permitting recovery of meat scraps from vertebral column' (Phillips *et al.* 2000, vol. 6, para. 3.165). That advice appeared to have been ignored by those responsible for designing the SBO controls (although MAFF's animal health officials told the Phillips Inquiry that they could not recollect receiving Bradley's note).

Two months later, however, in June 1989, MAFF's animal health officials learnt that an abattoir in the north west of England had stopped producing MRM from cattle bones because it could not guarantee that all central nervous system tissue would be removed from the vertebral column (Phillips *et al.* 2000, vol. 6, para. 3.584). They were also told by a large rendering company that it was 'totally impractical' to completely remove brain and spinal cord from a carcass and that MRM would inevitably contain spinal cord pieces

(Phillips *et al.* 2000, vol. 6, para. 3.591). Although officials recognised that some nervous tissue would be present in MRM they decided in September 1989 not to restrict the production or use of MRM. MAFF's note suggests that this was because there would only be minimal nervous tissue in MRM that would not present a significant risk, (Phillips *et al.* 2000, vol. 6, para. 3.592) but a note of the same meeting written by an official from the Department of Agriculture for Northern Ireland provides another far more revealing rationale:

> Mechanically recovered meat (MRM) – the possible danger raised by several of those consulted was recognised and during the discussion there was an expression of the illogicality of what was being done and in particular how easy it would be to have to concede the possible dangers of material other than those listed in the proposed ban. It was agreed not to raise it.

(Phillips *et al.* 2000, vol. 6, para. 3.593)

In other words, restrictions on the production and use of MRM would have made explicit the risks associated with peripheral nervous tissue and pieces of shattered or inadequately removed spinal cord explicit, but since nervous tissue was also present in normal cuts of meat, and could not practicably be removed from the carcass, and because cross-contamination with shattered spinal cord was inevitable, a ban on MRM might have thrown into question the safety of the entire carcase. Just as with officials' reasoning for extending an exemption for calf spinal cord to all calf offal, it seems that additional increases in risk were being sanctioned *despite warnings from the meat industry* in order to maintain a seemingly consistent and reassuring but misrepresentative rhetoric about the safety of beef. MAFF officials believed that such a narrative would help maintain stable markets and finesse pressures to introduce further and more expensive controls.

Ministers were initially unhappy about excluding MRM because they thought that it would inevitably include some nervous and lymphatic tissue (Phillips *et al.* 2000, vol. 6, para. 3.597). They were, however, persuaded to support the exemption after being told by the CVO, Keith Meldrum, in early November 1989, that the risks would be no greater than in the other cases where an exclusion from the ban had already been agreed, and that there would be no risk from pieces of broken spinal cord accidentally getting into the product (Phillips *et al.* 2000, vol. 6, para. 3.598).

On both points, however, there was no scientific evidence supporting Meldrum's claims. Officials had not bothered to conduct a risk assessment of MRM, and had not asked their scientific advisors to comment on the proposed decision, and so could not know how much nervous and lymphatic tissue might be included in products or whether, in practice, a spinal cord could readily be removed in its entirety from the carcass. The only evidence and advice then available on the inclusion of spinal cord was not based on any research findings either but it pointed strongly in the opposite direction. Ray Bradley told animal health officials on several occasions that it was possible that the spinal cord would be mutilated when the animal was split and could contaminate bone edges and end up in MRM (Phillips *et al.* 2000, vol. 6, para. 3.589 and 3.594). Furthermore, in September 1989, Ulster Farm By-Products Ltd, a rendering company, had written to MAFF's Animal Health Division pointing out that:

> It is totally impractical to remove in total on a commercial basis the brain and spinal cord. The carcass is usually split using a circular saw and this shatters the spinal cord and the sides of the beef, after being boned out, have the residual bone treated hydraulically to produce re-claimed meat that will include spinal cord pieces, etc.
>
> (Phillips *et al.* 2000, vol. 6, para. 3.591)

Bradley's advice went only to officials but not the Minister. Likewise, the letter from the rendering company was only read by senior veterinary and animal health officials.

New evidence and information in 1990

1990 was a critical year for BSE policy. Important information and evidence emerged, both as a result of research and surveillance activities and as a result of the experiences of those responsible for the practicalities of implementing and enforcing the SBO regulations. Below we discuss the ways in which the most important emerging evidence was interpreted and responded to.

We begin with one of the most significant developments, both scientific and political, to occur prior to March 1996, namely the discovery, beginning in the spring of 1990, that domestic cats were succumbing to a transmissible spongiform encephalopathy (TSE). That evidence, together with the later discovery that a number of wild cats in zoos had also contracted a TSE, was very important because it had not been possible, experimentally, to transmit scrapie to cats. If the feline TSE had been caused by exposure to the BSE agent, this implied not so much that the new disease was capable of jumping a new species barrier, via oral exposure, but more importantly, that the host range of BSE differed from that of scrapie. As one member of SEAC later put it: 'It demonstrated that you could no longer really plausibly argue that BSE was just scrapie in cows' (Phillips *et al.* 2000, vol. 6, para. 5.262). Yet the claim that BSE would not present a risk to humans was based on the hypothesis that BSE would behave exactly like scrapie. As far as humans were concerned, the cases in cats did not necessarily imply that humans were more at risk from BSE than they were from scrapie. The risk might be the same, it might be less, or it might be greater, but the analogy with scrapie could no longer be relied upon.

Mad Max

The first of 12 cats to be diagnosed with a TSE in 1990 was a Siamese, named Max, from the west of England. MAFF and the DoH officials learnt about 'Mad Max', as the media called the unfortunate cat, in May of that year after veterinarians from the University of Bristol passed details of their diagnosis to MAFF's Central Veterinary Laboratory.

The DoH official responsible for BSE told the CMO that either cats had always been susceptible but cases had gone unrecognised, or alternatively that 'a new agent, presumably BSE, is virulent in a way in which previous agents such as scrapie have not been' (Phillips *et al.* 2000, vol. 6, para. 4.501). She went on to say that although she thought the alternative scenario to be unlikely it was 'more worrying since it challenges the assumptions we have made for humans by analogy with scrapie' (Phillips *et al.* 2000, vol. 6, para. 4.501).

MAFF officials provided a far more reassuring assessment to Ministers, telling them that there was no necessary connection with BSE (Phillips *et al.* 2000, vol. 6, paras 4.499 and 4.502). Officials and Ministers decided that, rather than let details of the case leak out, MAFF would announce the discovery immediately (Phillips *et al.* 2000 vol. 6, paras 4.499, 4.502 and 4.499). In a briefing to the media, on 10 May 1990, the CVO, Keith Meldrum, dismissed the significance of the case, claiming that it was 'not entirely surprising', that 'there is no reasons or cause for concern at all', and that it had 'not changed the Government's assessment of the possible risk to humans from BSE' (Phillips *et al.* 2000, vol. 6, paras. 4.507 and 4.513 and vol. 5, para. 3.149).

Those claims dismayed some of Meldrum's veterinary colleagues. In a draft minute to a colleague, the CVLs's Head of Neuropathology noted that

> The comments made by the CVO on BBC 1 News at Six, 10 May 1990, were unfortunate, inappropriate and provocative. . . . The findings are preliminary but have potential agreed importance and should not, from virtually all viewpoints, have been represented as inconsequential.
>
> (Phillips *et al.* 2000, vol. 6, para. 4.518)

Despite the government's attempt to play down the possible significance of a feline TSE, critical scientists and the media leapt on the story. The *Sunday Times* reported Richard Lacey, a professor of microbiology, as saying that 'we now have two new mammals – cattle and cats – infected naturally for the first time by this agent. The likelihood is increased of the possibility of transmission to man from cattle' (Phillips *et al.* 2000, vol. 6, para. 4.522). Although

Meldrum responded to Lacey's claim as 'absolute nonsense' (ibid.) the next few days produced what the CMO later referred to as a 'rapidly escalating panic' (ibid., para. 4.542).

MAFF responded with two press releases on 15 May 1990. One quoted the Minister, John Gummer, saying that 'British beef is perfectly safe to eat. This is the view not only of our top scientists but also European Community experts' (MAFF 1990a). After describing the regulations that had been put into place, it also noted that '[t]hese actions fully protect the public from what is a remote and theoretical risk' (ibid.). The second press release stated that '[t]here is no reason to believe BSE will be any different from scrapie' (MAFF 1990b).

On 16 May, after briefly talking to three members of SEAC on the telephone, the Chief Medical Officer (CMO), Donald Acheson, also issued a press release in which he said: 'British beef can be eaten safely by everyone, both adults and children, including patients in hospital' (Phillips *et al.* 2000, vol. 6, para. 4.570). SEAC held an emergency meeting the following day. Its purpose was to endorse the CMO's statement by providing a letter which the CMO could use to advise the medical profession. That letter was not, however, produced at the meeting because some of the members wanted to provide a more detailed response than was possible at such short notice (Phillips *et al.* 2000, vol. 11, para. 4.100). The minutes of the meeting do, however, record SEAC as stating that '[i]n the present state of knowledge it would not be justified to state categorically that there was no risk to humans and it was not appropriate to insist on a zero risk' (Phillips *et al.* 2000, vol. 11, para. 4.99). Those comments were either not seen by Ministers or they were ignored because Ministers continued, subsequently, to insist that there was no risk from consuming beef. On 8 June 1990, for example, the Agriculture Minister told the House of Commons that there was 'clear scientific evidence that British beef is perfectly safe' (Gummer 1990).

In the weeks following its 17 May meeting, SEAC did not subsequently prepare a letter in support of the CMO's statement about the safety of beef. Instead the DoH secretary to SEAC drafted a letter, through a process involving SEAC and other MAFF and DoH officials. The first draft of the document was discussed by SEAC on 2 July 1990. Amendments were made by the DoH secretary in a second draft, dated 3 July 1990. This was then circulated to officials within MAFF and the DoH. Officials drew attention to 'considerable presentational problems' with the document and further drafts were subsequently prepared on 6 July and 10 July, but without the involvement of anyone from SEAC.

The head of MAFF's Animal Health Division, Robert Lowson, forwarded the 10 July version to Ministers and senior MAFF officials noting that '[t]he most *potentially inflammatory pieces of drafting in earlier versions have now been edited out'* (Phillips *et al.* 2000, vol. 11, para. 4.118; emphasis added). The document was also sent to Tyrell but was not subsequently modified. It was later sent to the CMO who forwarded it to all regional Directors of Public Health.

Both the 3 July draft and the final 10 July versions of SEAC's advice concluded that 'British beef can be eaten safely', thus endorsing the statement that the CMO had issued publicly in May 1990. Both documents noted, however, that BSE might not behave in exactly the same way as scrapie and neither version claimed that there was zero human exposure to the BSE agent. Nevertheless, whilst the final version only noted that 'very little BSE agent is expected to remain in the parts of the bovine carcass available for human consumption' (Lowson 1990) the 3 July draft had specifically pointed to the possibility of infectivity being present in specific tissues that were not covered by the SBO ban. Passages contained in the 3 July draft that were removed from the final version included the following:

> Traces [of the scrapie agent] have also been found in isolated experiments in liver, pancreas and bone marrow and in lung. . . .
>
> . . . Some of the edible offal [liver, pancreas and bone marrow] that have on rare occasions demonstrated low titres of infectivity are not included in the offal ban. . . .
>
> Such agent that does remain may lie in peripheral lymph nodes and possibly in major peripheral nerves, parts discarded in normal meat cutting, but which may still accompany some preparations of meat. . . .
>
> It is plausible for small amounts of BSE agent to be present, even after cooking, in those beef products that contain other than prime steak in a very small proportion of meals. . . .
>
> . . . No scientist is in a position to [provide an absolute guarantee of safety] for British (or Irish) beef.

(Tyrell 1990)

The effect of deleting what the head of MAFF's animal health division referred to as 'inflammatory pieces of drafting' was to draw attention away from the fact that residual levels of the BSE agent might remain in butchered meats, and thus to diminish the likelihood that MAFF would be challenged on both the scope of the SBO ban and its claims about the safety of beef. As the CVO, Keith Meldrum was able to subsequently claim: '[i]t isn't possible for BSE to enter the human food chain' (Meldrum 1992). Given that Ministers had not seen the early drafts of the paper, they too might not have been aware of the extent to which tissues other than those included in the SBO ban might contain the agent, and thus the options available for tightening the regulations.

The advice to the CMO also underplayed the potential significance of what by then was more than one case of a TSE in domestic cats. Although it was not at the time known if the cases had been caused by exposure to the BSE agent, that was a plausible scenario (later confirmed) whose significance went uncommented upon in the final document. The version of the paper discussed at the 2 July SEAC meeting had contained the phrase:

> If this is the start of a new cat epidemic it suggests this species could be sensitive to BSE in a way it has not been to scrapie. Both the epidemiology, and unsuccessful transmission attempts, suggest cats are not affected easily by scrapie.

> (Pickles 1990b)

In the 3 July and subsequent versions that phrase was omitted, although it is not clear if that omission was at the behest of SEAC members or officials. In its place was the following phrase, inserted by the DoH secretary:

> We do not yet know if the recent description of spongiform encephalopathy in a cat indicates transfer of scrapie or BSE to a new species or whether this is a feline disorder in its own right. In our view, this case does not increase the likelihood of BSE transmission to humans.

> (Phillips *et al.* 2000, vol. 11, para. 4.115)

An accurate description of the potential significance of the cat might have unsettled consumer confidence in the safety of beef, but it might also have indicated not only that there was scope for tightening the SBO regulations but also that proper compliance with, and enforcement of, the SBO controls would also be important.

Slaughterhouse practices and cross-contamination in 1990

As soon as the SBO regulations were introduced, concerns were raised about whether they could be, and were being, properly implemented and enforced. MAFF's attention was first properly drawn to those concerns by the Institute of Environmental Health Officers (IEHO), whose members were employed by local government and were responsible for enforcement of meat hygiene regulations in slaughterhouses. The IEHO sent MAFF's animal health officials a detailed letter, dated 1 February 1990, which concluded that the new SBO regulations were 'impractical and unenforceable' (Corbally 1990). Below we examine the government's response to two of the more important problems that had been raised by the IEHO.

Brain removal practices

One of the problems identified by the IEHO concerned an unanticipated effect of the SBO regulations on slaughterhouse practices. The new regulations introduced a commercial incentive for abattoirs to split cattle heads and remove the brain, before arranging for the 'head meat', such as tongue and cheek, to be harvested. Abattoirs usually sent cattle heads intact to butchers and specialist boning plants for removal of head meat. Under the SBO regulations, however, heads could not sent to butchers whilst the brain was still present. Boning plants, unlike butchers, were allowed to handle SBOs but they paid abattoirs a higher price for heads from which the brain had already been removed because they would not then have to deal with the costs of disposing of SBO materials. Abattoirs therefore began removing cattle brains by splitting their skulls with a cleaver or band-saw before dispatching the heads for extraction of the edible head meat. As the IEHO pointed out to MAFF, this practice risked contaminating the edible head meat with brain tissue. The IEHO recommended that MAFF should stipulate that all head meat should be removed at the slaughterhouse and that the splitting of cattle heads, in order to remove brains, should be prohibited (Corbally 1990).

MAFF's Secretary of State, John Gummer, was keen to amend the regulations but was told by officials that a departmental review of brain removal practices in slaughterhouses had concluded that there was no reason to do so because, even though brain tissue might contaminate cheek meat, it would do so 'only in tiny quantities' (Phillips *et al.* 2000, vol. 6, para. 4.168). Gummer was also told that

> If we were to amend the regulations to prohibit [head splitting] it would be likely to simply shift the argument from the splitting of heads to the splitting of spines where the same sort of issues could be raised.
>
> (Phillips *et al.* 2000, vol. 6, para. 4.172)

Thus it appears that officials were reluctant to adopt what was a relatively straightforward, cheap, and eminently sensible piece of advice, because it might have the effect of shifting attention to similar problems elsewhere. Unlike heads, cattle spines have to be split in order for slaughterhouses to handle and process carcasses and to comply with EC standards for intra-Community trade. Having claimed publicly that the SBO regulations were sufficient to prevent BSE infectivity from entering the human food chain, officials apparently reasoned that even ironing out unanticipated glitches with the new regulatory controls might give rise to pressure for additional more expensive and/or impractical controls.

Gummer was not convinced, however, and insisted that an independent expert provide him with advice on the risks of head splitting. That advice, from an academic veterinary surgeon, recommended that meat intended for human consumption should be removed before any cut was made to the skull, thus contradicting the advice from MAFF officials (Phillips *et al.* 2000, vol. 6, para. 4.175). Officials were still reluctant to ban head splitting. Instead they suggested to Ministers that MAFF should provide advice to abattoir inspectors, asking them either to ensure that meat was removed from the head before splitting of the skull or, if that were not possible, to minimise any contamination.

Ministers remained unhappy with their officials' proposal. Both Gummer and the junior Minister David Maclean insisted that if there were any doubt about the practice of head splitting, it ought to be banned (Phillips *et al.* 2000, vol. 6, para. 4.186). Officials reminded Ministers, however, that '[a ban] would provoke media interest out of all proportion to the minuscule nature of the problem' (Griffiths 1990) and that the 'Institute of Environmental Health Officers . . . would claim credit for having highlighted the problem and forced the government to act' (Griffiths 1990) Echoing the point made earlier to Gummer, Ministers were also told that:

> Amendment regulations would fuel debate on BSE generally and, inevitably, lead to demands for similar action on spinal cords. . . . A ban on splitting [spinal columns] would have grave consequences for the industry and for the export trade. Nor would it end with spinal cords. Concern would then be directed at nerve trunks and lymph nodes, which cannot be removed from carcasses.

> (Griffiths 1990)

Although those comments persuaded Ministers to agree with their officials, the IEHO, the organisation representing abattoir inspectors, wrote to its members in May 1990 recommending that removal of bovine brain should be 'expressly prohibited' (Phillips *et al.* vol. 6, para. 4.191). Officials' preferences were further undermined during a particularly heated Parliamentary debate on BSE on 21 May 1990, held in the wake of the media furore over Mad Max. Under pressure from opposition Members of Parliament, John Gummer promised Parliament that SEAC would be asked to review slaughterhouse controls. In doing so, SEAC were specifically asked to review MAFF's proposed guidelines on brain removal practices. SEAC responded by concluding that '[i]t was not consistent with [MAFF's policy] to permit the removal of the brain before head meat was harvested' (Phillips *et al.* 2000, vol. 6, para. 4.204). MAFF's guidance to abattoir inspectors was adjusted to reflect that advice but it took another two years before that advice was backed up with a legislative amendment to the SBO controls. In the meantime some abattoirs continued to split cattle heads prior to removing the head meat (Phillips *et al.* 2000, vol. 13, paras. 3.42–3.44).

Carcass splitting and mechanically recovered meat

A second problem that had been raised by the IEHO concerned the risks associated with producing MRM from bovine carcasses. We have already described how MRM was exempt from the SBO controls, even though senior

MAFF officials had been told by their scientific colleagues, and by representatives of the meat industry, that MRM would inevitably contain residual nervous tissue, and in particular pieces of spinal cord. Soon after the SBO regulations came into force, however, concerns about the safety of bovine derived MRM resurfaced.

In the first few months of 1990, the IEHO, the British Veterinary Association, the British Medical Association, several consumer groups and opposition Members of Parliament all voiced concerns about the safety of bovine-derived MRM (Philips *et al.* 2000, vol. 6, paras. 4.231–4.261). As the IEHO pointed out 'spinal cord could not be effectively removed in accordance with the Regulations' (Phillips *et al.* 2000, vol. 6, para. 4.124) and '... MRM could contain significant quantities of spinal cord tissue' (Phillips *et al.* 2000, vol. 6, para. 4.129). One of MAFF's junior Ministers had also visited a slaughterhouse and was reportedly 'very unhappy about MRM' after discovering that pieces of spinal cord were being left in the sides of beef (Philips *et al.* 2000, vol. 6, paras. 4.246–4.248).

We have already noted that on 21 May 1990, the Secretary of State, John Gummer, promised Parliament that SEAC would be asked to review slaughterhouse controls. The involvement of SEAC on this issue is curious. MAFF did not need technical advice on the problems of cross-contamination in abattoirs. The Department's network of officials, veterinarians and meat hygiene inspectors were best placed to know about slaughterhouse practices and, as far as MRM was concerned, they already knew that it was likely that pieces of spinal cord were ending up in the product. Furthermore, although SEAC might have usefully commented on the potential risks of small amounts of SBO entering the food chain, it did not have any expertise at all in relation to slaughterhouse practices. We believe Gummer's decision to ask SEAC to review slaughterhouse controls was motivated by the political benefits of involving external scientists rather than by their possession of superior technical or scientific skills. It was a means of shifting responsibility away from Ministers at a moment of political challenge.

Ministers and their senior officials recognised that SEAC lacked the relevant expertise to advise on MRM production methods, but rather than seek advice elsewhere, they decided that a paper would be prepared for SEAC by MAFF officials. Ministers later acknowledged that anything short of a clear endorsement from SEAC would be extremely problematic. On 5 July 1990, the junior Minister, David Maclean, wrote to John Gummer noting that MRM was a universally disliked product and that 'if [the chair of SEAC] is ambivalent about it, or says that some aspects are unsafe, then it will be impossible to defend the 'safe' aspects and we would, in all probability, lose the whole process' (Phillips *et al.* 2000, vol. 6, para. 4.252).

Despite the Ministers' concerns, the first draft of MAFF's paper, which had been written by officials from MAFF's Meat Hygiene Division, Food Standards Division and Food Science Division, gave explicit guidance to SEAC to impose restrictions on MRM production. The draft acknowledged that when carcasses were split inevitably pieces of spinal cord would contaminate the vertebral column which would then be used to produce MRM (Phillips *et al.* 2000, vol. 6, para. 4.342). The draft suggested four possible courses of action:

a) issue guidance to slaughterhouses on minimising contamination,

b) issue guidance to abattoir inspectors on spinal cord removal,

c) exclude bovine vertebrae in the production of MRM, or

d) exclude all bovine material in the production of MRM.

The draft paper argued that issuing guidance would be seen as recognising that there was a need for further action but without taking any enforceable steps, whilst excluding all bovine material would be widely opposed by the trade. It recommended that a prohibition on the use of bovine vertebrae in MRM production 'would solve any perceived problem while allowing trade in acceptable meat to continue' (Phillips *et al.* 2000, vol. 6, para. 4.280).

On 11 July 1990, MAFF's CVO, Keith Meldrum, told the authors of the first draft that the option of banning vertebral column was not without difficulty 'since we have allowed MRM to continue to be obtained for so long and we could be criticised that we are seeking a lower risk assessment than the facts warrant' (Phillips *et al.* 2000, vol. 6, para. 4.281; emphasis added). Meldrum told the authors to rewrite the paper explaining that MRM was obtained from 'totally healthy cattle in which the agent would either be totally absent from the brain or spinal cord or present in very low quantities indeed' (Phillips *et al.* 2000, vol. 6, para. 4.281). He also insisted that the paper put a more positive gloss on the options of issuing guidance to slaughterhouses and to inspectors and that there should be no overall recommendation.

Meldrum's comments illustrate the underlying concern that any tightening of regulations might throw into question the credibility of MAFF's antecedent policy. As Meldrum also told another official, responsible for producing the final version of the MRM paper: '[i]f we go further than to offer advice then [SEAC] is going further than the action we have proposed within the [State Veterinary Service] and presentationally it will appear [as] if our advice is faulty' (Phillips *et al.* 2000, vol. 6, para. 4.284).

When SEAC received the MRM paper, in November 1990, it did not contain any policy options or a recommendation. Instead, it just asked 'whether any action or guidance is required in relation to slaughterhouse practices, and whether any new RandD is needed' (Phillips *et al.* 2000, vol. 6, para. 4.289). SEAC concluded that 'provided all rules were properly followed and supervised, there was no need to recommend further measures on the grounds of consumer protection'(Phillips *et al.* 2000, vol. 6, para. 4.291).

As the head of MAFF's Animal Health Division later recalled, SEAC had provided that particular conclusion because the members did not feel able to advise about the extent to which regulations might have been 'properly followed and supervised' in practice. (BSE Inquiry Transcript 7 July 1998, pp. 124–5). Indeed, MAFF had not shared information with SEAC about the kinds of concerns about MRM that were being expressed by abattoir inspectors, officials or Ministers. SEAC was also unaware of the kinds of policy options that MAFF officials had been considering. Members of the committee had visited an abattoir, and had observed that it was possible to extract the spinal cord intact, but as the head of MAFF's Animal Health Division recalled: '[n]obody would have supposed that people would work normally with a group of government inspectors watching what they were doing, and nobody was under any illusion that that was what was happening' (Phillips *et al.* 2000, vol. 6, para. 4.352).

In response to SEAC's comments, officials told colleagues that 'no further action' on slaughterhouse controls was required (Phillips *et al.* 2000, vol. 6, para. 4.293). MAFF did not even issue guidance to abattoir operators or inspectors in order to emphasise the importance of spinal cord removal. Moreover MAFF also failed to check on how well or how poorly abattoir inspectors were enforcing the regulations, and failed to do so until 1995. SEAC's advice on slaughterhouse practices in 1990 was to produce complete closure on the issue of MRM contamination with nervous tissue for the next five years.

What is striking about that failure to pursue MRM contamination after SEAC had issued its advice was that SEAC had not just assumed good slaughterhouse practice and advised on the assumption that rules would be followed. Rather they had explicitly drawn attention to the fact that they were not in a position to know about the extent to which regulations were, or were not, being followed. The fact that MAFF officials had not responded to SEAC's caveat (and had not provided SEAC with evidence of the concerns about MRM) implies that they saw SEAC not as a body from which they required advice, but rather as a body that would provide legitimation to their prior policy commitments. In this case, SEAC's conclusion, despite the attached caveat, was sufficient to kick the MRM issue into the long grass.

Animal feed

The final development in 1990 that we scrutinise concerns evidence leading to a tightening of the ruminant-to-ruminant feed ban. In Chapter 5 we discussed how MAFF officials had decided that its ban on the recycling of ruminant protein would apply only to the diets of ruminants and not to other species, in order to maintain a market for ruminant slaughterhouse waste. That decision was taken despite having been told that a ruminant-to-ruminant feed ban would be unenforceable and despite recognising that they did not know whether animals such as pigs might be susceptible to BSE. We also described how the Southwood Working Party had wanted to extend the ban to cover the feed of pigs and other farm animals and how MAFF officials managed to persuade the members of the Working Party to drop that particular recommendation. We also noted that the Working Party represented its advice as if had been based solely on the grounds of an absence of risk, rather than a decision to acquiesce to MAFF's prior policy concerns.

After the Southwood Report was published, MAFF's failure to protect the entire animal feed chain was subject to criticism from TSE researchers, medical scientists and local government, especially after June 1989 when Ministers had announced the SBO ban for the human food chain (Phillips *et al.* 2000, vol. 5, paras 3.161 and 3.168). MAFF officials responded by stating that the Department was merely following the scientific advice of the Southwood Working Party. For example, a MAFF Press Release, dated 9 January 1990, stated that:

> There is no scientific justification to extend the ruminant feed ban to pigs and poultry. The Southwood Report acknowledged the importance of the feed ban for ruminants, but did not recommend that it be extended to pigs and poultry.
>
> (MAFF 1990b, emphasis added)

The animal feed industry, the rendering industry and the retail food industry were also unhappy with the fact that bovine offal was to be removed from the human food chain but not from animal feeds. In August 1989 the UK Agriculture Supply Trade Association, which represented animal feed manufacturers, told MAFF that it was going to recommend a voluntary ban on the use of SBO as an ingredient of animal feed (Phillips *et al.* 2000, vol. 5, para. 3.49). The note of a meeting between Ministers, officials and the UK Agriculture Supply Trade Association, held in October 1989 to discuss the animal feed's unilateral ban, reveals that:

> The Minister reacted forcibly. The Southwood Report provided no basis for such action. In making its proposals to ban these offals from entering the human food chain, the Government had gone slightly beyond the Southwood recommendations, but only for the purpose of administrative convenience. This would be made clear when final decisions on this matter were announced. The additional measures which UKASTA was proposing to take were not justified scientifically and would create a most unfortunate precedent for its members ... Mr Meldrum added that it was important to prevent a 'steam roller' effect of reacting to scares: if UKASTA reacted as

they proposed to do, pressure would arise to act on sheep offals, then a control programme for scrapie would be pressed for. Mr Packer suggested that pesticides could be the next in line for pressure on companies.

(Lebrecht 1989, emphases added)

Thus, not only were Southwood's self-censored concerns about the dangers of feeding ruminant material to farm animals portrayed as sufficient scientific justification not to take action, but the SBO ban in humans was again depicted as scientifically unnecessary. Furthermore, the problem with tightening regulatory restrictions was once again clearly perceived by MAFF officials as risking a loss of control of BSE policy, rather than in terms of the direct costs of extending the existing SBO ban in human food to animal feed. Despite the robust defence from ministers and officials, in November 1989 the UK Agriculture Supply Trade Association went ahead and instructed the animal feed industry not to accept meat and bone meal that had been produced using specified bovine offal (Phillips *et al.* 2000, vol. 5, para. 3.75). MAFF officials were furious.

A few months later, in May 1990, the issue of what should be permitted in animal feed predictably erupted once again after Max the Siamese cat was diagnosed with a TSE. This time, however, the pressure for a ban on the use in animal feed of bovine offal, or even all bovine protein, came not just from the feed industry and parts of the scientific community but also from the National Farmers Union, the Welsh Chief Medical Officer, the Food and Drink Federation, the House of Commons Agriculture Select Committee and even some of MAFF's own scientists (Phillips *et al.* 2000, vol. 5, paras 3.161, 3.168, 3.207 and 3.209). The Head of Neuropathology at MAFF's Central Veterinary Laboratory, Gerald Wells, recalled telling the Chief Veterinary Officer, Keith Meldrum, that he thought that the discovery of feline spongiform encephalopathy 'was probably of profound significance in relation to BSE and should lead to a complete ban on meat and bonemeal entering the animal food chain' (Phillips *et al.* 2000, vol. 5, para. 3.151).

In May 1990, SEAC indicated that it wished to discuss the composition of pig and poultry feed. The Secretary of State, John Gummer, decided that given that SEAC were going to look at the issue anyway he would make a formal request that they do so. MAFF's Permanent Secretary told Gummer that 'the issue would have to be very carefully handled. It would be appropriate for the Department to provide a background paper explaining our present policies and the reasons underlying these' (Phillips *et al.* 2000, vol. 5, para 3.173).

The background paper was ready in August 1990. It had an attached annex describing the 'crucial service' provided by the rendering industry (Phillips *et al.* 2000, vol. 11, para 4.314). The paper itself cited the Southwood Working Party's conclusions that no regulatory action was required in relation to pigs, poultry and pets. It also provided details of the Central Veterinary Laboratory's ongoing experiment to transmit BSE to pigs which, thus far, had not produced positive results. The paper concluded that despite the fact that cats had succumbed to a spongiform encephalopathy neither pigs nor poultry nor any other pet species had been shown to be susceptible to spongiform encephalopathies transmitted by ruminant material, and '[t]here does not therefore seem to be any current evidence on which to take a view different from the Southwood Working Party's'. The paper ended by 'invit[ing] [the committee] to endorse these conclusions' (Phillips *et al.* 2000, vol. 11, para 4.294).

The intention therefore was to get SEAC to provide seemingly scientific support for MAFF's preferred policy on animal feeds. MAFF had represented its policy as if scientifically justified in the face of criticism from a very broad range of stakeholders (a defence that continued after Gummer had asked SEAC for advice). The department had not previously asked SEAC to comment on the policy and would probably not have done if SEAC had not decided to look at the composition of pig and poultry feed. The characteristics of the paper MAFF provided to SEAC suggest that officials saw the committee as a political resource to justify an existing policy, rather than as providing independent scientific advice on which to construct policy. The Southwood Working Party's published conclusions about the risks of feeding ruminant material to pigs, which had previously been shaped by MAFF's policy objectives, were represented by MAFF as scientific conclusions, in order to persuade SEAC to endorse the same policy objectives. This was despite the fact that the animal feed industry had already voluntarily stopped using the specified bovine offals in their ingredients, and had already done so for nearly a year.

MAFF's background paper was never in fact presented to SEAC because it was overtaken by events. Four days after the background paper was ready, one of the pigs in MAFF's BSE transmission experiment was diagnosed with a TSE. Ministers had previously argued that if there was a positive result in this experiment the government would be faced with no option but to ban specified bovine offals from pig and poultry feed (Phillips *et al.* 2000, vol. 5, para. 3.199). At SEAC's next meeting, in September 1990, instead of being invited to endorse the earlier conclusions of the Southwood Working Party, the committee was invited to agree with a proposal to ban specified bovine offal in pig feed. SEAC agreed, but insisted that SBO be banned from the feed not just of pigs but of all species (Phillips *et al.* 2000, vol. 5, para. 3.220).

From 1990 until March 1996 evidence relating to the science and policy on BSE continued to accumulate. Much, although not all, of that evidence had been generated as a result of research, surveillance and monitoring activities funded and conducted by MAFF and the DoH. The final section of this chapter discusses the production of, and response to, that evidence up to 20 March 1996.

Research and monitoring: 1991–1996

Research and surveillance activities were self evidently important for BSE policy-making. Few of the uncertainties that existed in the late 1980s had diminished by the beginning of 1991. Amongst many other things, no one yet knew how or why BSE had appeared in the UK cattle herd, no one knew whether the disease was transmissible to humans and, if it did turn out to be transmissible to humans, no one knew what levels of exposure could be sufficient to cause infection. No one knew how much infectivity remained in the human food chain after SBO materials were removed, either in principle or in practice.

Almost all of the applied research on BSE, as opposed to basic research into the biology of TSEs, was funded by MAFF (Phillips *et al.* 2000, vol. 2, para. 6.3). The main exception was CJD surveillance, which was funded by the Department of Health and conducted by the CJD Surveillance Unit (CJD SU) in Edinburgh. As a consequence, MAFF exerted considerable control over which particular projects and lines of inquiry received funding and which did not. Although MAFF began funding research into BSE in 1987, initially conducting epidemiological investigations and commissioning a small number of transmission experiments, a systematic research programme did not begin until late 1990, primarily due to a lack of funding. Even then there were insufficient resources to begin investigating all the issues that had been identified as important by MAFF's expert advisors.

There is evidence that some senior MAFF officials appeared to view the purpose of research as demonstrating the truth of MAFF's assumptions rather than as an open-ended attempt to diminish or resolve some troubling uncertainties. In 1990 MAFF's CVO, Keith Meldrum, said

> There are so many unknowns with BSE that research is absolutely crucial and we have got to demonstrate without any doubt that BSE behaves exactly the same way in cattle that it does in sheep and goats. We believe it does; we have now to demonstrate that it does.

> (Prentice 1990)

It would be misleading to suggest that research projects were designed expressly for the purpose of supporting pre-existing government policy; as we describe below the results of some of the research commissioned by MAFF were instrumental in precipitating shifts in policy. Nevertheless, there were several important but politically sensitive research and surveillance topics and experiments that did not receive funding, at least not until after March 1996.

As well as controlling the level of funding and the direction of applied BSE research, MAFF's research programme was not open to external competition. Most of the research and surveillance activities funded by the department, at least in the period before March 1996, were conducted in two institutions: MAFF's own Central Veterinary Laboratory (CVL) and the Neuropathogenesis Unit (NPU), a public sector research institution set up in 1981 to study scrapie and other similar diseases which MAFF co-funded with the then Agriculture and Food Research Council. The fact that almost all applied BSE research was conducted within CVL and NPU had several consequences. It not only allowed MAFF to exercise control over the ways in which research findings were disseminated and represented but it also had the effect of inhibiting learning about the disease because the broader scientific community were effectively excluded from the research effort. Although some excellent scientists worked at CVL and NPU, the relevant competencies did not always exist in those institutions. Malcolm Ferguson-Smith, a member of the Phillips Inquiry Panel has noted, for example, that MAFF-funded experiments to test for the presence of BSE were based solely on highly expensive and time-consuming bioassays, when an existing technique known as western blotting (which allows detection of a *protein* in a sample by using an *antibody* specific to that protein) which can give results almost immediately was available and external scientists hold the competence to carry such programmes out (Ferguson-Smith 2001). There was also, for example, relatively little progress at CVL in developing a diagnostic test that could be used in live animals but other research groups were not encouraged, or able, to participate in research on that topic because MAFF had signed an exclusive agreement in December 1995 with a company called *Electrophoretics International* (which was owned by a Tory MP called Sir Michael Grylls) to develop a diagnostic test (Anon 1997). By adopting that tactic, MAFF had inhibited precisely the kind of competitive race between different research teams that would have given the teams of researchers a powerful incentive to develop a test as quickly as possible.

In practice, some effective tests were eventually developed, but the main efforts took place outside the UK. In Switzerland, where BSE was less common than in the UK, but more common than almost all other countries, in 1996 the federal government invested resources in a project based at the University of Zurich. By 1997 a test using the technique of western blotting was developed by the Zurich team. Together they formed a company known as Prionics that has subsequently developed and marketed BSE test kits. The test works by extracting and isolating proteins with target-specific antibodies, and then identifying them by fragmenting and staining the antibodies, and then separating the fragments on a two-dimensional gel under the influence of an electric field, since 'smaller proteins move faster than larger proteins' (Phillips *et al.* 2000, vol. 2, para 1.41).

Epidemiological surveillance and research was conducted entirely by a small group of veterinary epidemiologists within CVL. One of the UK's most eminent group of medical epidemiologists, lead by Roy Anderson at Oxford University, repeatedly approached MAFF to offer assistance with research into BSE but were refused access to CVL's data base until after March 1996. Anderson has since claimed that the epidemiological expertise in the CVL was far poorer than that available in the medical field, and that if his team had gained access to BSE data it would have been able to show that the scale of the epidemic would probably be larger than officially predicted and that controls on the animal feed chain were ineffective (Anderson 1998). Anderson also claimed that improved advice on how best to limit the size of the epidemic could have been provided, and that if that advice (to slaughter affected herds rather than just affected animals) had been followed at the end of 1989, approximately 330,000 animals infected with the BSE agent would not have entered the human food supply (Anderson 1998).

In the remainder of this section we discuss four key topics in which research, surveillance and monitoring were important, describing the kinds of evidence that emerged and the ways in which that evidence was interpreted, disseminated and responded to. Those topics by no means constitute all the relevant areas of BSE research. They are, however, pivotal to understanding the evolution of BSE policy, in relation to the protection of public health, and they illustrate the nature of the relationships between science and policy in BSE policy decision-making.

Host range and transmission characteristics of BSE

Evidence about the host range and transmission characteristics of BSE was important for several reasons. In particular, it provided a check on the government's claim that BSE was simply scrapie in cows and thus would probably behave just like scrapie and not pose a risk to human health.

By the end of 1990, there was already evidence that the host range and transmission characteristics of BSE was distinct from conventional sheep scrapie. As we noted in Chapter 5, CVL researchers had discovered in 1988 that BSE could not be transmitted experimentally to hamsters, even though hamsters were known to be readily susceptible to scrapie (Phillips *et al.* 2000, vol. 2, para. 3.51). In 1990, researchers at the NPU also discovered experimentally that a line of sheep, which was believed to be resistant to scrapie, had contracted BSE (Phillips *et al.* 2000, vol. 2, para. 3.51). Beginning in the late

1980s, TSEs were also discovered in a variety of zoo species and domestic animals that had presumably been fed material contaminated with the sheep scrapie agent but had never before been diagnosed with a TSE. These include several exotic ungulates and species of wild cat. We have already discussed the discovery of a novel TSE in domestic cats, in 1990; a species that is not susceptible experimentally to infection from scrapie. All of this evidence indicated that BSE was not simply 'scrapie in cows'.

In public, the fact that the evidence indicated that BSE behaved in quite distinct ways from scrapie was not made explicit by British policy-makers, who continued to insist that the source of BSE was probably scrapie infected sheep protein and that, like sheep scrapie, BSE was unlikely to present a risk to humans. For example, the CVO told journalists in 1994 that

> We believe that BSE must have come from scrapie initially, and scrapie has not been a risk to man in two hundred plus years here in the UK. And the probability is that BSE is the same, and will not in fact be [a] threat to man.

(Channel 4 Television, 1994)

The accumulating evidence that BSE did not behave like scrapie was not, however, missed by the UK government's expert advisors. In 1991, for example, one SEAC member noted in the medical literature that there was evidence that the BSE agent exhibited distinct transmission characteristics from scrapie in sheep, and that it was therefore essential to minimise human exposure to the pathogen (Will 1991). SEAC was not, however, asked to provide a risk assessment on BSE, nor was it asked to comment formally on the safety of beef following the 1990 letter to the CMO that had been produced by SEAC and its secretariat.

One of the ways in which MAFF was able to maintain its public narrative that BSE was almost certainly 'scrapie in cows' was by ensuring that no other groups of scientists became involved in assessing the possible risks from BSE. In 1990 Donald Acheson, the CMO, had tried to insist that the Director of the Public Health Laboratory Service (PHLS) – the established disease surveillance institution in the UK for new and emerging diseases – should be appointed onto SEAC, but MAFF officials resisted those efforts. As Deirdre Hine, the Welsh Chief Medical Officer later recalled, '[Donald Acheson] told me that the basis of the consistent opposition to the involvement of the PHLS was the anxiety that their involvement would be tantamount to admitting the possibility of a human health risk' (Phillips *et al.* 2000, vol. 11, para. 4.28).

One experiment, in particular, namely an attempt to feed scrapie-infected brain tissue to cows, would have helped to clarify the government's key assumption that scrapie-contaminated carcasses provided the original source of BSE. In 1987 scientific staff at MAFF's Central Veterinary Laboratory proposed that such an experiment take place (Phillips *et al.* 2000, vol. 2, para. 6.1437). Similarly, in June 1988, immediately after his committee's first meeting, Southwood wrote to the MAFF Permanent Secretary asking that an experiment be undertaken to test if meal infected with scrapie could cause BSE in cattle (MAFF/DoH 1989, para. 11, pp. 3–4). The government's first BSE research advisory committee, under the chairmanship of Dr David Tyrrell, had also argued in 1989 that 'we need to be sure that the disease really came from sheep' (Tyrell Committee, 1989, p. 5, para. 33). Despite the advice, the experiment was not viewed by MAFF as a priority and it was not until 1997 that MAFF eventually commissioned research directly to test that pivotal assumption (Phillips *et al.* 2000, vol. 2, para. 7.11).

Another important aspect of the transmission characteristics of BSE concerned the susceptibility of sheep to the disease. As we noted previously, in 1989 Ray Bradley had warned that BSE might have *passaged* into sheep via infected animal feed and that sheep meat might consequently pose a risk to human health. Experiments were clearly needed to assess if the infection had occurred in the UK's sheep flocks, especially after the NPU had demonstrated that 0.5 g of BSE-infected material could cause BSE in sheep (Phillips *et al.* 2000, vol. 2, para. 3.167). Research into the putative occurrence of BSE in sheep did not begin, however, until June 1997 but several years later it was discovered that cows brains were used in the experiments, in the mistaken belief that they were samples from sheep's brains (Anon 2001). In November 2001 the British government announced a new set of experiments. The effective delay by then corresponded to over 12 years.

An empirical check on the SBO ban

In deciding which bovine tissues should be included in the SBO ban, MAFF scientists and officials had had to rely on analogies with the scrapie infectivity levels that had been found experimentally in various sheep tissues, because pathogenesis or tissue infectivity data from cattle infected with BSE did not then exist. As we noted earlier, those tissues that, in sheep, were found to have the highest levels of scrapie infectivity, and which also had no commercial value and were practical to remove, were selected for the SBO ban.

In 1989, when the SBO ban was being formulated, Ray Bradley, Head of Pathology at CVL repeatedly told senior animal health officials in MAFF that pathogenesis or tissue infectivity studies were desirable in order to provide some empirical check on whether the appropriate tissues had been selected, particularly in regards to those tissues that had been exempted from the ban

(Phillips *et al.* 2000, vol. 6, paras 3.405 and 3.410). Although it was highly likely that nervous and lymphatic tissues would contain the highest level of infectivity (as with all TSEs) there was no reason to expect that BSE would spread in cattle in exactly the same way as scrapie did in sheep. Furthermore, some sheep tissues that might be expected to contain infectivity, such as stomach, had not been tested for the presence of scrapie (Phillips *et al.* 2000, vol. 6, paras 3.420). As Bradley noted in a comment on MAFF's proposal to exclude tripe (i.e. stomach) from the ban: 'it is important to measure the infectivity in these tissues as soon as possible' (Phillips *et al.* 2000, vol. 6, para. 3.451). Nearly two years earlier, in December 1987, Bradley had argued that it was important to determine which bovine tissues contain the agent and in what concentrations (Phillips *et al.* 2000, vol. 2, Para. 6.142). Furthermore, in June 1989 the Tyrell Committee had recommended that '[t]here is an urgent need to determine BSE infectivity titres in a large variety of bovine tissues' MAFF/DoH 1990, p. 13.

CVL staff had wanted to begin infectivity studies, and other experiments, in January 1988 but lack of funds and staff prevented those experiments from starting (Phillips *et al.* 2000, vol. 2, para. 6.178). Eighteen months later there was still no progress, but once the Tyrell Committee had completed its report in June 1989, a bid was made by MAFF to the Treasury in order to fund the studies identified as priorities by the Tyrell Committee (which including the infectivity studies). That bid was rejected by the Treasury in August 1989 and MAFF were forced to cut non-BSE research work to finance the studies recommended by Tyrell (Phillips *et al.* 2000, vol. 2, para. 6.192).

Tissue infectivity studies of BSE infected cattle thus began in late 1989 at the Neuropathogenesis Unit, using mice as the recipient species with exposure via simultaneous inoculation into the brain and abdomen. The ability of the NPU to perform tissue transmission studies was, however, limited in any one year, due to funding constraints (Phillips *et al.* 2000, vol. 2, para. 7.51). Thus beginning in late 1989, only 30 transmission studies were possible, another 30 could be initiated in the second year, and 20 in the third year (Phillips *et al.* 2000, vol. 2, para. 6.193).

Preliminary results from the tissue infectivity studies first became available in 1992. They indicated that spleen, lymph nodes, semen, white blood cells and muscle all failed to produce disease in the mice (Phillips *et al.* 2000, vol. 2, para. 3.208). Further results became available in 1993 and these also indicated that peripheral nervous tissue, spleen, lymphoid tissue had failed to produce disease in the mice (ibid., para. 3.211). Apart from brain and spinal cord, no other bovine tissues appeared to contain infectivity.

There were two main shortcomings with the tissue infectivity studies, in addition to the delay in beginning the experiments. The first was that infectivity levels rise and fall over the duration of the incubation period, and they do so in different ways in different tissues. It was therefore possible that infectivity might peak and then fall before tissues were isolated for the infectivity study, especially in non-neural tissues. Ideally, therefore, a pathogenesis study, rather than a tissue infectivity study, would be required to obtain a robust understanding of the infectivity of different bovine tissues because pathogenesis experiments measure possible infectivity in tissue types at different points in time.

A second shortcoming was that the tissue infectivity studies involved transmission across a species barrier, in this case from cattle to mice. The problem was not just that infectivity might be present but undetectable, given the limits of sensitivity of the mouse bioassay. In addition, the species barrier between cattle and mice was unknown and thus the sensitivity of the experiment was also unknown. Transmission studies from cattle to cattle (i.e. without any species barrier) would have provided a more sensitive method of identifying the presence of infectivity in different cattle tissues. The Tyrell Committee had described cattle titration studies as 'prohibitively expensive on a routine basis' and had not recommended that they be conducted (Tyrell 1989, p. 12). Nevertheless, although they were more expensive, and longer in duration than cattle to mice studies, they would have been immensely informative.

The absence of a pathogenesis study – the first shortcoming – was not resolved until December 1991 when the CVL began a pathogenesis study using mice as the recipient species (Phillips et al. 2000, vol. 2, para. 3.212). Forty-four tissue types, taken at various intervals from cattle that had been deliberately fed with infected bovine brain, were studied for infectivity. The first animals were killed two months after exposure and then others subsequently at four month intervals. In June 1994, infectivity was reported in the ileum (small intestine) of an animal that had been slaughtered six months after eating the infected brain. The presence of infectivity could not therefore be ruled out at any time between 2 and 6 months after exposure. Ileum was one of the tissues included in the SBO ban, but the ban as a whole did not apply to calves aged less than 6 months. That result led, on the basis of a recommendation from the CMO, to a tightening of the SBO ban in November 1994 to include ileum and thymus in animals aged under 6 months. Thymus was included, not because infectivity in that tissue had been reported, but because it was sold for human consumption as 'sweetbread' (unlike calf brain, spinal cord, spleen and tonsils which were not designated as SBOs). No further tissues in the pathogenesis experiment were shown to contain infectivity, prior to March 1996. We note, however, that the experiment was ongoing and that in 1998 additional tissues that were not covered by the initial SBO ban (for example, bone marrow, retina and dorsal root ganglia) were also found to contain infectivity. That evidence, and the UK government's reaction, is discussed in Chapter 8.

The species barrier problem – the second shortcoming with the tissue infectivity studies – does not appear to have been discussed within MAFF until January 1992 (Phillips *et al.* 2000, vol. 2, para. 7.34) although independent scientific critics had raised the problem in the previous year. (Dealler and Lacey 1991). In January 1993 MAFF began a comparative bioassay in which the infectivity of bovine brain, spleen and lymph nodes was compared by inoculation into both mice and calves (Phillips *et al.* 2000, vol. 2, para. 3.218). Preliminary results became available in November 1995 and they indicated that the cattle assay was 1000 times more sensitive than the mouse bioassay (ibid., para. 3.219). The implication was that negative results from the mouse bioassays could not be taken as evidence of the absence of infectivity.

Although bovine brain, spleen and lymph nodes were tested in the 1993 cattle bioassay no other tissues were tested until after March 1996 (Phillips *et al.* 2000, vol. 2, para. 3.219). It is stunning that a cattle bioassay to test for the presence of infectivity in widely consumed tissues such as bovine muscle and liver did not begin until more than a decade after BSE was first reported. As the Phillips Inquiry noted in 2000, '[t]he true infectivity of cattle tissues remains to be determined' (Phillips *et al.* 2000, vol. 2, para. 3.224) and that remains the case and will remain so for many years. Although cattle bioassays of a wider variety of tissues began in 1996 and 1998, they are not due to be completed until 2013 and 2014 (FSA 2003).

Whilst pathogenesis and tissue infectivity experiments were important in determining which tissues deserved to be included in the SBO ban, a risk assessment, based on either historical or current human exposure to the BSE agent, would have required not only data on the levels of infectivity in different tissues, but also the numbers of subclinically infected animals that were entering the human food chain. Such information, together with data from an appropriately designed pathogenesis study, might have enabled quantitative estimates of the amount of infectivity that humans consumed. A range of scenarios, as to the level of risks posed to humans, might then have been calculated, depending on different assumptions about the size of the species barrier between cattle and humans.

Estimating the number of subclinically infected animals that were entering the human food chain was, however, a sensitive topic for MAFF and, in fact, it was not until November 2001, that the UK government announced that it would test 250,000 cattle to discover the extent of undiagnosed disease (DEFRA 2001). In 1989, however, the Tyrell Committee had recommended that MAFF should conduct a survey of cattle brains routinely sent for slaughter in order to monitor the incidence of unrecognised infection (MAFF/DoH 1990, p. 10, para. 5A1f). Such a survey was not initiated by MAFF although

CVL scientists did calculate the number of infected but asymptomatic cattle entering the food chain from some epidemiological data. Those estimates were nevertheless kept secret. As the Head of Epidemiology at CVL acknowledged in 1994, in correspondence with an academic scientist: 'the decision has been made by the powers that be that no quantitative estimate [of subclinical infection] is made public' (Phillips *et al.* 2000, vol. 11, para. 5.150).

Enforcement of the SBO ban

Earlier in this chapter we discussed the serious concerns about compliance with the SBO controls that had been raised in 1990 by the Institute of Environmental Health Officers, whose members were responsible for enforcement of the SBO controls. We showed how their specific concerns about cross-contamination from carcass splitting and brain removal did not lead to any significant changes in the rules governing the processing of carcasses in abattoirs, nor did they lead to any efforts to ensure that meat inspectors paid particular attention to the proper removal of SBOs.

At that time, responsibility for enforcement of controls in abattoirs largely fell to Environmental Health Officers who were employed by local authorities. Meat hygiene standards in many British slaughterhouses were poor. Abattoirs operated on tight margins, and paid their staff – who were typically poorly trained and employed on piecework – low wages. Many also failed to meet minimum EC regulations and consequently were not permitted to produce meat for export. Local government was frequently unable or unwilling to enforce to an adequate level of hygiene. Environmental Health Officers were sometimes physically assaulted if they attempted to enforce standards, and local authorities were sometimes unwilling to jeopardise local employment where the design and operation of plants was unsatisfactory (Phillips *et al.* 2000, vol. 6, paras 4.70–4.76). Proper enforcement of the SBO controls was very unlikely to have been achieved, partly because of insufficient numbers of inspectors (Phillips *et al.* 2000, vol. 2, para. 4.322), and partly because the practice of carcass splitting caused inevitable cross-contamination and could trap pieces of spinal cord behind bone. The latter required inspectors to use an axe to remove the residual pieces, or return the carcass to the saw, and in practice few inspectors believed that 100 per cent compliance with the SBO regulations was necessary and they were reluctant to slow down the production line to achieve full compliance (Phillips *et al.* 2000, vol. 2, para. 4.325).

MAFF had a monitoring role too, but for slaughterhouses that produced meat for the domestic market that only consisted of an annual visit by an employee of the State Veterinary Service. Between 1989 and 1995, MAFF's

State Veterinary Service did not properly monitor the extent of compliance with the SBO regulations in slaughterhouses. In particular, whilst Veterinary Officers may have checked to see if SBOs were being properly disposed of, they were not concerned to ensure that SBOs were properly removed from the carcass (Phillips *et al.* 2000, vol. 6, paras 4.330, 4.333 and 5.151). Not surprisingly, with only occasional visits and no attempts to check carcasses, no significant problems with compliance with the SBO ban were identified by MAFF's State Veterinary Service in the period from late 1989 to the spring of 1995.

It was not until April 1995 that systematic efforts were made to check compliance with the SBO regulations. That development was provoked by a major institutional change to the arrangements for enforcement in abattoirs. In April 1995, a new Meat Hygiene Service (MHS) within MAFF was established in response to the need to ensure that all slaughterhouses complied with EC regulations, which was a requirement of the European Single Market of 1993 (Phillips *et al.* vol. 6, paras 5.85–5.149). The MHS took over local authorities' previous duties for the enforcement of regulations in slaughter houses.

Immediately following the launch of the MHS, a major benchmarking exercise was taken to assess hygiene standards within the meat industry. It took much of the year to complete but the results contrasted markedly with the impression that had been gained over the previous five or six years. The notes from a single member of the initial inspection team show that in 11 of the 57 slaughterhouses that he visited, spinal cord was not properly removed (Phillips *et al.* 2000, vol. 6, para. 6.49). In the overall exercise, more than 40 per cent of abattoirs failed to fully comply with SBO regulations (Swann 1998, para. 14). One senior veterinary official later explained that the survey had identified failures to properly remove spinal cord, failure to remove thymus, failure to separate spleen, failure to stain SBO, failure to mark SBO containers, deficiencies in paperwork and failure to remove SBO spillage from abattoir floors. The benchmarking exercise noted that some plants were designed in such a way that removal of SBO was difficult. This specifically applied to spinal cord removal where inability to reach one section of the spine resulted in retention of 4–6 inches of spinal cord. The exercise also identified widespread resentment at the cost of SBO controls and discovered that both plant owners and veterinary staff were invariably of the opinion that BSE was an animal disease only, and that as a consequence the SBO regulations were often not taken seriously (Swann 1998, paras 14, 18 and 19).

The benchmarking exercise was not completed until the end of 1995. Meanwhile from June 1995, MAFF's Veterinary Officers had begun to make regular unannounced visits to slaughterhouses. The first round of inspections, in June 1995, by the SVS did not identify failures to properly remove SBO from meat intended for human consumption, but it did discover, as one senior MAFF official put it, 'widespread and flagrant infringement of the regulations requiring staining of SBO' (Phillips *et al.* 2000, vol. 6, para. 6.83). This implied that tissues such as brain and spinal cord were being routinely processed for animal feed, rather than being disposed of. A second round of inspection visits the following month identified a handful of failures to remove SBOs from material for human consumption. That discovery prompted, for the first time in August 1995, explicit instructions to inspectors to check whether spinal cords and other SBOs were completely removed from carcasses (Phillips *et al.* 2000, vol. 6, para. 6.119). Further inspections in August, September, and October 1995 continued to reveal failures to remove spinal cord from carcasses. In September and October inspections had identified 17 instances in 16 different slaughterhouses of failure to remove spinal cord from carcasses (ibid., para. 6.193).

Greater efforts to monitor regulatory compliance in 1995 also reflected growing concern about vCJD cases. By then there were growing concerns about cases of CJD both in young people and in farmers. Agriculture Ministers and officials began to insist that the MHS achieve 100 per cent compliance (Phillips *et al.* 2000, vol. 6, para. 6.162). The failures to remove SBOs were communicated in writing to the Cabinet, but in a way that, contrary to the wishes of the CMO, attempted to imply that none of the SBOs had actually entered the human food chain. As one DoH official put it at the time,

> This is indicative of the unwillingness of some MAFF officials to accept the lapses in SBO controls as an issue of genuine public health concern, as opposed to one about the undermining of public confidence in the safety of British beef.
>
> (Phillips *et al.* 2000, vol. 6, para. 6.181)

SEAC were told about the failures properly to remove spinal cord in slaughter-house on 23 November 1995. One member was 'appalled' because of the assurances previously given to SEAC that there was very little chance that spinal cord would remain in the carcass (Phillips *et al.* 2000, vol. 6, para. 6.221). SEAC recommended in response that the use of bovine vertebrae should no longer be permitted in the production of mechanically recovered meat.

Young people with CJD

The CJD Surveillance Unit had been set up in 1990 with Department of Health funding to check for changes in the incidence, or atypical cases, of CJD after recommendations to do so by both the Southwood Working Party and the Tyrell Committee in 1989. In late 1993, a suspect case (later confirmed) of CJD in a 16-year-old girl was reported to the CJD Surveillance Unit in Edinburgh.

CJD is extremely rare in young people. A second case in an exceptionally young person was identified by the Unit in May 1995, and a third in August 1995. By the end of September 1995, four more cases in people under the age of 50 had been referred to the CJD Surveillance Unit. A further seven cases were referred by the end of December 1995, although by that point only three of the total number of referred cases had been confirmed as CJD (Phillips *et al.* 2000, vol. 8, para. 5.77).

The referrals and confirmed cases provoked strong concerns within both SEAC and the DoH. In September 1994 the CMO had wanted to 'strengthen the clinical membership of SEAC' because of increased human health concerns over BSE (Phillips *et al.* 2000, vol. 11, para. 4.22). As a consequence, Professor John Pattison, Dean of University College London Medical School, was appointed to SEAC in November 1994. Pattison became chair of SEAC a year later in November 1995, at which point he decided to appoint additional members. These were Professor Jeff Almond, a virologist and microbiologist, Professor John Collinge, Head of the NeuroGenetics Unit at St Mary's Imperial College School of Medicine, Dr Michael Painter, a consultant in communicable disease control, Professor Peter Smith, an epidemiologist and statistician from the London school of Hygiene and Tropical Medicine, and Ray Bradley who had recently retired as Head of Pathology at MAFF's Central Veterinary Laboratory. All five of the new members attended their first SEAC meeting on 5 January 1996.

Two of the confirmed cases of CJD in teenagers had been published in the medical literature in October 1995 and although SEAC released a statement noting that 'it is not possible to draw any conclusions' from those cases (Phillips *et al.* 2000, vol. 6, para. 6.251), the development profoundly worried many in the scientific community. On 1 December 1995, an eminent neuropathologist, Sir Bernard Tomlinson, President of the British Association for the Advancement of Science and a former advisor to Department of Health, stated on BBC radio, that:

> Until we can say quite positively there really is no evidence now that BSE transfers to humans, until we can say that, I believe we've got to pay that price and all offal should be kept from public consumption. But I certainly don't eat any longer beef pies, for instance, or puree, I wouldn't eat a burger.

> (Phillips *et al.* 2000, vol. 6, para. 6.273)

Thomlinson was by no means the first or last to express such doubts about the safety of British beef, prior to 20 March 1996, but he was one of the most authoritative, influential and eminent experts to contradict the Government's reassuring narrative. Other senior scientists also began publicly acknowledging the risks, indicating that they thought there was growing evidence of transmission to humans (e.g. Penman 1995).

The response of some Ministers was to assert their previous reassurances with ever-greater vigour. On 3 December 1995, the Secretary of State for Health, Stephen Dorrell, agreed during a television interview that there was 'no conceivable risk' of anyone eating beef being infected with BSE (Phillips *et al.* 2000, vol. 6, para. 6.280), and on the same day the Secretary of State for Agriculture, Douglas Hogg, was reported as agreeing with the statement that British beef was perfectly safe to eat (idid., para. 6.279). Hogg did admit, however, that 'I cannot on the evidence before me give a categoric guarantee that it cannot be transmitted. We believe it cannot be and the scientific evidence suggests it cannot be' (ibid.).

On 7 December 1995, MAFF Ministers and officials decided to draft a set of questions for SEAC, not for the purpose of advising on policy, but with the intention of distributing the answers in a letter to the media in an attempt to quell the media furore. The intention was to provide SEAC with the questions at its next meeting on 5 January 1996. In the interim the questions were shown to the Meat and Livestock Commission (MLC) (Phillips *et al.* 2000, vol. 6, para. 7.8). On 3 January, two days prior to the SEAC meeting, the Director General of the MLC, Colin Maclean, wrote to Richard Kimberlin, a member of SEAC, who, unbeknownst to the rest of SEAC, was a paid consultant to the MLC (Phillips *et al.* 2000, vol. 6 para. 7.42). Maclean's letter to Kimberlin listed the questions that MAFF was planning to pose and enclosed a draft set of answers written by the MLC's public relations firm. The letter explained:

> We agree that we need succinct answers to these questions and my colleagues in our PR company . . . have drafted the sort of questions (Appendix A) they would like to see (although they cannot put words into SEAC's mouth!) However, this should give you some feel for what we would initially like.

> (Phillips *et al.* 2000, vol. 6, para. 7.10)

Three of MAFF's questions had asked 'Is beef safe?', 'Are beef products safe to eat?', and 'Are the protective measures for the public sufficient?' Maclean's letter noted that in relation to the three question 'unequivocal 'yes' answers are preferred' (ibid., para 7.11). Maclean's letter also noted that 'an ideal way forward would be for SEAC members to write a letter saying that they have not changed their eating habits' (ibid., para. 7.12) and he supplied a draft letter which he suggested that Kimberlin arrange for SEAC to send to *The Times*.

MAFF's questions were put to SEAC in January 1996. Responsibility for producing draft answers was allocated to certain members and they were supplied in time for SEACs next meeting in February 1996. The answers provided to the three questions listed in the previous paragraph were prepared by two members: Kimberlin and Jeff Almond who had just joined the committee. As shown below in Table 6.1, Kimberlin's answers, which he presented without disclosing that he had been approached by the MLC on this issue, essentially reproduced those that had been drafted by the MLC's public relations firm. Almond's answers appear in contrast far more measured and reasonable.

SEAC were never required to decide on a single set of answers to send to Ministers, and subsequently to the media, because the events leading up to

Table 6.1 The safety of beef: questions and answers

MAFF:	'Is beef safe?'
MLC:	'Yes. We have no doubt about the fact that the beef on sale in the high street is safe to eat.'
Kimberlin:	'Yes. We have no doubts that the beef on sale in the high street is safe to eat.'
Almond:	'We should not take the view that beef *is safe until proven dangerous*. In my view to do so would be wrong ethically and morally. To do the opposite, i.e. to assume that beef *is dangerous until proven safe* is also difficult because the corollary would be the destruction of the national herd. . . . Both of the two italicised propositions above are unpalatable. Therefore the only practical option is to adopt the middle ground (as Southwood commendably did) which is to assume a risk, ie, that all carcasses are infected, and then minimise that risk by removal of all SBOs'
MAFF:	'Are beef products, e.g. offal such as liver, and hamburgers, sausages and meat pies, safe to eat?'
MLC:	'Yes. The Government has banned specified offal from the manufacture of all beef products and controls are rigorously applied. Beef products on sale in the high street are therefore perfectly safe to eat.'
Kimberlin:	'Yes. The only tissue from which there might be a theoretical risk due to BSE are the so called specified bovine offals (SBOs): but these tissues have been banned from all human food products since January 1990'
Almond:	'As regards hamburgers, sausages, meat pies, these are likely to have carried a higher potential risk than prime beef in that they were more likely to contain portions of spinal cord that had been improperly removed. The recent ban on the use of the spinal column for MRM goes some way to alleviate this concern.'
MAFF:	'Do the protective measures in place fully meet all the recommendations that SEAC has made?'
MLC:	'Yes. The Precautionary measures established by the Government protect the public from any remote, theoretical risk from BSE even though no link has been demonstrated between BSE and CJD'
Kimberlin:	'Yes'
Almond:	'In light of our discussions last time (and my own 'inspection') this is clearly not the case. Some abattoirs are not effectively removing the spinal cord. They continue to smear much of this tissue across other parts of the carcass during sectioning and butchering.'

Sources: Phillips *et al.* 2000, vol. 6, paras 7.11 and 7.18–7.26

20 March 1996 overtook the discussion. At the same February meeting SEAC was told by Robert Will of the CJD Surveillance Unit that five individuals aged under 30 had now been diagnosed with CJD, and that all five cases showed an unusual pathology. As Will emphasised: 'the crucial issue is not simply the young age or pathology of recent cases but the short time scale in which 5 cases in individuals under 30 years had occurred' (Phillips *et al.* 2000, vol. 6, para. 7.141). John Collinge was of the opinion that five cases in people under 30 years in less than a year 'must be very significant in statistical terms', and that the cases were likely to represent BSE transmission to humans (ibid., paras 7.142 and 7.143). The view of the CJD Surveillance Unit at that point, however, was that it was premature to decide whether the cases were linked with BSE (Phillips *et al.* 2000, vol. 6, para. 7.141).

The MAFF secretary to SEAC failed to convey the concerns to Ministers expressed by some of the committee members at the February meeting, that the cases of CJD in young people might represent transmission to humans. Instead, the minute from the Secretary discussed the presentational problems that planned scientific publications on the cases might invoke. It noted, for example, that 'I also need to alert the Minister to the fact that Dr Will, the Deputy Chairman of SEAC and Head of the CJD Surveillance Unit, is preparing two scientific papers. Both are potentially tricky and will need careful handling' (Phillips *et al.* 2000, vol. 6, para. 7.149). Meanwhile MAFF officials continued to prepare briefing material on BSE, including a leaflet entitled *British Beef and BSE: The Facts* which continued to maintain that there was no evidence of a link between BSE and CJD and which asserted that beef was safe. DoH officials were, however, reluctant to be associated with the leaflet. As the deputy CMO put it on 29 February: 'We should not follow MAFF's hyberbole of reassurance' (Phillips *et al.* 2000, vol. 6, para. 7.72).

At SEAC's next meeting on 8 March 1996, the committee was told that the CJD Surveillance Unit was confident that they had a identified a new variant of CJD in young people. Since 1965 there had only been 17 cases of CJD in patients under 30 worldwide, but the recent cases in the UK were all pathologically distinct (Phillips *et al.* 2000, vol. 6, para. 7.211). SEAC members argued that the cases were unlikely to have been identified merely because of increased referrals, or that the new variant had previously been unrecognised. Rather, a novel factor had precipitated the disease, and BSE was a likely explanation (Phillips *et al.* 200, vol. 6, paras 7.213–7.215).

On 13 March the chair of SEAC, John Pattison, met senior MAFF and DoH officials to discuss the implications of the CJD Surveillance Unit's conclusions. Pattison noted that, in light of the epidemiological data on BSE, SEAC could consider removing cattle aged over 24 or 30 months old from the human food chain, but that this was a very complicated question in view of the economic consequences. Pattison asked for guidance on the limits of SEAC's considerations. MAFF's Permanent Secretary, Richard Packer told Pattison that if SEAC made a recommendation, the Government was likely to follow it, and that while economic considerations were secondary, any recommendation should be balanced, and that changes to the rules had to be proportionate (O'Donoghue 1996).

Later that day Packer later told Douglas Hogg, the Secretary of State for Agriculture, that elements in SEAC were considering recommending a ban on the consumption of beef aged over 24 months but that 'it is far from clear that the cost of such a measure would be proportionate to any reduction in risk' (Phillips *et al.* 2000, vol. 6, para. 7.250). Packer noted, however, that the economic consequences of SEAC recommendations would be academic if statements were released by SEAC and the CMO acknowledging the possibility of transmission to humans (ibid.). Hogg subsequently told Packer that MAFF should avoid seeking to influence the conclusions to which SEAC would come and that before making a public statement or taking action 'we [need] clear advice from the Committee as to the facts and the steps which the Government should take' (Strang 1996). Thus, the policy judgement about how to respond to evidence of possible transmission to humans was delegated to SEAC.

On 16 March SEAC held an emergency meeting in order to provide advice to Ministers. The members revisited the evidence of a novel variant of CJD and agreed to advise Ministers that exposure to BSE, before the introduction of the SBO ban in 1989, was the most likely explanation at present. SEAC were less successful in agreeing on policy measures. As we have emphasised on several occasions, understanding the science of BSE could not, by itself, imply particular policy recommendations. Amongst other things, the level and significance of both historical and current exposures to the BSE agent were uncertain, and thus a judgement needed to be made about the significance of current risks from UK beef. Judgements were also required about the proportionality of any further control measures. Yet the costs, political consequences and practicalities of different courses of action were not issues that training in virology or epidemiology, for example, could illuminate. The minutes of the 16 March meeting record Jeff Almond stating that:

> If one set out to eliminate any potential theoretical risk from BSE then it would be necessary to destroy the entire national herd of cattle, however, various control measures could reduce any risk to a minimal level. Ultimately a decision on whether a zero or minimal risk was acceptable was a political one.

> (Phillips *et al.* 2000, vol. 6, para 7.265)

SEAC could not arrive at an agreed set of recommendations. Some members considered that no further restrictions were necessary whilst others were of the view that total eradication was the only answer (Phillips *et al.* 2000, vol. 11, para. 4.629).

On 18 March the Secretary of State for Agriculture, Douglas Hogg, wrote a note to the Prime Minister proposing a series of interim measures in advance of SEAC's advice. This comprised, at a minimum, a prohibition on the sale of beef and beef products from animals aged over 30 months. Hogg explained that 30 months was chosen because infectivity increases with age and because 30 months was already enshrined in EC legislation in respect of exports, it was enforceable because 30-month old animals could be identified from the animals' teeth, and because most prime beef came from animals below this age and might allow the beef industry to continue (Packer 1996). Earlier that day Hogg had met John Pattison and Pattison had told him that SEAC would expect about 5000 infected animals aged over 2 years and 24,000 infected younger animals to reach the human food chain. Pattison said that the older animals were likely to be at least ten times more infectious that younger ones and that '[a]ction on older animals [either a complete ban or the removal of all bones lymphatic nodes and nerves] was therefore likely to take out at least half the potential problem' (Phillips *et al.* 2000, vol. 6, para. 7.293).

Hogg's note to the Prime Minister also suggested the possible withdrawal of all beef products from the shelves and raised a worst case option of ordering the complete slaughter and restocking of the national herd, given the likely damage of a public announcement that BSE could affect humans for the UK cattle industry. Finally, Hogg recommended setting up a Public Inquiry into the government's handling of BSE to be chaired by a High Court Judge (Phillips *et al.* 2000, vol. 6, paras 7.306–7.308).

By 19 March, it was clear that Hogg's Ministerial colleagues did not support the introduction of interim measures, prior to advice from SEAC. Ministers were anxious, however, to make a public statement about the connection between BSE and the new variant of CJD before the news reached the media, but did not want to make such a statement in the absence of advice from its committee. SEAC was therefore encouraged to meet and provide advice as rapidly as possible and a meeting of the committee was arranged for later that day. The main options discussed by SEAC were to slaughter the entire herd and restock, slaughter all cattle aged over 30 months, or de-bone beef from animals aged over 30 months.

The meeting resumed on the morning of 20 March and SEAC were asked to provide advice by 10.30 am in time for a Ministerial announcement in Parliament later that day. SEAC agreed a statement on the morning of 20 March. It noted that:

> The Spongiform Encephalopathy Advisory Committee have considered 10 cases of CJD which have occurred in people aged under 42 ... Although there is no direct evidence of a link, on current data and in the absence of any credible alternative the

most likely explanation at present is that these cases are linked to exposure to BSE before the introduction of the ban on specified bovine offals in 1989. This is a cause of great concern.

(Phillips *et al.* 2000, vol. 11, para. 4.632)

SEAC's statement also noted that it was 'imperative' that the existing measures were properly enforced. It made two key additional recommendations: That carcasses from animals aged under 30 months must be de-boned in licensed plants under supervision from the Meat Hygiene Service and the trimmings classified as SBO, and that the use of mammalian meat and bone meal in the feed of all farm animals must be prohibited. SEAC concluded that if those recommendations were carried out 'the risk from eating beef is now likely to be extremely small' (Phillips *et al.* 2000, vol. 11, para. 4.632).

Steven Dorrell, the Secretary of State for Health, outlined SEAC's statement in the House of Commons that afternoon, and announced that the Government would be following SEAC's recommendations.

Bibliography

Anderson, R. (1998) Statement to BSE Inquiry No. 9c, annex 1, in Phillips *et al.* 2000, op. cit.

Anon (1997) *The Economist*, 22 February, p. 25.

Anon (2001) 'Bungled BSE experiments due to refrigerator mix-up', *New Scientist*, 30 November.

Bradley, R. (1989) 'BSE: Disposal of brains and spinal cords from aged-cull cattle and sheep', Minute dated 12 April 1989 to A. J. Lawrence, *BSE Inquiry Year Book* Reference No. 89/04.12/1.1–1.5 in Phillips *et al.* 2000, op. cit.

BSE Inquiry Transcript (1988) Oral hearings, Day 43, 7 July 1998, pp. 124–5, in Phillips *et al.* 2000, op. cit.

Capstick, C. (1990) Secretary's Meeting with CMO – Friday 22 June 1990, Minute dated 20 June 1990. *BSE Inquiry Year Book* Reference No. YB90/6.20/15.1, in Phillips *et al.* 2000, op. cit.

Channel 4 Television (1994) *Dispatches: BSE – the human link*. Broadcast on 25 January 1994.

Cockburn, C. (1989) BSE: Use of offals in meat products, Minute, *BSE Inquiry Year Book* Reference No. 89/06.02/51–5.10, in Phillips *et al.* 2000, op. cit.

Corbally, M. (1990) Letter to Animal Health Division of MAFF, from Institute of Environmental Health Officers, 1 February 1990.

Dealler, S. and Lacey, R. W. (1991) 'Transmissible spongiform encephalopathies: The threat of BSE to man – a reply to K. C. Taylor', *Food Microbiology*, **8**, 259–62.

DEFRA (2001) *Government expands BSE testing programme*, News Release 233/01, 13 November 2001.

Ferguson-Smith, M. (2001) 'A sorry tail of BSE blunders', *The Times Higher Educational Supplement*, 2 November, 21.

FSA (2003) 'Research Projects MO3', at http://www.food.gov.uk/science/research/meat_hygiene_research/m03programme/m03projilist/

Griffiths, M. J. (1990) 'BSE: Splitting Heads', Minute dated 2 May 1990 to M. Hill, MAFF. *BSE Inquiry Year Book* Reference No. 90\05.02\1.1–1.2, in Phillips *et al.* 2000, op. cit.

Gummer, J. (1990) *Hansard*, 8 June 1990, column 906. The Stationery Office, London.

Lawrence, A. (1989) BSE, Minute dated 29 March 1989. *BSE Inquiry Year Book* Reference No. YB 89/3.29/3.1, in Phillips *et al.* 2000, op. cit.

Lebrecht, A. J. (1989) Minister's Meeting with UKASTA: 2 October 1989, minute datated 4 October 1989. *BSE Inquiry Year Book* Reference No. YB 89/10.04/5.1–5.2, in Phillips *et al.* 2000, op. cit.

Lowson, R. (1989) Briefing for Incoming Ministers – Animal Health, minute dated 25 July 1989. *BSE Inquiry Year Book* Reference No. YB 89\07.25\5.1–5.5, in Phillips *et al.* 2000, op. cit.

Lowson, R. (1990) BSE : paper on the safety of beef. *BSE Inquiry Year Book* Reference No. YB90\07.13\5.1–5.13, in Phillips *et al.* 2000, op. cit.

MAFF/DoH (1989) *Report of the Working Party on Bovine Spongiform Encephalopathy*. London: Ministry of Agriculture Fisheries and Food/Department of Health.

MAFF/DoH (1990) *Consultative Committee on Research into Spongiform Encephalopathies, (the 'Tyrell Report')*, Interim report. Ministry of Agriculture, Fisheries and Food, London.

MAFF (1990a) *British Beef Is Safe, Gummer*, News Release 185/90, 15 May 1990, London: Ministry of Agriculture Fisheries and Food.

MAFF (1990b) *Bovine Spongiform Encephalopathy (BSE)*, News Release 184/90, 15 May 1990, London: Ministry of Agriculture Fisheries and Food.

Meldrum, K. (1992) *Radio Times*, 31 May 1992.

Metters, J. S. (1989) BSE: Action proposed by MAFF Ministers on bovine offal, minute dated 9 June 1989. *BSE Inquiry Year Book* Reference No. YB 89/6.9/5.1–5.4, in Phillips *et al.* 2000, op. cit.

O'Donoghue, K. (1996) BSE, minute dated 15 March 1996. *BSE Inquiry Year Book* Reference No. YB96/3.15/2.1–2.4, in Phillips *et al.* 2000, op. cit.

Packer, R. (1996) Draft Minute for the Minister to Send to [The Prime Minister], YB 96/3.18 8.1–8.6.

Penman (1995) 'Top Scientists adds to BSE warnings', *Independent*, 4 December 1995, p. 4.

Phillips, Bridgeman, J. and Ferguson-Smith, M. (2000) *The BSE Inquiry: Report: evidence and supporting papers of the Inquiry into the emergence and identification of Bovine Spongiform Encephalopathy (BSE) and variant Creutzfeldt-Jakob Disease (vCJD) and the action taken in response to it up to 20 March 1996*. London: The Stationery Office.

Pickles, H. (1990a), 'Bovine Spongiform Encephalopathy', minute dated 1 June 1990. *BSE Inquiry Year Book* Reference No.YB 90/6.01/3.1–3.2, in Phillips *et al.* 2000, op. cit.

Pickles, H. (1990b) 'Safety of Beef', draft dated 15 June 1990, *BSE Inquiry Year Book* Reference No. YB90/6.15/19.1, in Phillips *et al.* 2000, op. cit.

Prentice (1990) *The Times*, 22 January 1990.

Southwood Working Party (1999) Witness Statement No. 1D, in Phillips *et al.* 2000, op. cit.

Stagg, S. (1989a) Southwood Report – BSE, Letter dated 24 February 1989, *BSE Inquiry Year Book* Reference No. YB89/02.24/14.1, in Phillips *et al.* 2000, op. cit.

Stagg, S. (1989b) Minute on 'BSE: Use of Offals in Meat Products', dated 7 June 1989, *BSE Inquiry Year Book* Reference No. YB 89/6.07/7.1, in Phillips *et al.* 2000, op. cit.

Strang, W. G. G. (1996) 'BSE and CJD', Minute to K. O'Donoghue, YB96/3.15/3.1–3.2 in Phillips *et al.* 2000.

Swann (1998) Statement No. 158 to the BSE Inquiry, in Phillips *et al.* 2000.

Tyrrell, D. (1990) Opinion on the Public Health Implications of Eating Beef and the Epidemic of BSE, Draft of 3 July 1990, *BSE Inquiry Year Book* Reference No. YB90\07.03\13.1–13.13, in Phillips *et al.* 2000, op. cit.

Will, R. G. (1991) 'The spongiform encephalopathies', *Journal of Neurology Neurosurgery and Psychiatry*, **54** (9), 761–3.

Chapter 7

BSE policy in continental Europe

Although BSE began in the UK, and was (and remains) primarily a British problem, it also spread to other countries, especially in Continental Europe, as a consequence of trade in both animals and feedstuffs. This chapter discusses the policy responses to BSE in European jurisdictions outside the UK, prior to March 1996. It focuses, in particular, on the response of the European Commission. We show how, for the Commission, BSE was primarily seen as a threat to the functioning of the internal market and to the economic welfare of the farming and food industries. Consequently, the Commission only proposed and established regulations on BSE in order to ensure that all Member States were willing to continue importing British meat and cattle products, and even then it did so reluctantly. The Commission also contrived to represent its policies as robustly supported by the best scientific advice. This is the tactic that, as we have seen, was adopted in the UK.

For many individual Member States, BSE was also primarily seen as a threat to domestic farming and meat industries rather than as a threat to public health. One consequence of those policy orientations was that 20 March 1996 marked the beginning of a political crisis not just in the UK, but for the European Commission and for many Continental Member States too.

The pathogenic and political dispersion of BSE to continental Europe

Until the existence of BSE in British cattle was publicly acknowledged by MAFF, in late 1987 and early 1988, the countries with which the UK traded animals and animal feedstuffs had no reason to suspect that British exports might be contaminated with a novel pathogen. Consequently none of them imposed any trade restrictions, and BSE was transmitted beyond the UK, mainly through contaminated meat and bone meal (MBM) and animal feeds containing MBM. The agent was then recycled within national herds, thus allowing the disease to become established in several different jurisdictions. Many veterinary and agricultural officials in continental European countries felt justifiably aggrieved at MAFF for having knowingly allowed BSE to reach other countries.

As soon as MAFF publicly acknowledged the existence of BSE several countries imposed controls on the import, from the UK, of live cattle and/or MBM to try to prevent the spread of BSE to their jurisdictions. The timing and extent of those restrictions varied considerably. Germany, Ireland and France prohibited imports of British MBM in 1989, for example, whereas some other countries, such as Portugal, did not act for another year or two. The European Commission did not impose an export ban on UK MBM until March 1996.

There was also considerable variation in the timing of domestic regulatory restrictions. For example, in 1989 and 1990, prior to discovering any cases of, BSE, the Netherlands, Austria, Sweden and Denmark banned the use of ruminant derived meat and bone meal for use as cattle feed. Other European countries, for example, Germany, Belgium, Greece, Italy, Luxembourg and Spain, had no feed ban in place until the EU-wide ban on mammalian proteins for ruminants was introduced in 1994 (Court of Auditors 2001).

Not surprisingly, the reported incidence of BSE varied between different countries. Prior to March 1996, BSE had been reported and confirmed in the domestic herds (i.e. not including animals that had been imported from the UK) of four European countries: the Republic of Ireland, France, Portugal and, outside the EU, Switzerland. The relevant figures, up to March 1996, are given in Table 7.1.

A few cases of BSE were also reported in several other jurisdictions. but these were all in animals that had been imported from the UK (notably Germany with four cases, Denmark with one case and Italy with two cases). All those jurisdictions, and the remaining European countries, believed their domestic herds to be free of BSE. As we will discuss in Chapter 8, however, after March 1996, and especially since 2000 and the introduction of a Europe-wide rapid post mortem monitoring regime, many European countries have discovered that the pathogen was present in their domestic herds too (Office Internationale des Epizooties 2003). This suggests that BSE was in fact more widespread in continental Europe in the years prior to March 1996 than was recognised at the time.

Table 7.1 Number of reported BSE cases in the domestic herds of the Republic of Ireland, France, Portugal and Switzerland in years 1989–1996

	1989	1990	1991	1992	1993	1994	1995	1996
Ireland	10	13	15	16	16	18	15	73
Switzerland	–	2	8	15	29	64	68	45
France	–	–	5	–	1	4	3	12
Portugal	–	–	–	–	–	12	15	31

Source: Office Internationale des Epizooties, 2003.

BSE policy-making structures in the European Commission

Although responsibility for food safety policy-making has fallen historically to national governments, in the process of establishing the European Economic Community and completing the internal European market it became a Community-wide responsibility, with the European Commission playing a central role. Historically, free trade within Europe had been hampered by a complex range of non-tariff barriers that arose as a consequence of the differences between the national rules governing products such as food and drinks. The Commission had at least two reasons for trying to ensure the achievement and maintenance of uniform food safety standards for intra-Community trade. First there were presumed to be considerable economic benefits, in terms of reduced costs and increased efficiencies, to be derived from the integration of the European market. Second, it was widely presumed in the Commission and in the food industry that regulatory differences between Member States worried and/or confused consumers about the quality and safety of the food supply (Byrne 2000).

The adoption of common health standards for animals and meat intended for export to other Member States were amongst the earliest acts of the European Economic Community. Following the introduction of the Single European Act in 1987, however, several additional Directives were adopted to complete the internal market in animals and animal products. Their aim was to ensure that veterinary checks should be carried out at the place of dispatch only and not at the Community's internal borders. Responsibility was placed on Member States to ensure that animals and products intended for intra-Community trade conformed to Community rules. Each Member State was required to notify other Member States and the Commission of any outbreak in its territory of an animal disease likely to constitute a serious hazard to animals or human health and to implement any control or precautionary measures provided for in Community rules (Council Directives 89/662/EEC and 90/425/EEC). In such cases the Commission was empowered to adopt any measures considered necessary in addition to those already taken by the Member State concerned. These Directives enabled the Commission to adopt measures to ensure co-ordination of action among Member States and, if necessary, to take measures restricting the export of animal products from any Member State.

The European Commission and two of its advisory committees were the most important European bodies with responsibility for BSE policy-making. Although the Council of the European Union (made up of ministerial representatives of the Governments of Member States) was and remains the principal legislative and decision-making body of the EU, it adopts legislation on the basis of proposals submitted to it by the Commission. Prior to 2000, responsibility for developing regulatory and legislative proposals on BSE fell to two Directorates General of the Commission: DG-VI, which was responsible for agricultural and fisheries, and DG-III which was responsible for industry, and after 1992 for the internal market. In practice DG-VI took the lead responsibility on BSE.

DG-VI and DG-III acted on the advice of two key advisory committees. One of these, the Standing Veterinary Committee (SVC) was explicitly concerned with policy matters and comprised representatives from each of the Member States, typically senior officials from the agriculture departments of their home country. Draft legislative measures that had been proposed by the Commission would be submitted to the SVC, which would then provide an opinion on the draft. If a qualified majority of the SVC voted in favour of the Commission's proposal, the Commission would adopt it. If the opinion was unfavourable, or no opinion was delivered, the Commission would submit its proposed measure to the Council of Ministers. The SVC representatives generally expressed the views of their individual governments, and were therefore expected to incorporate national veterinary policy interests into their deliberations and recommendations.

The second committee to advise the European Commission was known as the Scientific Veterinary Committee (ScVC). It was primarily (or ostensibly) a scientific body, responsible for advising the Commission and the Standing Veterinary Committee on all scientific and technical problems concerning animal health and veterinary public health. Its normal practice was to reach decisions by consensus rather than by taking votes. The members of the ScVC were veterinary scientists, appointed by the Commission on the basis of nominations from the Member States but the Commission was responsible for convening the ScVC, drawing up its agenda and providing the secretariat.

In practice the ScVC provided not just scientific advice but also policy advice and specific policy recommendations. As with the UK committees on BSE, key policy decisions about the acceptability of uncertainties and risks have, in practice, been made within the ScVC, though they were routinely represented as if they were purely scientific judgements. It is also important to appreciate that although the ScVC was nominally comprised of individuals appointed on the basis of their veterinary expertise, in practice many members worked in the official veterinary services of the Member States. It would therefore be unreasonable to discount the possibility that members of the ScVC might bring their domestic policy considerations to bear on decisions about the nature and acceptability of risks and the attendant uncertainties.

In practice, the BSE subgroup of the ScVC was almost always chaired by a British veterinary official and about half of the subgroup's members were British. The minutes were also drawn up by a temporary Commission official of British nationality who used to work in MAFF (European Parliament 1997a, p. 10). On matters relating to BSE the ScVC tended, not surprisingly, to reflect thinking within MAFF. The Commission had no additional sources of scientific expertise on TSEs to draw upon.

European Policy on BSE: 1987–1990

Once the UK government had made the emergence of BSE public, in late 1987, the European Commission might have been expected to respond on two issues: prevention of the further spread of the animal disease to the herds of other countries and protection of European citizens' public health.

The protection of animal health

Three measures were important in minimising the spread of BSE to, and within, the rest of Europe: controls on exports of live UK cattle, controls on exports of UK MBM and controls on the composition of ruminant feed within individual jurisdictions. As regards the first of those measures, in July 1989, some 18 months after learning about BSE, the European Commission banned the export of live cattle from the UK that had been born before July 1988 (the date when the UK's ruminant feed ban was introduced).

European Commission action in relation to the remaining two measures was extraordinarily delayed. The most important measure available to the Commission to prevent further spread of BSE was to ban exports of ruminant protein and ruminant derived MBM from the UK to other Member States. The UK had acknowledged that MBM was the probable vector of BSE in July 1988 when it banned the use of ruminant protein in ruminant feed within the UK. Despite the fact that UK feed manufacturers responded to the loss of their domestic market by increasing exports of MBM, no measures were taken by the European Commission to restrict UK exports of ruminant-derived animal feed until March 1996.

In July 1989, the Commission had asked the UK to ban exports of ruminant derived MBM, after prompting from the Standing Veterinary Committee, but the UK did not do so (European Parliament 1996a, p. 10). The Commission subsequently prepared a draft Decision banning exports of UK MBM, but in early 1990 the Commission's Legal Service had ruled that the Commission could not do so under the Directive proposed by the Commission (European Parliament, 1997a, p. 29). Alternative means of incorporating the proposed Decision into Community law were not, however, sought (ibid. p. 30).

As well as failing to impose controls on exports of UK MBM, the European Commission also failed to insist, until 1994, that Member States other than the UK prevent the widely adopted practice of recycling ruminant protein to other ruminants. If BSE was present but undetected in those countries, that restriction would have been vital to prevent further recycling and amplification of the disease. The Commission had wanted to introduce a European-wide measure banning the feeding of ruminant meal to ruminants in late 1989, but the Standing Veterinary Committee had not provided unanimous support for that proposal (European Parliament 1996a, p. 9). Instead, the Commission's ScVC advised in January 1990 that all Member States should take whatever action was deemed appropriate in their own countries (ibid.).

The protection of human health

Before the summer of 1989 there were no efforts, either from the European Commission or individual Member States, to restrict exports of bovine carcass meat and meat products from the UK to the rest of the European Community or, on the basis of the assumption that BSE might already be present in the domestic herds of non-UK countries, to restrict bovine tissues entering the food chain within individual jurisdictions.

In August 1989 West Germany announced that it would only allow imports of UK beef that had been certified as originating from BSE-free herds and only if brain, spinal cord and other internal organs had been removed prior to export. The UK had recently announced, but not yet introduced, a 'specified bovine offal' (SBO) ban, and Germany stated that it was entitled to take unilateral measures until such time as Community-wide measures had been introduced that protected the entire European public (Anon 1989a).

Initially, the German government was persuaded by the Commission to postpone unilateral action, on the grounds that the need or otherwise for adopting Community measures on BSE would depend on the UK's forthcoming SBO controls (Lawrence 1989a). The British delegation to the ScVC maintained that there was no danger of BSE to human health; indeed it asserted in September 1990 that even the decision to slaughter and destroy clinically affected animals (let alone the SBO ban) was a 'purely precautionary to ensure that public confidence was maintained' (Lawrence 1989b).

By October 1989, however, the German government had decided that it would still go ahead with unilateral restrictions on UK beef. German veterinarians were not convinced by the claim that there was no risk of BSE to human health (Lawrence 1989b). At a meeting of the Standing Veterinary Committee, held on 24 October 1989, the British delegation claimed that the German government's request for certification to accompany beef exports was 'totally unreasonable and unjustified' since the UK could not prove a negative (i.e. that meat came from a BSE-free herd) and because there was no risk to human health which, the UK suggested, was a claim that had been endorsed by the Southwood Working Party (Lawrence 1989c). British Ministers condemned the German action as motivated only by a desire to protect its own market rather than by any concern over health, whilst the British CVO told the media that what the Germans were doing was 'scientifically unsound' (Hornsby 1989).

The UK delegation had not accurately represented the conclusions of the Southwood Working Party. Southwood and his colleagues had concluded that it is 'most unlikely that BSE will have any implications for human health. Nevertheless, if our assessments of these likelihoods are incorrect, the implications would be extremely serious' (MAFF/DoH 1989, para. 9.2). The Southwood Working Party had not asserted or concluded that there was no risk to human health. Given that the UK government's scientific advice (and indeed the scientific evidence) did not indicate a zero risk, a policy response that sought to introduce controls, no matter how precautionary, could not have been 'unscientific'. Policy judgements in those circumstances were instead concerned with identifying acceptable levels of uncertainty and risk. The UK CVO's rhetorical attack on the German position could therefore be seen as inappropriate. Since much of Britain's print media have an almost inexhaustible appetite for portraying Germany in an unfavourable light, the UK government's position was sympathetically spun by many of the newspapers; a pattern that has been repeated frequently in subsequent years.

Following the 24 October 1989 meeting of the SVC, a senior MAFF official told his colleagues privately that the ScVC would soon meet and that it would be an appropriate forum to 'educate' the Commission and other Members States about BSE (Lawrence 1989c). Since Member State representatives took the advice of the SVC very seriously he concluded '[o]ur input is therefore extremely important' (ibid.) The centrality of the tactic of trying to ensure that the perspective provided by MAFF's vets dominated the conclusions of the SVC was clear.

On 6 November 1989 West Germany banned imports of British beef, given that consignments could not be certified as coming from herds of BSE-free origin (Erlichman 1989). On the same day the Commission organised a meeting of scientific experts on TSEs in order to provide answers to a pre-selected set of questions on both veterinary and human health aspects of BSE. That group served, in effect, as an ad hoc subcommittee providing advice (on both scientific and policy matters) to the ScVC that met on 27 November 1989. The record does not indicate who proposed the list of questions but the document with which to answer those questions was primarily provided by British veterinary officials and British scientific advisors to the UK government (Anon 1989b). The document noted that the British offal ban (which had just come into force) was a legal device to prevent offals from being used in baby foods, and was intended to reassure the public; the implication being that it was not a measure to safeguard public health (Anon 1989b, p. 17). The UK delegation's account of why the SBO ban had been introduced was once again not accurate.

At the 6 November 1989 meeting there was a consensus that the possibility that BSE might be pathogenic to humans was remote, but that it could not be ruled out. The participants also agreed that it would therefore be prudent to observe recommendations to reduce human exposures to the BSE-pathogen to what was referred to as an 'acceptable' level (Anon 1989b, p. 18). As far as the risks of oral transmission of BSE to human consumers were concerned, the participants agreed that, given that clinical cases of BSE and all the 'specified bovine offals' were removed from the human food chain: 'the risk to humans has been reduced well below an *acceptable* level capable of maintaining *the present level of public health* in regard to transmissible spongiform encephalopathies' (Anon 1989b, p. 19; emphases added).

The conclusions of that closed and unaccountable meeting of experts were presented to the ScVC on 27 November 1989. The ScVC reached a slightly more precautionary conclusion than their specialist advisors, to the effect that

Meat derived from animals in countries in which BSE is widespread is not considered to be a *(significant)* danger to public health. As a precautionary measure *every* attempt should be made *to prevent* the inclusion of *large* quantities of lymphatic and nervous tissue from products intended for human consumption.

(Bradley 1989; emphases added)

The UK government's note of that meeting emphasised that the word 'significant':

Was not in the original draft and by contact with Mr Marchant in Brussels [the Commission official responsible for convening the meeting and an ex-employee of MAFF] we are attempting to have it removed since it is inconsistent with the present and accepted scientific data.

(Bradley 1989)

The word may have been inconsistent with MAFF's preferred representation of the possible risks, but there were no data with which it was inconsistent.

Given that the available evidence provided no reason for assuming that BSE infectivity would be confined to those tissues that the UK's SBO regulations were intended to exclude from the food supply, we believe British attempts to create the impression that the evidence supported an assertion of absolute safety were misleading. When the ScVC next met (on 8 January 1990) its conclusions were identical to those of the previous meeting (Phillips *et al.* 2000, vol. 6, para. 4.431). The word 'significant' had been retained so the efforts of MAFF officials have the word deleted were unsuccessful. Nonetheless, the ScVC did not endorse the restrictions that were being imposed by Germany, nor is there any indication that consideration was given to any other kinds of restrictions. MAFF may therefore not have been able to persuade the participants that the risks were zero, but UK officials did persuade the committee that the risks were acceptably low, and therefore that the German restrictions were disproportionate and unnecessary.

In light of the ScVC's conclusions the Commission took the view that the UK's SBO ban was sufficient to protect public health and that normal cutting procedures would meet the ScVC's view that obvious lymphatic and nervous tissue should be removed (Phillips *et al.* 2000, vol. 6, para. 4.432). The Commission also threatened to start infringement proceedings against Germany if it did not lift its restrictions on UK beef (Lowson 1990). By mid-January, however, the German government had modified its requirement that all UK exports of beef be certified from BSE-free herds. Instead, it wanted all bones and visible lymphatic glands to be removed from all beef exports (Lowson 1990) That would have enabled trade with Germany to resume, but it was still more restrictive than the proposed Community-wide rules that would have only insisted on the removal of specified bovine offals.

On 7 March 1990, the Standing Veterinary Committee met to discuss a draft Directive prepared by the Commission that sought to ban the export from the UK of those SBOs that had already been banned for human consumption within the UK. The German delegation sought an additional EC-wide provision, namely that the UK should only be allowed to export boneless beef if all conspicuous nervous and lymphatic tissues had been removed. The Commission and the UK argued that the position on beef had already been resolved by the ScVC (Lawrence 1990a). Commission officials suggested, as a compromise, that a provision be included which would enable the UK to export beef so long as conspicuous nervous and lymphatic tissue were removed, but omitting the requirement that all the meat had been de-boned (Lawrence 1990b).

At a subsequent meeting of the Standing Veterinary Committee (on 13 March 1990) the UK delegation warned that adopting such a compromise risked drawing media and public attention to BSE, but that MAFF wanted no further publicity for BSE. The issue of cost was not mentioned, and thus opposition to the measure from the UK was presumably only because it would have made explicit that fact that scientists were concerned about the safety of bovine tissues which could not be entirely removed. In the face of that argument, the Commission officials withdrew their compromise proposal (Lawrence 1990b). Thus, on the 9 April 1990, a European regulation came into force banning exports of SBOs from the UK (Decision 90/200/CEE). The European Commission therefore adopted a policy on BSE that was not particularly restrictive, but that particular policy only lasted a month and a half.

Mad Max

In May and early June 1990, a press furore erupted after it was revealed that a domestic UK cat (Max) had been diagnosed with a novel feline spongiform encephalopathy. As noted in Chapter 6, the discovery was significant because it indicated that BSE was transmissible to other species via a feed-borne route and because it implied that BSE might have an unpredictable host range, given that repeated attempts to transmit scrapie to cats through the feed route had been unsuccessful. Several Member States, including France, Italy and West Germany, banned imports of all UK beef.

The European Commission condemned the bans as illegal, and the Agriculture Commissioner threatened to take infringement proceedings against the offending Member States (Palmer and Myers 1990). In early June, in an attempt to resolve the dispute, a meeting of the Council of Agricultural Ministers was held. Immediately prior to that meeting, the ScVC also met. The Committee decided that there was no new information upon which to modify its previous opinion. Why the emergence of a feline spongiform encephalopathy did not count as new evidence has never been explained, although MAFF's position was that the case had no bearing on any other species. The ScVC asserted that:

> ... meat derived from bovine animals in countries in which BSE occurs is not considered to be a danger to public health. Nevertheless, as a precautionary measure, every attempt must be made during the cutting process to remove obvious nervous and lymphatic tissues from products to be supplied to the consumer. These tissues, where removed, must not be put into products for human consumption.
>
> (SVC 1990)

Compared to the ScVC's January statement, this version omitted the word 'significant'. On the other hand, it had replaced 'should' with 'must' and the term 'normal cutting process' had been changed to 'cutting process'. Those marginal adjustments indicate the several policy issues that were disputed.

The Commission's Assistant Director-General for Agriculture (Mr Legras) was sufficiently concerned that his staff prepared a draft Directive proposing that the UK could only export beef meat to the rest of the Community if both the bones and the lymphoid and nervous tissues had been removed, as the German government had been demanding. The official who drew up the Draft Directive had proposed to expand the ScVC's advice to include the removal of bones because he thought that the draft Directive 'would have allowed a better implementation of the recommendation of the Scientific Veterinary Committee' (European Parliament 1997b, Annex 18). His underlying reasoning assumed that removing bones would have had the effect of removing a greater proportion of nervous tissue from meat than would have been possible using normal cutting methods. When, however, the Agriculture Commissioner was presented with the draft Directive at the Council meeting of 6 and 7 June, the reaction was 'hostile'. The officials who had drafted the new proposal were not even able to discuss it because they were 'excluded from the meeting room' (European Parliament 1997b, Annex 18). That exclusion has never been explained, but the obvious presumption is that their proposals were unacceptably precautionary.

At the Council meeting of 6/7 June 1990, Agriculture Ministers reached a compromise on trade in beef and calves from the UK. Their decision required the UK to certify that all boneless beef for export to Member States had 'obvious nervous and lymphatic tissue' removed. It also required certification that bone-in-beef for export came from farm holdings where BSE had not been confirmed in the previous two years. Once that had been agreed, France, Italy and West Germany lifted their bans on British beef.

In the UK MAFF officials initially argued that the Council Decision was best implemented by guidelines rather than by legislation because a formal ban would be considered 'contentious' and 'derisive' (Phillips *et al.* 2000, vol. 6, para. 4.441). MAFF's Ministers thought, however, that adding the major lymphatic tissue to the SBO ban might be a more appropriate way of implementing the Council Decision. They were, however, persuaded by officials not to follow a legislative route on the grounds that the European Commission Decision:

> Was largely for presentational purposes. . . . A statutory provision would however increase public concern as it would be assumed that such removal had not been the normal practice and could lead to pressure for the removal of all such material from meat, which would be impossible to implement as lymphatic material is throughout the carcass and is exposed wherever meat is cut.

> (Phillips *et al.* 2000, vol. 6, para. 4.450)

Thus, once again in the UK it appears, incremental adjustments to regulations were avoided because of a concern not to undermine the narrative that the risks from consuming beef were, and always had been, negligible and that risks were being properly controlled.

Three months later, on 12 September 1990 an extraordinary meeting of the ScVC (with additional invited experts) was organised, in response to a request from the West German government, to reassess the Council Decision. All the representatives at that meeting, except for the UK scientists, agreed that henceforth beef meat from the UK should only be exported to other EC countries if it came from herds that had previously been shown to be clinically free of BSE and that had not previously been fed with meat and bone meal (European Parliament 1997b, Annex 39). No decision could be reached at that meeting of the ScVC, and a proposal emerged to convene a further extraordinary meeting of the Standing Veterinary Committee to facilitate a decision.

Six days later on 18 September 1990, the Commissioner for Agriculture (MacSharry) gave the Director General for Agriculture (Legras) a written instruction insisting: 'BSE: stop any meeting' (European Parliament 1997a, p. 23; European Parliament 1997b, Annex 20). On 9 October, a representative of the Agriculture Commissioner told a meeting of the SVC that 'It is necessary to keep cool so as not to provoke unfavourable market responses. Do not talk about BSE any more. This item should not appear on the agenda' (European Parliament, 1997b, Annex 22). Furthermore, that meeting concluded that: 'the BSE affair must be minimised by using disinformation. It is better to say that the press has a tendency to exaggerate' (ibid.) The approach of the Agriculture Commissioner therefore appears very close to that adopted by MAFF ministers, namely the primary objective was the maintenance of market stability.

European policies: 1990–1996

In the four years or so from late 1990 to the summer of 1994, there were no further European Community controls on BSE. The Commission's veterinary checks on UK slaughterhouses were also suspended, in response to pressure from MAFF officials (European Parliament 1997a, p. 28). The last inspections to be conducted (in June 1990) had, however, revealed failures to separate carcass meat from nervous and lymphatic tissues, problems with identification of the origin of animals arriving at slaughterhouses, and a lack of systematic ante mortem inspections (European Parliament 1996b, p. 12). With no information about the extent of compliance with European Commission regulations, there was little scope for the Commission to consider altering the existing legislation. Meanwhile, however, three more European countries – Switzerland, France and Portugal – discovered BSE in their domestic cattle herds, as had the Republic of Ireland in January 1989.

BSE Policy in Ireland, Switzerland, France and Portugal

Ireland was the first country, outside the UK, to recognise BSE in its domestic herd and the Irish Department of Agriculture, Food and Fisheries responded by introducing a slaughter and compensation policy, along the same lines as had been introduced in the UK the previous year (van Zwanenberg 1999). By August 1990, after some 20 cases of BSE had been reported, the Irish Government introduced a ban on using domestically produced MBM in ruminant feed, after the EC's ScVC had announced that countries should assume that MBM was the agent of transmission of BSE and that national authorities take appropriate temporary action. At the same time, powers were introduced to slaughter all the animals in a herd in which a case, or cases, of BSE had been discovered. The slaughtered animals were then sold for human consumption if they were found, on the basis of an ante mortem examination, not to be exhibiting clinical signs of BSE. Given that the animals were entering the human food chain the policy was not about providing additional safeguards to public health; rather, the rationale for the slaughter programme, as Agriculture Department officials and the media later acknowledged, was one of customer confidence and a desire to protect export markets (van Zwanenberg 1999). No additional significant domestic regulations were introduced until early 1996, although the Irish government continued to implement EU legislation during that period. As in most other European countries with BSE in their domestic herds, the Irish government had not yet thought it appropriate to remove the theoretically most infectious cattle organs from the human food chain. BSE was seen predominantly as an animal health problem, and a threat to trade interests rather than a threat to public health. Indeed, the Irish Government's Food Safety Advisory Committee had produced a short report on BSE for the Minister of Health and the Minister for Agriculture and Food in late 1989, the summary of which had stated only that '[t]here is no evidence that Bovine Spongiform Encephalopathy (BSE) or Scrapie is transmissible to humans' (Food Safety Advisory Committee 1989). No formal recommendations were made.

Switzerland, which lay outside the EU, banned imports of British cattle, MBM, and bone-in beef in June 1990 in the aftermath of the disclosure that a domestic British cat had succumbed to a TSE. Five months later, in November 1990, the first case of BSE in a Swiss cow was reported and over the next five years Switzerland reported the highest incidence of BSE of any non-UK country. In contrast to the Irish response to domestic BSE, the Swiss authorities not only insisted, from November 1990 onwards, that affected cattle had to be destroyed and that MBM should no longer be fed to ruminants, but also that brain, spinal cord, eyes, tonsils, spleen, thymus and intestines of cattle aged more than six months were removed and destroyed from all animals (Barbier and Janet 1999). That measure reflected a far greater concern with the protection of human health than was apparent in EU Member States with low levels of BSE.

France banned the use of UK-derived MBM in ruminant feed in August 1989, although, as the French media later pointed out, that move, even if fully complied with, was already too late to prevent infection of French herds. During the first six months of 1989, for example, the UK had exported over 8000 tons of MBM to France (Joly *et al.* 1999). In July 1990, France prohibited the use of all MBM in cattle feed. after the EC's ScVC had advised that countries should assume that MBM was the agent of transmission of BSE and take appropriate temporary action. The following year, in February 1991 a French cow was diagnosed with BSE. Four additional cases were diagnosed that year, followed by a relatively small number of cases in most of the subsequent years to 1996 As in Ireland, and many other European countries with relatively low levels of domestic BSE, the government did not consider it necessary to remove the 'specified bovine offals' from the human food chain, at least not until after March 1996.

Although the first cases of BSE in Portuguese cattle were not reported until 1994, the disease had been diagnosed in several cattle that had been imported from the UK between 1990 and 1993, but the Portuguese Ministry of Agriculture kept that information confidential (Gonçalves and Gonçalves 1999). The media exposed the fact that the cases had been kept secret in the Spring of 1993, giving rise to a widely publicised political controversy. In response, public hearings were organised by the Portuguese Parliament but a Parliamentary committee concluded that government scientists had not performed sufficient tests to confirm that BSE was in fact the disease responsible for the deaths of the affected cattle, despite the fact that the researchers had relied on widely accepted histopathological methods of diagnosis. The Parliament concluded, therefore, that BSE 'did not exist in Portugal' (Gonçalves and Gonçalves 1999). In 1994, the presence of BSE in the domestic herd was eventually admitted, after BSE was diagnosed in several Portuguese animals. Portugal implemented European BSE regulations, but prior to March 1996 no additional measures were adopted to control the disease.

Germany and Commission Policy after 1994

The absence of any Commission legislation to BSE from 1990 to 1994 came to an end after the German Government submitted papers to the Council of Ministers in late 1993 demanding a prohibition on exports of UK cattle older than three years. The Germans was responding to a recommendation from its *Bundesgesundheitsamt* (BGA or Federal Health Office) that a ban should be imposed on the import of cattle products from the UK. Although Germany had not discovered any cases of BSE in its domestic herd, its government was far more proactive than most other Member States in seeking to impose restrictions on imports of British beef, and in the process provoked frequent tensions with both the UK and the European Commission.

The German response to BSE was partly a means of protecting its domestic markets by reassuring consumers that infected beef would not enter German food chains, but also because several of its expert advisors took a quite sceptical view of British claims that there was no evidence of any risk to human health from BSE. In the autumn of 1989, for example, the German delegation in Brussels had refused to accept the UK's assertion that there was no danger of BSE to human health and that UK policy measures were primarily a means of ensuring that public confidence was maintained (Lawrence 1989b). Instead its policy regime recommended unilateral restrictions on UK beef, in recognition that a potential hazard existed and that it could be lowered by insisting, for example, on the removal of as much nervous and lymphatic tissue as possible. Unlike Ireland, Switzerland, France and Portugal, however, where Ministries of Agriculture were primarily responsible for BSE policy, responsibility for BSE policy in Germany (and more generally the control of animal health) was shared between health and agriculture ministries. Nevertheless, despite the vigorous attempts to control imports of British beef, the German government did not move as swiftly on the domestic front. For example it failed to ban the use of domestic MBM in ruminant feed until March 1994.

In December 1993, an international symposium on Transmissible Spongiform Encephalopathies was held at the *Bundesgesundheitsamt* (BGA). The symposium considered evidence indicating that the pathogen responsible for BSE was distinct from the scrapie pathogen, and that BSE was transmissible to several different animal species via a food route. The BGA subsequently recommended that a ban should be imposed on the import of live cattle and cattle products from the UK, and from other BSE-affected countries (Dressel 1999).

Germany subsequently asked the Council of Ministers to prohibit exports of UK cattle older than three years and in February 1994 attempted to secure a complete EC/EU-wide ban on exports of British beef. That attempt failed, but by April 1994, the German cabinet began discussing the imposition of a unilateral ban on all British beef. It set a deadline for the end of May 1994 for the European Commission to take tougher measures to restrict UK beef exports, namely that all exported beef should come from animals under three years old which also came from herds which had been free of BSE for four years or more.

One of the German government's concerns was that it was not possible, in practice, to remove all the nervous and lymphatic tissue from meat as was supposed to happen under the prevailing rules (Ratcliffe 1994). The (private) view of the UK government was that the German proposals (in particular the removal of more and more of the parts of cattle carcasses that might contain the infectious agent, such as bones and nervous and lymphatic tissues) would not only increase costs unacceptably to the meat trade, but it would also, as a UK official put it, 'be an implicit acknowledgement that we had been potentially "poisoning" the UK population up until now' (Render 1994). Once again the UK resisted incremental regulatory changes for fear that its existing narrative of safety would be undermined.

On 28 June 1994 the German government introduced a 6-month restriction on imports of British beef. Only animals aged under three years old and from certified BSE-free herds could be imported. The following month, the ScVC met to discuss BSE and concluded that the existing controls should be tightened so that shipments of un-boned beef would have to come from herds that had been free of BSE for six years, rather than two years, as had previously been the case. Those recommendations were formally adopted in a Commission Directive of July 1994 and the German government withdrew its proposed unilateral measures.

There were further tensions over the rules governing the export of British beef in the latter half of 1994. The German government wanted a more precise and stricter set of rules governing the trimming of nervous and lymphatic tissues. In October and November 1994 the ScVC agreed on a text that was not acceptable to the German delegation. The German government threatened to reactivate its draft legislation imposing a unilateral ban if the rules were not changed (SVC 1994). The Directorate General for Agriculture, DG-VI, attempted to intervene in the disagreements within the ScVC by writing to the German Ministry of Health and asking it to ensure that dissenting German scientists do not express their opinions in public (European Parliament 1997a, p. 27).

On 22 March 1996, two days after the British government announced a probable link between BSE and a new variant of CJD, the European Commission's ScVC met to discuss the implications of the dramatic development for European consumers. The Committee concluded that no regulatory measures beyond those already announced by the British government would be required (European Parliament 1997c, p. 78). Three days later, however, in yet another abrupt volte-face the European Commission proposed an indefinite ban on the export of all British beef and beef products anywhere in the world, so as to prevent re-importation back into the EU. Faced with a collapse in consumer confidence, and thus demand for beef, across the continent, a complete ban was the only available means of stabilising the market. The proposal was accepted by the SVC with only the UK objecting (European Parliament 1997c, p. 78).

Summary

The European Commission's policy approach on the topic of BSE, until March 1996, was like that in the UK, framed by an agricultural perspective. The main concern of policy-makers was to try to ensure that public anxiety and impediments to the free flow of trade were avoided and thereby to diminish the adverse impact of BSE on the economic welfare of the farming and food industries.

Starting in 1990, and repeatedly since then, the Commission only proposed tighter regulations and/or enforcement on BSE after several Member States had unilaterally imposed restrictions on their importation of meat and cattle products. The Commission frequently responded to those initiatives by criticising them as unnecessary, unscientific and as protectionist, even though in reality they had emerged as a consequence of different views about whether the possible but unquantified risks of consuming certain bovine tissues were acceptable given the costs, practicalities and public relations consequences of imposing stricter controls.

The similarities between the approach of the Commission and that of MAFF are striking, especially in the light of the extent to which UK officials and the print media complained about intransigent continental Europeans. The Commission, like MAFF, tried to ensure that as little public and media attention as possible would be drawn to BSE, to ensure that consumers retained their confidence in the safety of the food supply and the probity of the policy-making process, given that their confidence could be reflected in changing levels of consumer demand. Even though there was some contention at the Scientific and Standing Veterinary Committees, and at the Council of Ministers, about the extent and significance of the risks that BSE posed, the Commission attempted to play down scientific dissent and disagreement. Furthermore, the Commission contrived to represent its policies as robustly supported by the best scientific advice. MAFF officials played a key role in persuading Commission officials to adopt that approach.

The domestic policy regimes of individual European Member States were, however, a different matter. As long as BSE could be represented as an alien threat that could and should be excluded, BSE policy-making was relatively simply. The policy of trying to keep your competitor's diseases out of your herd and population did not require scientific proof that the disease would be fatal; it was sufficient for it to be unwelcome. Thus, for example, Germany was one of the few States to acknowledge that BSE was a potential public health problem, but with no known domestic cases, Germany could focus on protecting its borders from imports of contaminated animal feed, live animals and meat. Notably, Germany did not put in place precautionary controls on its own domestic beef supply in case the disease was already present although undetected. For those countries where BSE had been reported in the domestic herd, the policy challenge was substantially more complex. Ireland, Portugal and France opted for the strategy of treating the disease as an animal health but not a public health problem.

Given the policy orientation of the European Commission and Member States with BSE in their domestic herds, the 20 March 1996 announcement marked the beginnings of a political crisis, not only for the UK, but for all those jurisdictions that had gambled with public health that BSE would turn out to be innocuous to humans. Member States without reported cases of BSE, such as Germany, were not immune either, but their problems only really began to emerge a few years later after BSE was found to be prevalent in the domestic cattle herds or virtually every European Member State.

Bibliography

Anon (1989a) Meat imports into the Federal Republic of Germany from the United Kingdom, Telex Message. *BSE Inquiry Year Book* Reference No. 89/08.21/8.1, in Phillips *et al.* 2000.

Anon (1989b) *Bovine Spongiform Encephalopathy: Risk to animal and public health.* A resume of the private experts, opinions expressed at an EC meeting on 6 November 1989 in Brussels. BSE Inquiry Year Book Reference No. YB 89/11.6/6.2, in Phillips *et al.* 2000.

Barbier, M. and Janet, C. (1999) *BSE and the Swiss National Action System*, Report for the BASES project and for the European Commission, DG XII, July 1999. Economie et Sociologie Rurales, Université Pierre Mendès France: INRA.

Bradley, R. (1989), Extended report of meeting with representatives of community institutions or of major governments, Scientific Veterinary Committee, YB 89/11.28/5.1, in Phillips *et al.* 2000.

BSE Inquiry (1998) Transcript, 6 November 1998, in Phillips *et al.* 2000.

BSE Inquiry (1999a) *The Central Veterinary Laboratory 1985–1989*, Revised Factual Account No. 4, para. 234, in Phillips *et al.* 2000, op. cit.

BSE Inquiry (1999b) *Revised Factual Account No 5. 'The Early Days'*, in Phillips *et al.* 2000. op. cit.

Byrne, D. (2000) See, for example, comments of Commissioner David Byrne in European Commission (2000) *Food Law from Farm to Table – Creating a European Food Authority*, 8 November 2000, Doc. IP/00/1270. European Commission, Brussels.

Commission Decision of 9 April 1990 concerning additional requirements for some tissues and organs with respect to Bovine Spongiform Encephalopathy (BSE), Official Journal L 105/24 of 25. 4. 1990.

Commission of the European Communities (2000) *White Paper on Food Safety*, COM(1999) 719 final. 12 January 2000. European Commission, Brussels.

Council Directive 89/662/EEC of 11 December 1989 concerning veterinary checks in intra-community trade with a view to the completion of the internal market. Official Journal L 395 of 30. 12. 1989.

Council Directive 90/425/EEC of 26 June 1990 concerning veterinary and 200 technical checks applicable in intra-community trade in certain live animals and products with a view to the completion of the internal market. Official Journal L 224 of 18. 08. 1990.

Court of Auditors (2001) 'Special Report No 14/2001, Follow up to Special Report No 19/98 on BSE', *Official Journal of the European Communities*, C 324/1 20 November 2001.

Dealler, S. (1996) *Lethal Legacy*. London: Bloomsbury Publishing.

Dressel, K. (1999) *BSE and the German National Action System*, Report for the BASES project and for the European Commission, DG XII, July 1999. Munich, Munich University: Institut für Soziologie der Ludwig-Maximilians.

Erlichman, J. (1989) 'German ban on 'suspect' UK beef is confirmed', *Guardian*, 7 November 1989, p. 2.

European Parliament (1996a) *Replies from the Commission to Questions From the Committee Members*, Temporary Committee of Enquiry into BSE, 18 September 1996, PE 218.980, European Parliament, Brussels.

European Parliament (1996b) *Working Document*, Temporary Committee of Enquiry into BSE, 18 September 1996, PE 218.979. European Parliament, Brussels.

European Parliament (1997a) *Report on Alleged Contravention or Maladministration in the Implementation of Community Law in Relation to BSE*. Part A, PE220.544/fin./A, 7 February 1997, European Parliament, Brussels.

European Parliament (1997b) *Report on Alleged Contravention or Maladministration in the Implementation of Community Law in Relation to BSE*. Part A – Annexes, PE220.544/fin./Ann, 7 February 1997, European Parliament, Brussels.

European Parliament (1997c) *Report on Alleged Contravention or Maladministration in the Implementation of Community Law in Relation to BSE*. Part B – Work of the Committee on Inquiry and Basic Data, PE220.544/fin./B, 7 February 1997, European Parliament, Brussels.

Food Safety Advisory Committee (1989) *Bovine Spongiform Encephalopathy, Report to the Minister for Health and the Minister for Agriculture and Food*, December 1989. Department of Agriculture, Dublin, Republic of Ireland.

Gonçalves, M. E. and Gonçalves, L. (1999) *BSE and the Portuguese National Action System*, Report for the BASES project and for the European Commission, DG XII, July 1999. Lisbon: Instituto Superior de Ciências do Trabalho e da Empresa.

Griffin, J. M. *et al.* (1997) 'Bovine spongiform encephalopathy in the Republic of Ireland', *Irish Veterinary Journal*, 50 (10), 593–600.

Hornsby, M. (1989) 'German action a restraint of trade', *The Times*, 2 November 1989, p. 2.

Joly, P. B., Le Pape, Y., Barbier, M., Estades, J., Lemarié, J. and Marcant, O. (1999) *BSE and the French National Action System*, Report for the BASES project and for the European Commission, DG XII, July 1999, INRA, Economie et Sociologie Rurales, Université Pierre Mendès France available at http://www.grenoble.inra.fr/Docs/pub/A1999/BASEFRA.pdf.

Lawrence, A. (1989a) Standing Veterinary Committee (SVC) Meeting on 5 September: BSE, Memo to Mr Lebrecht, MAFF, YB 89/9.6/9.3, in Phillips *et al.* 2000.

Lawrence, A. (1989b) Public health SVC 13 September: BSE, *BSE Inquiry Year Book* Reference No. YB 89/09.15/5.1, in Phillips *et al.* 2000.

Lawrence, A. (1989c) BSE – SVC meeting on 24 October, Memo, *BSE Inquiry Year Book* Reference No. YB 89/10.25/6, in Phillips *et al.* 2000, op. cit.

Lawrence, A. (1990a) SVC 7 March, *BSE Inquiry Year Book* Reference No. YB 90/3.8/1.1, in Phillips *et al.* 2000, op. cit.

Lawrence, A. (1990b) BSE: Standing Veterinary Committee Meeting on 13 March, *BSE Inquiry Year Book* Reference No. YB 90/03.14/9.1, in Phillips *et al.* 2000, op. cit.

Lowson, R. (1990) BSE: Standing Veterinary Committee (SVC), *BSE Inquiry Year Book* Reference No. YB 90/1.18/1.1, in Phillips *et al.* 2000, op. cit.

MAFF/DoH (1989) *Report of the Working Party on Bovine Spongiform Encephalopathy.* London: Ministry of Agriculture Fisheries and Food/Department of Health.

Ministry of Agriculture Fisheries and Food/Department of Health (1989) *Report of the Working Party on Bovine Spongiform Encephalopathy.* 3 February 1989. Ministry of Agriculture, Fisheries and Food, London.

Office Internationale des Epizooties (2003) see data at http://www.oie.int/eng/info/en_esbmonde.htm

Palmer, J. and Myers, P. (1990) 'EC court action likely on beef', *Guardian*, 5 June 1990, p. 1.

Ratcliffe, E. (1994) BSE: Parliamentary Secretary's meeting with German delegation: 26 May. *1994*, Minute, BSE Inquiry Year Book Reference No. YB 94.5.27/5.1, in Phillips *et al.* 2000, op. cit.

Render, T. J. (1994) BSE: Secretary's Meeting with German officials: 24 May 1994. Minute to Mr Eddy, Ministry of Agriculture Fisheries and Food, dated 25 May 1994, BSE Inquiry Document No. YB 94/5.24/7.1–7.7, in Phillips *et al.* 2000, op. cit.

SVC (1990) Joint meeting of Animal and Public Health sections of the scientific veterinary committee, Brussels 6 June 1990, BSE Inquiry Document No. YB 90/06.06/12.8, in Phillips *et al.* 2000, op. cit.

SVC (1994) Standing Veterinary Committee, 8 November 1994, BSE, Minute, See *BSE Inquiry Year Book* Reference No. YB 94/11.09/3.1, in Phillips *et al.* op. cit.

Trichopoulou, A. *et al.* (2000) European Policy on Food Safety, report to the STOA Programme of the European Parliament, Athens, September 2000. European Commission, Luxembourg.

van Zwanenberg, P. (1999) *BSE and the Republic of Ireland's National Action System*, Report for the BASES project and for the European Commission, DG XII, July 1999. SPRU, University of Sussex.

Chapter 8

The aftermath of 20 March 1996

The announcement that BSE was the most probable cause of 10 cases of a new variant of CJD in young British citizens precipitated a major political crisis for the British government. Ministers and senior officials insisted, following SEAC's advice to de-bone animals aged under 30 months, that the UK beef currently on sale was safe, but they struggled to maintain a credible narrative. After the repeated official reassurances about the safety of British beef, statements such as those from the chair of SEAC that the number of future cases of CJD was 'totally unpredictable' shocked European citizens (MacIntyre, Hunt and Arthur 1996). With news of the link between CJD and BSE splashed across the front pages of the word's media, beef sales plummeted across Europe. Within days of the UK Government's announcement, the UK's trading partners had imposed unilateral export bans and within a week a worldwide ban had been imposed by the European Commission on all UK exports of beef, cattle and cattle products.

In the weeks and months that followed, the perception that BSE was primarily a British problem underwent a dramatic change. Individual Member States, faced in some cases with very dramatic effects on domestic consumer demand, were forced to reappraise their own policies, especially after more and more jurisdictions started to discover BSE in their domestic herds. The European Commission also began to be significantly more involved in the management of BSE. Initially, its focus was on dictating UK policy, but it also began formulating a pan-European framework for dealing with the disease.

Although the diminution of the key uncertainty in BSE policy had very significant political consequences it did not have as profound an impact on the ways in which policy on BSE were made as one might have expected. Ministers continued to overemphasise the completeness and reliability of knowledge about the disease and still routinely failed to acknowledge that they were taking any political decisions in relation to BSE.

Before more significant changes to the ways in which BSE policies were made and represented could take place, other kinds of broader political and institutional changes were required. These were eventually catalysed by the election in 1997 of a Labour government and the subsequent Phillips Inquiry in the UK, and by an Inquiry into EU policy on BSE conducted by the European

Parliament. Those institutional and political changes are the subject of the next chapter. Here we briefly describe some of the major shifts in BSE policy, both in the UK and in continental Europe, which occurred in the three or four years after March 1996.

The British policy response

The British government's immediate policy response to the discovery of a new variant of CJD in young people was to announce that carcasses from animals aged under 30 months were to be de-boned in licensed plants. As we noted in Chapter 6, that policy decision had been delegated to SEAC who had advised accordingly. SEAC had also advised that all mammalian meat and bone meal should be banned from the feed of all farm animals, and had concluded that exposure to BSE, before the introduction of the SBO ban in 1989, was the most likely explanation for the new type of CJD, and that once the new recommendations had been introduced 'the risk from eating beef is now likely to be extremely small' (Phillips *et al.* 2000, vol. 11, para. 4.632).

Although, in light of SEAC's advice, Ministers and senior officials insisted that British beef could be eaten with 'confidence' and that they personally would continue to eat it (MacIntyre, Hunt and Arthur 1996), BSE rapidly became a major political crisis for the British government. Beef sales plummeted by more that 50 per cent in the first week and the major fast food chains stopped using UK beef. All EU Member States imposed unilateral bans on imports of British beef (Wintour, Bowcott and Bates 1996). Within days, MAFF officials learnt that British food retailers were no longer prepared to purchase beef from animals over 30 months of age. The National Farmers Union and the Institute of Grocery Distributors were also pushing for a government-financed cull in the face of rising job losses and plummeting consumer demand. On 3 April 1996, Ministers bowed to those commercial pressures and announced that instead of de-boning cattle over 30 months, as advised by SEAC, it was going to slaughter and destroy all cattle older than 30 months.

On 27 March, the European Commission responded to plummeting beef sales across the Continent by prohibiting British exports of live cattle, beef, beef products, and mammalian-derived meat and bone meal to anywhere in the world – Commission Decision 96/239/EC (European Commission 1996). An export industry worth an estimated £520 million a year had evaporated overnight (House of Commons 1996, p. 118). The export ban was deeply disappointing for the UK government, not only because of the loss of the export market, but because it also implied that the Commission did not consider the UK's immediate policy response to be adequate.

Many of the members of the British government were already highly antagonistic towards the EU as a political entity. Ministers claimed that the ban was politically motivated rather than based on scientific evidence (Anon 1996). At a time when domestic confidence in the British government's ability properly to manage food-safety risks was vulnerable, it argued to its domestic audience that the refusal of continental European countries to accept British beef was the product of anti-British prejudice and of narrow nationalistic trade protectionism on the part of foreign governments, and was totally devoid of any scientific legitimacy (Hogg 1996; Wintour 1996). The conservative mass-circulation newsprint media largely reinforced that message (Neyer 2000).

Ministers asserted that if there had ever been a significant risk from eating British beef, then it had occurred during the mid- to late 1980s. Now that the regulations had been tightened, Ministers frequently claimed that British beef was as safe as any other European beef safe or, if they were being less careful, that British beef was simply safe.

The persuasiveness of the British government's new reassurances after March 1996 was not evident in continental European countries, and in the United Kingdom's other potential export markets, and for good reasons. The key policy-relevant uncertainty as far as BSE was concerned had been markedly diminished. It appeared likely that transmission of the cattle disease to humans was possible. Nevertheless there remained many other uncertainties which made it very difficult to be certain as to how safe UK beef (and indeed beef in other countries where BSE existed) actually was.

Knowledge about the actual level of human exposure to the BSE agent from British cattle, even given the SBO ban and the ban on use of animals over 30 months old for human food, was unclear. It was certainly far smaller than it had been prior to March 1996, and substantially less than in the late 1980s; yet no one could reliably estimate the actual level of contamination.

First, the number of subclinically infected animals aged under 30 months in 1996 was not known, but it was unlikely to be zero. The limit of 30 months was chosen not because it would be impossible for infectivity to be present in animals younger than 30 months old but because it markedly diminished the proportion of infected animals entering the human food chain. Ministers frequently represented that decision as legitimated by, and only by scientific considerations relating to public health because they frequently asserted that all beef entering the human food chain, post March 1996, was safe. It was in fact a bureaucratic artefact, based on hybrid science–policy judgements that were represented as if legitimated by scientifically established thresholds.

Second, although infectivity had been demonstrated experimentally in relatively few bovine tissues by 1996, all of which should have been removed from bovine carcasses prior to entering human food chains, the tests that had been conducted and completed were not sufficiently sensitive to rule out the presence of relatively low levels of the BSE agent. For example, infectivity had not been found in muscle tissue, but the experiments at that time had all been conducted by inoculating bovine tissue into mice rather than to animals of the same species.

No only were the numbers of infected animals entering the human food chain and the level of BSE agent remaining in those animals unknown. In addition, no one knew how much of the BSE agent would be sufficient to transmit the disease to humans. Whilst scientists could be confident that British beef was substantially less of a risk than it had been prior to March 1996, the absolute, as opposed to the relative, remaining level of risk was unknown.

The embargo on British beef

The European Commission's world-wide ban on exports of British beef and all cattle products infuriated the British government. Ministers threatened to disrupt a broad range of business at the European Council of Ministers, unless barriers to continental imports of British beef were rapidly dismantled (Wintour 1996). In April 1996 the government also decided to challenge the legality of the Commission's ban in the European Court of Justice (a challenge that was later rejected by the Court). The British government also tried to emphasise what it represented as the dangers of foreign beef and the safety of the domestic supply. Much of that belligerence may have been for domestic consumption, but it contributed very little to resolving disputes.

The Commission insisted that the export ban would be maintained until the UK eradicated BSE. The term 'eradication' had been largely absent from UK policy rhetoric until that point. In June 1996, a summit of the European Council, held in Florence, backtracked on the demand for total eradication and agreed a framework of action that would be required of the UK prior to any lifting of the export ban. This included, amongst other things, rigorous implementation of the UK regulations, a selective cull of cohorts of older animals which were considered at greater risk of BSE, removal of meat and bone meal from feed mills and farms and subsequent cleansing of premises and equipment, improved checks on slaughterhouse practices for removing specified bovine material from carcasses, and the introduction of a passport system for all cattle and the creation of a computerised cattle tracking system.

Some of the conditions were responded to fairly quickly. For example, in June 1996 a Feed Recall Scheme was launched, the aim of which was to collect and dispose of any MBM and feed containing MBM which was still on farms, at feed mills or at feed merchants. New legislation was also introduced in August 1996 which prohibited the possession of MBM on premises where livestock feeding stuffs are kept, and set out conditions for the cleansing and disinfecting of places, vehicles and equipment where MBM had been produced, stored or used. August 1996 was subsequently taken to be the date at which the ruminant feed ban was fully effective, and animals born after that date were presumed not to have contracted BSE from contaminated feedstuffs.

By October 1997, the UK had proposed a Date-Based Export Scheme, applicable to animals born after 1 August 1996, together with proposals for a cull of the offspring of BSE cases of animals born after August 1996. The cull was premised on the assumption that after 1 August 1996 all risks of feed borne transmission ceased, with maternal transmission representing the only remaining route of infection. Evidence that there was vertical transmission of BSE between dam and calf had emerged in July 1996, as interim results from MAFF's cohort study emerged (Wilesmith *et al.* 1997). The offspring cull would therefore remove animals born after that date that may have been infected by their dams

The end of the export ban was finally announced by the European Commission in July 1999, by which time over 4 million cattle had been slaughtered under the various eradication schemes. The Commission acknowledged that BSE had not yet been eradicated in the UK, but it argued that beef did not represent a risk to health. One of the causes of the delay was the inability of the UK to track the offspring of cows that had succumbed to BSE. Since the late 1980s, the importance of establishing a centralised and computerised animal identification record keeping system had been repeatedly emphasised by the UK government's advisors, partly because it would have supported research in veterinary epidemiology, but perhaps more importantly, in the event that evidence emerged that BSE could be transmitted vertically (as it indeed did), it would be possible to trace the offspring of any cow which developed BSE, so that those offspring could be withdrawn from the human food supply. A decision fully to establish a centralised records system was not finally made until December 1996, and data were not finally entered into the official database until the autumn of 1998.

Domestic policy developments

In addition to the efforts of the UK government to persuade the European Commission to lift the export embargo, there were a number of important domestic developments, primarily in reaction to the emergence of new scientific evidence that infectivity could be present in tissues that were not otherwise restricted by the SBO ban. For example, in late 1997, evidence emerged that that infectivity had been detected in nervous tissues known as dorsal root ganglia (located in the vertebrae), the trigeminal ganglia (located in the skull), the retina, and in the bone marrow (Phillips *et al.* 2000, vol. 2, para. 3.215). In January 1998 the UK Government added bone, dorsal root ganglia and lung to the list of SBOs. Prohibited bovine tissues now included: the entire head excluding the tongue, but including the brains, eyes, trigeminal ganglia and tonsils; the thymus; the spleen and spinal cord of animals aged over six months; the vertebral column, including dorsal root ganglia, of animals aged over thirty months; the intestines from the duodenum to the rectum of bovine animals of all ages (The Specified Risk Material Order 1997, S.I. 1997/2964).

The policy response in continental Europe

On 22 March 1996, two days after the UK Government had announced that BSE had probably transmitted to humans, the Commission's Scientific Veterinary Committee concluded that no additional measures were required for the protection of European citizens' health, on the grounds that there was no evidence of a link between BSE and CJD (Neyer 2000, p. 5). Three days later, however, faced with a utter collapse of the beef market, that advice was rejected by the representatives of the Member States when the Standing Veterinary Committee voted, by 14 to 1, to ban UK beef. From that moment on the European Commission began to take a more proactive role in the development of Member States' BSE policies. Nevertheless, it was not until 2000, after a series of institutional and procedural changes to EU food safety policy-making, and the discovery of BSE in several more continental European countries' domestic cattle herds, that a common EU policy really began to take shape.

Initially, in the wake of the March 1996 disclosure, the Commission funded a BSE research programme, extended its activities in the assessment of risk, and stepped up inspection of BSE controls in individual Member States. As far as common legislation was concerned, however, the main area in which the Commission was active, before 2000, was in the development of a common epidemiological surveillance and monitoring strategy.

Surveillance and monitoring

From April 1998, all Member States were required to implement a monitoring system and to test, by histopathological examination of the brain, all cattle older than 20 months displaying behavioural or neurological symptoms. Cases of BSE had of course already emerged in a number of different European countries prior to March 1996, and there was no reason why other Member

States should not have BSE in their domestic herds too. The Commission's Food and Veterinary Office soon reported weaknesses in the surveillance systems of several countries and concluded that BSE probably existed in Germany, Italy and Spain – which had yet to report BSE cases – and was probably under-reported in others that already had reported domestic cases of BSE (Court of Auditors 2001, para. 21).

All Member States were naturally concerned to protect their own domestic beef industries and those that had no reported cases in their domestic herds acted by trying to prevent imports of infected meat and animals and by reassuring their own population that their territory was free of the disease. The strategy backfired dramatically in several jurisdictions in late 2000 and early 2001. New rapid post-mortem tests had become available, and by January 2001 the European Commission was insisting that Member States' monitoring programmes use the new tests on all animals over 30 months that were destined for human consumption (European Commission 2002).

Initially, France reported a rising incidence of BSE cases, but cases in the domestic herds of Germany, Italy and Spain were also reported for the first time, triggering a second major EU-wide crisis over BSE. Consumption of beef and beef prices fell rapidly, by 25 per cent between October 2000 and January 2001 (Court of Auditors 2001, para. 14). Individual Member States responded with unilateral bans on imports of beef from the affected countries, forcing the European Commission to intervene in an attempt to maintain stability. The Commission introduced a temporary ban on, and the use of, MBM for all farm animals and proposed that all animals aged over 30 months should be tested. It also began purchasing animals for destruction and taking beef into intervention storage in order to maintain prices.

Protecting the feed and food chains

Common European-wide controls on the animal feed and human food chain were not introduced until more than four years after the British announcement that BSE might be transmissible to humans. It was not until the majority of Member States realised that they too had BSE problems of their own, in the wake of the second BSE crisis of 2000, that agreement was reached.

EU-wide controls on the animal feed-chain had in fact been in place since 1994 when a ban on the use of mammalian meat and bone meal in ruminant feed had come into force. After March 1996, however, those regulations were not tightened and so mammalian meat and bone meal continued to be allowed for use in feed for non-ruminant farm animals. This was despite the fact that it was by then obvious, from experience in the UK, that a ruminant feed ban on its own was problematic because there was a problem of potential cross-contamination, for example in feed mills, between ruminant and non-ruminant feed, as well as a risk that farmers might feed non-ruminant feed to cattle. The EC's Food and Veterinary Office reported on several occasions that there was a significant risk of contamination of ruminant feed by mammalian meat and bone meal. In December 2000, in the mist of the second BSE crisis, the European Council temporarily banned the use of animal proteins in feed for all farmed animals. That ban was made permanent as of January 2001.

There were no EU-wide controls on the human food chain, aside of course from the ban on all exports of British beef and beef products. It was clear, however, that with BSE reported in the domestic herds of Ireland, France, Portugal and Switzerland, the disease was not solely a British problem. Proposals to introduce EU-wide restrictions on the consumption of 'specified risk materials' (SRMs), analogous to the specified bovine materials that had been prohibited in the UK, were introduced by the Commission in October 1996 (European Commission 1996). Those proposals were overwhelmingly rejected by the SVC, with only France and the UK voting in favour.

With no majority in the SVC the Commission put the proposed ban to the European Council but it was again rejected. The SRM measures were proposed once again by the Commission in July 1997, but they were rejected and postponed four times. The problem of securing acceptance was primarily that countries such as France (and the UK) that already had a domestic BSE problem had introduced unilateral controls and wished to see a common policy, whilst those countries that considered themselves free of BSE were opposed to the measures recommended by the Commission. Common controls were eventually introduced in October 2000, after the majority of Member States realised that they too had BSE problems of their own.

Bibliography

Anon, *Guardian*, 26 March 1996, p. 1.

Court of Auditors (2001) Special report No. 14/2001, *Official Journal of the European Communities*, 20 November.

European Commission (1996) Commission Decision 96/239/EC.

European Commission (2002) *Report on the Monitoring and Testing of Bovine Animals for the Presence of Bovine Spongiform Encephalopathy (BSE) in 2001*. Brussels: European Community.

Hogg, D. (1996) *Hansard*. 3 April 1996, column 407, The Stationery Office, London.

House of Commons, Agriculture and Health Select Committees Report (1996), The Stationery Office, London.

MacIntyre, D., Hunt, L. and Arthur, C. (1996) Ministers admit possible link between mad cow disease and human deaths, *Independent*, 21 March 1996, p. 1.

Neyer, J. (2000) 'The regulation of risks and the power of the people: lessons from the BSE crisis', *European Integration Online Papers*, 4 (6) http://netec.mcc.ac.uk/WoPEc/data/Articles/erpeiopxxp0049.html.

Phillips, Bridgeman J. and Ferguson-Smith, M. (2000) *The BSE Inquiry: Report: evidence and supporting papers of the Inquiry into the emergence and identification of Bovine Spongiform Encephalopathy (BSE) and variant Creutzfeldt-Jakob Disease (vCJD) and the action taken in response to it up to 20 March 1996*. London: The Stationery Office.

The Specified Risk Material Order (1997) S.I. 1997/2964.

Wilesmith, J. W., Wells, G. A. H., Ryan, J. B. M., Gavier-Widen, D. and Simmons, M. (1997) 'A cohort study to examine maternally-associated risk factors for bovine spongiform encephalopathy', *Veterinary Record*, **141**, 239–43.

Wintour, P. (1996) 'Major goes to war with Europe', *Guardian*, 22 May 1996, p. 1.

Wintour, P., Bowcott, O. and Bates, S. (1996) Ministers defy beef outcry, *Guardian*, 26 March 1996, p. 1.

Chapter 9

BSE and the partial reform of food policy-making

The BSE crisis that erupted in London in March 1996, and other food safety scares and crises concerning for example *salmonella, E.Coli* 0157, food additives and GM foods, led to waves of institutional reform in numerous jurisdictions, not only in the UK. The amplitude of the shock waves varied with the direction in which they travelled, and the speed of transmission also varied, particularly as a function of the extent to which they encountered resonant conditions. By the end of 2003, however, fundamental institutional structural and procedural changes had been made to food safety policy-making (and in other areas of science-based risk policy-making) in for example the UK, France, Germany, Ireland, Greece, Austria and at the European Commission.

In the UK, MAFF was widely held to have been centrally responsible for almost all of the policy failures over BSE. Many commentators, including politicians and scholars, recognised that in the UK, even before March 1996, the contradictory remit under which MAFF laboured was unsustainable. MAFF aspired to promote the commercial interests of the farming and food industries, but ultimately it inflicted massive damage on those interests while simultaneously failing to protect public health and the interests of consumers. Having failed all of its constituencies, MAFF had to be changed, and eventually (in June 2001) after the debacle of the Food and Mouth Disease epidemic of 2001 it was replaced by the Department for the Environment, Food and Rural Affairs (DEFRA). For the first time since the end of the Second World War, a European country had no Ministry of Agriculture. Having failed to serve any of its constituencies MAFF was first butchered to create the Food Standards Agency and then abolished.

New food safety policy-making institutional structures were also established in, for example, France, Germany and at the European Commission, and all of those institutions are expected by the governments that created them to take responsibility (amongst other things) for 'rebuilding trust' and 'consumer confidence' in both food safety and public policy-making (Krebs 2003; EFSA 2003b). A highly influential group of senior policy-makers across Europe assumed (and some continue to assume) that trust would return once the new institutions had been established and became fully operational because the new institutions will be 'independent' and 'transparent'; although it has not always been clear of whom, and what, experts and policy-makers should be independent, nor how 'openness' is to be interpreted. From the perspective of one relatively conservative group of protagonists and commentators, policy-making mechanisms have been, and remain, fundamentally sound, it is just that their soundness was not, and has not yet been, recognised; with greater openness trust will be re-established. Another, rather more astute group of commentators assumes that openness and transparency constitute such a radical break with tradition that they are bound to produce marked shifts in policy outcomes.

UK

It was in the UK that change, in the aftermath of March 1996, came first and where it has been most radical. The history of BSE policy-making, sketched in the previous chapters, as well as numerous other food safety policy failures, was almost universally seen to have deprived MAFF of its institutional legitimacy (Lang *et al.* 1996, 1997). When Tony Blair became Prime Minister and took responsibility for food safety policy-making away from MAFF and passed it to the Food Standards Agency there were very few complaints from anyone outside of MAFF (MAFF 1997b).

Even before he became Prime Minister, Tony Blair realised that he had radically to restructure the UK's food policy-making institutions. In the run-up to the General Election of May 1997 the Labour Party had already indicated that it envisaged creating a Food Agency, but almost no progress had been made by the shadow ministerial team or the staff of the Labour Party in articulating the shape of any reforms that were envisaged (Strang 1995).

The final straw that led to the break-up of MAFF and provoked Blair into forcing the pace of change emerged on 6 March 1997, when it was reported that MAFF had failed to disclose even to fellow ministers at the Scottish Office information about unacceptably poor standards of hygiene in Scottish abattoirs. The report had revealed that abattoirs were a 'breeding ground for *e.coli*' (Blitz and Kampfner 1997).

That evening, by which time a Labour victory at the forthcoming General Election seemed a certainty, Tony Blair, without waiting for his shadow team to deliver its policy proposals, summoned Professor Philip James. James was the Director of the Rowett Research Institute in Aberdeen and one of the UK's leading public health and nutritional policy experts. Blair asked James to provide him as a matter of urgency (i.e. in time for the forthcoming election in early May) with detailed proposals on how a Food Standards Agency should be designed, established and operated, but especially to indicate how regulation could be separated from sponsorship (James 1997a, p. 9).

One of Tony Blair's first meetings, after arriving in Downing Street in May 1997, was with Philip James. James delivered a 55-page document, which had been prepared in just seven weeks. When (later that day) the Prime Minister invited Jack Cunningham to take the post of Secretary of State at MAFF, he handed Cunningham a copy of the James report and told him to implement it rapidly (MAFF 1997a). As previously requested, James provided detailed proposals on the creation of a Food Standards Agency (FSA). James proposed relocating responsibility for food safety policy away from MAFF, and transferring it to the Department of Health, which would act on the advice of a new FSA.

James argued that

> The catalogue of food scares that has faced the British public in the last ten years has eroded – some would say destroyed – confidence in the current system. The problem is not just one of public perception. Many public interest groups and chairmen of expert scientific committees, as well as companies in the food producing, processing and retailing fields, consider that there are real failings in the present system.
>
> (James 1997a, p. 14)

James therefore did not accept the analysis that suggested that consumer confidence and public trust could be achieved just by making the existing policy-making processes transparent, but he did assert that

> An agency is needed which puts the public interest first and is seen to be removed from political pressure and interference from vested interests . . . An agency must be open and transparent in all its work.
>
> (James 1997a, p. 16)

Much of the analysis that James developed concentrated on trying to ensure the separation of responsibility for regulating the food and agricultural sectors from responsibility for their sponsorship, and on the creation of an integrated regulatory regime to cover 'the whole food chain, from the plough to the plate' (James 1997a, p. 16). James also emphasised the importance not just of food safety but also of issues concerning nutrition given that the mortality, morbidity and economic costs of poor nutrition were substantially greater and more serious than those arising from microbiological and chemical risks (James 1997a, p. 11). Much of the debate that followed the publication of the James Report concentrated on the issue of whether or not the Agency's responsibilities and terms of reference should include nutrition, or whether it should be confined to safety issues, leaving responsibility for nutrition with the Department of Health. James argued that public health required an integrated food policy that could create incentives for the food and farming industries not just to produce safe foods but also nutritionally desirable ones. The complexities of the history and future of the relationships between science and politics in policy-making were not a major focus of the debate in the immediate aftermath of the publication of James' proposals.

The James report said very little about the kinds of advice it envisaged the FSA providing to ministers. In particular it provided no indication of whether the FSA should provide Ministers with prescriptive policy advice or with advice on a range of policy options, between which Ministers could then choose. James did, however, stipulate that: 'Ministers . . . would be accountable for policy decisions which they made in response to advice from the Commission' (James 1997a, p. 28). which suggests that the FSA should not decide for Ministers which policies they should adopt.

The James Report was not couched in terms of a vocabulary of 'risk assessment' and 'risk management', and those expressions rarely emerged in the subsequent debates about the creation of the FSA. James' analysis represented the FSA as having a hybrid science-based policy advisory role, but argued too that it was necessary to provide the FSA, and its advisors, with functional independence from Ministers and vested commercial interests. He also envisaged that the FSA and its expert scientific advisors would have some direct public accountability, as well as indirect accountability via Ministers and Parliament. James recommended that the FSA's scientific advisors should meet in public and provide full declarations on any 'current and former interests' (James 1997a, p. 24, para. J).

Between the publication of the James Report in May 1997 and the sub-sequent delivery of the government's White Paper on The Food Standards Agency in January 1998, a team of Ministers and officials from the DoH and MAFF elaborated and refined James' ideas, and in some respects shifted them in significant directions. James had argued that the FSA should be a 'non-departmental public body' with executive powers (James 1997b, p. 2, para. 5 of minutes; cf. MAFF 1998, para. 6.1). When the draft legislation establishing the FSA emerged in January 1999, the FSA had been re-characterised as a 'non-ministerial departmental body' (Rooker 1999). The difference between the two is considerable. A non-departmental public body provides expert advice to Ministers but does not act as if it were a Minister. A non-Ministerial departmental body, on the other hand, is like a ministry but without the direct and routine involvement of Ministers.

When the White Paper was published, the agriculture and health Ministers repeatedly asserted in numerous fora that once the FSA was established, policies would be decided by elected representatives rather than by unaccountable officials, although Ministers would, for the first time, be advised by the independent, science-based and consumer-focused FSA (Rooker and Jowell 1997). The White Paper was not couched in the decisionist vocabulary of risk assessment and risk management but, encouraged by ministerial remarks, it was widely interpreted as implying that the FSA would provide expertly-informed assessments of risks, and that it could recommend possible actions that Ministers might choose to take. The FSA was also expected to indicate to Ministers and the general public the extent of the uncertainties complicating their assessment of the risks and to indicate the scope and grounds for exercising a precautionary approach from the consumers' point of view (MAFF 1998, Chapter 2). It was not generally envisaged that the FSA would act to shield Ministers from responsibility for deciding policy, but that is the way it turned out. The White Paper did not define the FSA as either a non-departmental public body or as non-Ministerial departmental body. On that issue, the White Paper made no comment.

One important distinctive feature of the 1998 White Paper on the creation of the FSA was that Ministers provided some explicit guiding principles. Principle 1, which states that '[t]he essential aim of the Agency is the protection of public health', introduced some clarity into the FSA's role of a sort that never characterised MAFF. Principle 2 states that '[t]he Agency's assessments of food standards and safety will be unbiased and based on the best available scientific advice, provided by experts invited in their own right to give independent advice'. Whilst that principle emphasised the crucial role of scientific expert advisors and their independence, it failed to indicate what kind of advice (scientific or policy advice or both) that the FSA should provide.

One important difference between the proposals made by Philip James and the eventual outcome, first set out in the White Paper, was that James had argued that the remit of the FSA should cover the entire food chain from the 'plough to the plate' as James put it. In the White Paper a different division of responsibilities was proposed. The White Paper stipulated that the FSA's remit would give it full responsibility for all regulatory issues concerning food, once the food had left the farm, but that MAFF would retain primary responsibility for regulatory policy-making in respect to all on-farm matters. In practice, MAFF was left with primary responsibility for regulatory policy-making covering four aspects of food safety namely: pesticides, veterinary medicines, genetically modified foods and BSE. In respect to all of those responsibilities, MAFF was supposed to act on the basis of advice from the FSA, and the FSA was supposed to provide 'oversight'. Ministers and officials talked in terms of a 'double-lock mechanism' but on-farm food safety policy-making remained within MAFF's remit. MAFF's retention of responsibility for BSE policy was interpreted by some as a profound shortcoming in the reform process, while others saw it rather as a form of punishment that MAFF was going to have to continue to endure.

In March 1999, the UK government issued a *Consultation on Draft Legislation* that included a draft *Food Standards Bill* (MAFF 1999). In that document, for the first time the FSA was described as 'a non-ministerial government department' (MAFF 1999, p. 3, para. 13). At the Second Reading of the FSA Bill in June of that year, the then MAFF Secretary of State (Nick Brown) said to the House of Commons:

> The Food Standards Agency is being established as the principal authority in Government on food safety and standards matters. It will be the chief source of policy advice to Ministers and other public authorities. Its functions will include drafting and making recommendations on legislation, negotiating in the European Union and internationally on behalf of Ministers, and providing the necessary information and assistance to support decision making. In carrying out that role, the agency will operate from day to day at arm's length from Ministers. However, responsibility for making legislation and ultimate democratic accountability remain, very clearly, with Parliament.

(Brown 1999)

That account indicated that the FSA was expected to recommend legislation and regulations, that is to say that it was expected to provide Ministers with prescriptive policy advice rather than leaving it to Ministers to take the crucial policy decisions. Between the publication of the James Report and the Draft Bill, the FSA had been transformed from an advisory body into a policy-making body.

The FSA took up its responsibilities on 1 April 2000. Late the previous year, the government announced that its first Chairman would be Professor Sir John Krebs. John Krebs came to the FSA from his previous post as Research Professor of Zoology at the University of Oxford. Krebs' appointment was fascinating precisely because he was a scientist, but was being asked to take political responsibility for a non-ministerial government department. The Board of the FSA was expected to become the UK's food safety policy-making body, on behalf of the government, with a Chairman who was a formidable scientist but someone with no public constituency or roots in the consumer or public health movements. Ministers chose a scientist because they wanted the FSA's policy judgements to be seen as being scientifically legitimate.

It was difficult to discern, in advance of the FSA becoming operational, precisely how the creation of the FSA would modify the division of labour between government Ministers, civil servants and expert advisors in the process of deciding food safety policy. The text of the legislation establishing the FSA gave few clues, and Parliamentary debates contributed little enlightenment. The crucial unknown was how that division of labour would evolve.

When Krebs was appointed as FSA Chair, he was invited to meet the Secretary of State at the Department of Health (Frank Dobson) who explained to Krebs in straightforward terms how he envisaged the division of labour between the FSA and the DoH. Dobson said to Krebs that: 'I will never hesitate to use you as my shield' (personal communication, 7 June 2001, Gresham College London). The clear implication of that confidential guidance, not pre-figured in any of the legislation or Parliamentary debate, was that the Department of Health wanted the FSA Board to take full responsibility for food policy-making, and only to provide Ministers with ready-made decisions. The institutional location, powers and remit of the FSA suggest that it was designed as much to protect Ministers from having to take responsibility for food policy-making as it was to protect consumers from food-borne risks. Since the Food Standards Agency became operational, UK Ministers have made few conspicuous contributions to food policy-making. Their role has mostly been confined to applying a bureaucratic 'rubber stamp' to decisions that the FSA has taken. One important exception has been that when in July 2003 the Board of the FSA recommended phasing out the restriction on the consumption of cattle over 30 months of age, Ministers decided to adopt a more cautious and precautionary policy.

As a consequence, all of the crucial elements that go into routine food policy-making have had to be internalised in the FSA. All relevant types of considerations, both scientific and technical, and economic, social and cultural factors and judgements have been actually or potentially on the FSA's agenda. The FSA has responsibility for gathering scientific and other forms of evidence, and for obtaining expert advice and risks assessments and for making risk management policy decisions. As John Krebs has acknowledged, 'The Food Standards Agency is, in a real sense, a child of the BSE crisis' (Krebs 2003). The FSA Board understood that learning the lessons of the BSE saga and crises meant that the legitimacy of policy-making processes, and the acceptability and sustainability of policy decisions, depended upon clarifying and reconfiguring the relationship between science and policy-making. Given that the FSA was designated as a non-Ministerial department of government, and in the light of Dobson's guidance to Krebs, the option of locating responsibility for risk management policy-making in the DoH, while the FSA provided well-informed expert risk assessments, was not available. If the relationships between science and politics were to be reconfigured, that reconfiguration had to be accomplished within the FSA. The structure of the FSA, and its relationship to the DoH, cannot be straightforwardly mapped on to any of the theoretical models sketched in Chapter 2. The FSA was, and is, an irredeemably hybrid science–policy body.

The FSA Board has come to see itself as a risk management decision-making body. It endeavours to act on the basis of robust advice from scientific and other relevant groups of experts to whom it sometimes looks to provide risk assessments. The Board of the FSA appreciated the necessity to reconfigure the structures and procedures that it inherited from MAFF, and a process of evolution is under way, but the FSA has not chosen to subdivide itself into separate scientific and policy-making divisions. FSA has no internal divisions or 'Chinese walls' to insulate or separate scientific deliberations from the political aspects of policy-making. The FSA Board has, however, committed itself to making policy in a transparent fashion. If transparency were to be achieved, it would entail that the interactions between scientific and political deliberations would become open to inspection, and the issue of scientific and democratic legitimacy of food safety policy decisions would have to be confronted.

In practice, the FSA Board has been struggling to change many aspects of the policy-making culture that it inherited from MAFF. Many of the former senior MAFF officials have taken early retirement, or been shifted to other departments. Some bright and able officials have been recruited, but a broad swath of mid-level officials, especially those with some scientific expertise, are working at the FSA and dealing with the same policy topics for which they were responsible in MAFF. The FSA has been a site of internal struggle between the new guard and the old guard. The *ancien régime* has not been entirely displaced despite the best efforts of some Board Members and senior officials. The direction in which the evolution has moved, and the extent of that movement, will be discussed in this book's final chapter, but it has generally been easier to identify the direction in which the Board are trying to change the institution's culture than it has been to discern what the Board envisages as an eventually stable solution.

The extent to which, and the ways in which, policy-making can be judged to be legitimate depends crucially on its various forms of accountability. The FSA is not structured in a way that readily facilitates separate lines of scientific and democratic accountability. Openness and transparency will be necessary but not sufficient conditions for scientific accountability. Lines of democratic accountability are, however, hard to discern. Ministers are accountable to Parliament, but Ministers are not taking the decisions. The FSA Board is accountable to Ministers at the DoH, but Ministers have not been exercising any conspicuous oversight, and since Ministers have taken no decisions they have not been called upon to justify or defend those decisions before Parliament.

While the FSA's accountability to Ministers has been partial and maybe even marginal, the FSA has tried to operate in a way that has provided many more opportunities for it to be directly accountable than was ever the case under MAFF's regime. The FSA's procedures and website provide numerous ways through which it can engage with, and be accountable to, stakeholders, external experts and the general public, and those ways are not mediated by Ministers. The Board of the Food Standards Agency meets in public, and those meeting are broadcast on the World Wide Web. The FSA Board has indicated to all its expert scientific advisory committees that it expects them (sometimes) to meet in public too, and to place as much of their evidence in the public domain as possible. In this way, the FSA Board is endeavouring to demonstrate that its policy-making processes are accountable and legitimate.

Reform of food safety policy-making at the European Commission

At the Commission, the BSE crisis of March 1996 produced a political earthquake of a similar magnitude to that in the UK. For the Commission, as with the UK government, BSE was not the only difficult food safety problem that had to be managed: other scares concerned for example the contamination of animal feedstuffs with dioxins and diesel wastes, while disputes between Member States over the acceptable safety of beef hormones and food irradiation had been intractable. By the late 1990s, moreover, the challenge of GM foods had undermined the sustainability of the Commission's traditional ways of managing risk policy-making. In several important respects, the challenge that BSE (and other food safety issues) posed for the European Commission was even more difficult than that which had confronted the UK government after 20 March 1996.

Sales of beef fell, in percentage terms, far more rapidly in neighbouring continental European countries, after March 1996, than in the UK, although in those countries where more pork was eaten, beef had accounted for a smaller proportion of total meat consumed. The Commission could just about manage to cope with instability in the beef sector, as long as it was confined to the British Isles, but once instability spread across the continent, it became far harder and more costly.

The European Commission that was in place in the mid- and late-1990s had inherited a regime under which the Common Agricultural Policy (or CAP) accounted for approximately 50 per cent of the EU's total budget (Black 2003). Even before the BSE crises of 1996 and the late 1990s, the CAP was under attack from numerous directions. Within the Commission, albeit outside of the Commission's Directorate-General for Agriculture, the CAP is seen as a huge and unsustainable burden, because its scale of expenditure prevents the other Directorates-General from taking a wide range of initiatives that they are keen to pursue.

Pressure to reform the CAP and to cut subsidies to the European agricultural system came from outside the EU as well as from within. During the protracted negotiations, under the Uruguay Round of the General Agreement on Tariffs and Trade, leading to the establishment of the World Trade Organisation in 1994, the European Community (as it then was) undertook substantially to diminish agricultural subsidies and barriers to the importation of agricultural products from outside of Europe, in exchange for improved access to the domestic markets of developing countries. The US gave similar undertakings.

By the time of the BSE crisis of March 1996, the EU had continued to discuss reducing subsidies, but few significant agreements had been reached, and no substantial action had been taken. The agricultural crises that began in March 1996 undermined the economic viability of many livestock farms, and European agricultural subsidies rose in response. Subsequently, the Bush administration in the USA abruptly raised subsidies to US farms, and negotiations at the WTO are moving at a glacial pace. The post-March 1996 crisis in agricultural economics reinforced the consensus at the Commission that food safety policy-making in Europe had to be reformed.

An investigation into the BSE crisis by a committee of the European Parliament showed that the Commission had reproduced many of the failings of MAFF, in its handling of BSE policy-making (European Parliament 1997). It argued that the possible risks had been ignored or seriously understated and that the Commission had adopted a policy of 'disinformation' in its dealings with the European Council and other stakeholders. It concluded, moreover, that BSE policy-making at the Commission had been at least as concerned with maintaining stability in agricultural markets as it had been with protecting public health. The publication of that critical report reinforced the pressure on the Commission to transform – and be seen to transform – how food safety policy-making was managed. In response, in April 1997, the Commission issued a Green Paper on Food Safety (European Commission 1997).

The European Commission, and the governments of many Member States argued that the BSE crisis had provoked an EU-wide collapse in the confidence of consumers in the safety of the food supply, and the probity of the policy-making process, and that unless the Commission got a firm grip on food safety issues, individual Member States could and would take independent unilateral actions that would disrupt the single internal market, and undermine confidence in EU-wide measures.

The publication of the Green Paper lead to a first round of reforms. It resulted in the relocation of responsibility for the scientific advisory system, from DG-III, responsible for industry, to what was then known as DG-XXIV, which had responsibility for consumer protection and public health. That change produced a partial separation of responsibility for scientific advice from that for regulatory policy-making, but it left the latter located in the Directorate General that was also expected to promote the economic interests of the food industry. That arrangement was in effect, however, a preliminary move, before a deeper process of reform was accomplished.

By 1997, the Commissioner for DG-XXIV, Hans Reichenbach, had become impatient with the slow pace of reform and so convened a trio of leading public health policy experts to advise on what the next steps might be (James, Kemper and Pascal 1999). Reichenbach's trio comprised Professor Philip James from the UK (author of the original proposals for the FSA), Fritz Kemper from Germany and Gerard Pascal from France. They were asked to undertake a re-analysis of the organisation of scientific advice in the light of the last two years experience with the new system of expert recruitment and working procedures. That report triggered a process resulting in the transfer of responsibility for food safety policy-making into (what had been) DG-XXIV, where the secretariats of the scientific advisory committees were already located, and which was renamed as the Directorate General for Health and Consumer Protection or DG-SANCO.

DG-SANCO then took the lead within the Commission, in preparing a White Paper that emerged in January 2000, proposing the establishment on a European Food Authority (European Commission 2000). The White Paper asserted that:

> Assuring that the EU has the highest standards of food safety [...] is a key policy priority for the Commission. This White Paper reflects this priority. A radical new approach is proposed. This process is driven by the need to guarantee a high level of food safety. [The document explained]: The establishment of an independent European Food Authority is considered by the Commission to be the most appropriate response to the need to guarantee a high level of food safety. This Authority would be entrusted with a number of key tasks embracing independent scientific advice on all aspects relating to food safety, operation of rapid alert systems, communication and dialogue with consumers on food safety and health issues as well as networking with national agencies and scientific bodies. The European Food Authority will provide the Commission with the necessary analysis. It will be the responsibility of the Commission to decide on the appropriate response to that analysis.

> (European Commission 2000, Executive Summary, p. 3)

The publication of that document marked a watershed at which techno-cratic narratives seem to have been abandoned by DG-SANCO (and by some but not all of the rest of the Commission) in favour of the post-1996 official orthodoxy of a Red Book decisionist model. The White Paper proposed creating a new institution (the European Food Authority or EFA) separate from and at arms' length of, DG-SANCO. The EFA would provide DG-SANCO with 'independent scientific advice' and 'dialogue with consumers', while DG-SANCO would 'decide on the appropriate response'. That rhetoric resonates readily with a model of the division of labour between 'risk assessment' and 'risk management'. The White Paper argued that the scientific experts in the EFA should be 'independent', but it failed to clarify of whom or what they needed to be independent. The White Paper also emphasised a need for transparency without clarifying how the Commission interpreted that concept (European Commission 2000, pp. 15–16, para. 35).

The EFSA has suggested that while its Board will routinely meet in public, its expert advisory committee will only be expected to meet in public sometimes (EFSA 2003c). Similarly, the EFSA has indicated that it will try to 'ensure wide access to documents in its possession' (EFSA 2003c) without explaining whether all documents will be accessible while the EFSA is deliberating, or only after it has completed its deliberations, and delivered its advice.

The text of the White Paper, and the intentions of the Commission, were difficult to interpret because the document also stated that: 'the Commission believes that the scientific work currently undertaken by the scientific Committees related to food safety should be a core part of the proposed authority' (European Commission 2000, para. 45, p. 18). That remark suggests a continuation of the traditional practices rather than a radical break, since historically (ostensibly scientific) committees such as the Scientific Committee for Food effectively decided important policy issues, with DG-III and subsequently DG-SANCO providing routine endorsements, and bureaucratic rubber stamps. It became clear, moreover from the comments of representatives of most Member States, European Commission officials and representatives of food industry trade associations, that there was a widespread expectation that the EFA would provide not just scientific advice but also policy advice (Trichopoulou et al. 2000).

It was therefore unclear what impact the establishment of an EFA will have in practice on the relationship between science and politics. Apart from DG-SANCO and the EFA being expected to focus primarily on the protection of public health and the interests of consumers, there is little evidence that DG-SANCO envisages providing the EFA with much in the way of guidance, or to invoke the vocabulary of the co-evolutionary model, of upstream framing conditions. It was not even clear whether risk managers in DG-SANCO envisage providing the EFA with an indication of the range of policy options they foresee employing.

In the period between the publication of the Commission's White Paper in January 2000 and the eventual passage through the European Parliament of the legislation to establish an EFA in 2002, most of the debate was focused on a very different, but also very important issue. Just as in the UK, very powerful voices argued that the remit of the EFA should be confined to issues of food safety, such as BSE and chemical contamination, but should not extend to issues of nutrition such as obesity and diet-related cardiovascular disease. The large food manufacturing companies, especially those responsible for marketing high-calorie food products containing large amounts of fats and carbohydrates, were particularly keen for the new body to focus on food safety, but their side of the argument was joined by some experts who argued that although nutritional and dietary matters, such as over-consumption and epidemics of cardiovascular disease and obesity, were very important, it would be difficult enough for the Authority to get a grip on, and to deal effectively with, microbiological and chemical contamination, without having its effort diffused over too many issues.

In the event, during the legislative process in 2002, the European Parliament decided that a European Food Safety Authority (i.e. an EFSA rather than the EFA previously envisaged) would be established. At the time of writing, September 2003, the EFSA is in an embryonic form, and very few decisions have been taken about it, and even fewer have been taken by it. On the EFSA's website the Authority describes itself, and it relationship to the Commission and other political authorities, in strictly orthodox 'Red Book' decisionist terms. 'The Authority will primarily be a scientific risk assessment body; the responsibility for risk management or decision making remaining with the EU's political institutions: the European Commission, the Council of EU Ministers and the EU Parliament' (EFSA, 2003b). It will be fascinating to see how in practice the EFSA actually operates because, while the documents represent the EFSA as a body with a purely scientific remit, all the indications from both EFSA and DG-SANCO are that they expect the *status quo ante* to continue in the sense that the EFSA will be expected to continue providing the kind of prescriptive policy advice that European Commission food policy committees have provided since they were first established in the mid-1970s. One key difference, however, is that the EFSA, and its advisory committees, will be expected to conduct their deliberations in a more open and accountable fashion (EFSA 2003c). It remains to be seen how far it will be possible to reconcile those historical practices with aspirations for independence and for transparency.

The challenge facing EFSA

The European Food Safety Authority, even with its relatively restricted remit, along with DG-SANCO, is confronted by a crucial difficulty that does not confront individual Member States in the same way or to the same extent. EU Member States, or to be more precise their National Competent Authorities (or NCAs) such as the UK's FSA and its French counterpart the Agence Française de la Sécurité Sanitaire des Aliments (AFSSA) have considerable independence of each other. The UK Food Standards Agency is expected by the UK government, and by British stakeholders, to make autonomous and independent judgements about what is, and what is not, acceptably safe. The FSA is not under pressure from within the UK to align its judgements with those of the French, the German, the Greeks or the Finns. Similarly the NCAs of most of the UK's fellow EU Member States are under no domestic pressure to agree with the FSA. In the event of a dispute between Member States about the safety and acceptability of some food product or process, each national jurisdiction will try to ensure that its NCA prevails. The constituencies to which NCAs are supposed to be accountable are always domestic and some disputes are inevitable.

The EFSA, however, is in a predicament that differs markedly from each and all of the Member States' NCAs. From the perspective of the Commission and the EFSA, the existence and continuation of disagreements between NCAs over scientific or policy issues concerning food safety represents a severe threat. Commissioner Byrne, who had responsibility for DG-SANCO, repeatedly argued that consumer confidence is undermined by disagreements between national jurisdictions. Consequently, the challenge facing the EFSA is not just to conduct scientific risk assessments, and maybe also to provide DG-SANCO with science-based policy advice, but it will also be expected to provide sufficiently authoritative judgements to ensure that they are shared by the NCAs in all Member States.

Given the reverberations of the BSE crises, and for example different national assessments of the safety and acceptability of genetically modified crops, as well as the domestic expectations for the new NCAs, the EFSA's task will be an exceptionally difficult one. Once scientific expert advisors operate in transparent ways, with the evidence on the basis of which they reach their conclusions in the public domain, the uncertainties characterising the scientific evidence and understanding will also be evident. This will create the conditions under which different NCAs may be seen to disagree, in ways that may be both scientifically and democratically legitimate. The conditions for unanimity, consensus and convergence may therefore be undermined rather than reinforced.

Once the EFSA is fully operational, it will struggle to ensure that all the NCAs of the separate Member States speak with one voice on scientific and policy matters. Without that unanimity, however, the Commission's attainment and maintenance of an integrated and unified European market will be jeopardised.

The incentives for the NCAs, however, are likely to be significantly different from those of the EFSA. If all the NCA's consistently fall in line with the EFSA, then their *raisons d'être* will evaporate. That may indeed be the ultimate aim of some officials at the European Commission and perhaps even at the EFSA, but that aim is not yet widely shared amongst most Member States. Historically, Portugal has been the only Member State whose government consistently preferred Brussels-based advice to that of their domestic experts (Gonçalves and Gonçalves 1999). The creation of the EFSA may be as likely to contribute another voice to the prevailing cacophony as to result in EU-wide harmonisation. The ambition of the European Commission was to create an institution that would be the 'first among equals', and to try to get all the national experts to speak with one voice, and to provide uniformity, but how far that can be accomplished remains to be seen.

France

In France, BSE was just one of a lengthy and complex series of public health controversies that provoked institutional reform. Other foci of hotly-contested debates about public health and safety included a scandal concerning contaminated blood products which resulted in the prosecution of several Ministers and officials for culpable negligence (Joly *et al.* 1999). Public health scares were also concerned with bacterial contamination of unpasteurised dairy products with organisms including *Listeria monocytogenes*, *Salmonella* and *E.Coli* 0157 (Goulet *et al.* 1995; Desenclos *et al.* 1996). These controversies culminated in 1998 in a wave of institutional reform, of which the creation of the Agence Française de la Sécurité Sanitaire des Aliments (AFSSA or the French Food Safety Agency) was one important part.

In French policy-making circles, the problems underlying the crises and scandals (including BSE) were widely assumed to have arisen as a consequence of the provision of poor quality scientific advice, compromised by its lack of independence from vested interests and by a lack of procedural transparency (Hirsch *et al.* 1996). As a consequence, the institutional location and role of AFSSA was informed more by a Red Book-type decisionist analysis that emphasised the desirability of separating science from policy-making than by an analysis emphasising the desirability of separating responsibility for regulation from that for industrial sponsorship. Thus, AFSSA, unlike the UK's FSA, is not just accountable to the Ministry of Health; it is also accountable to the ministries of Agriculture and Consumer Affairs. The opportunities for tensions between AFSSA's responsibilities for regulatory policy and the Ministry of Agriculture's responsibility for sponsoring farming interests remain.

A distinctive feature of the French reform process has been the introduction of, and an ostensible reliance on, an explicit institutional separation of the functions of 'risk assessment' and 'risk management'. That contrast is, moreover, officially represented as if it were identical to the separation of science from politics. The official narrative was that they had not been properly or clearly distinguished under the antecedent regime.

Formally, AFSSA is mandated to provide ministers with science-based risk assessments in relation to all categories of food or feed products destined for humans or animals (Joly et al. 1999; Hirsch 2001). It is also mandated to assess risks to consumers arising from animal diseases, and the use of veterinary or agrochemical products and from GM foods and crops. In relation to all those aspects of food policy-making, AFSSA is nominally responsible for risk assessment but not for risk management decision-making, which is supposed to lie with ministers. There is, however, one exception. For historical reasons, specific responsibility for risk management policy-making in relation veterinary medicines was assigned to AFSSA.

In practice, however, AFSSA's remit is being interpreted both by the Agency itself and by the ministries that it serves in a more ambiguous and ambitious fashion. In the event, in France as in the UK, Ministers expect their agencies to take responsibility for many, if not for all, policy decisions, even while they label those agencies primarily as scientific rather than as political bodies. AFSSA and the FSA have both been politically obliged to take responsibility for almost all policy judgements about food safety, even though they have no political constituencies and their accountability to their citizens is rather indirect. The risk in such an arrangement, from the point of view the agencies, is that if food scandals and crises were to occur, blame might more readily attach to the agencies rather than to the Ministers they serve.

The ambiguities in the role of AFSSA has made it into a difficult institution for which to take responsibility, but those ambiguities have also created some scope for institutional autonomy. AFSSA, as an institution, has responded by exercising considerable discretion, by sometimes providing prescriptive policy advice while at others providing only a scientific discussion of the possible risks. For example, in the context of the UK–French dispute about the acceptability of UK beef exports, discussed in Chapter 8, AFSSA offered several opinions about the safety of British beef. AFSSA chose to provide scientific opinions but no policy recommendations, even though Ministers (especially the Minister of Agriculture) had previously indicated that they wanted a specific prescriptive policy recommendation. AFSSA has, therefore, exercised a significant degree of discretion and autonomy, and on occasions, such as over BSE controls, has obliged Ministers to take responsibility for some difficult policy decisions, rather than making those policy decisions for, and on behalf of, Ministers. Ministers have not, however, always been grateful.

In other contexts (putting aside the field of veterinary medicines for which AFSSA is explicitly supposed to take responsibility for risk management) AFSSA has provided Ministers with policy recommendations. In effect, risk management policy decisions are being taken within the agency, and passed to Ministers for their routine rubber stamps. In practice, senior officials in AFSSA have concluded that the Agency cannot always be neutral on risk management issues, and that it must take policy considerations into account in formulating advice, and that sometimes it should provide specific policy recommendations.

The legislation under which AFSSA was established, indicated that the Agency was expected to be 'transparent', although how that notion of transparency was to be interpreted in practice was unclear. AFSSA has interpreted the obligation to be open as requiring that judgements, advice and recommendations to Ministers should be published, and they are, although AFSSA has not published the advice it receives from its scientific expert committees. Since the relationship between the available scientific evidence, or those parts of it that are taken into account, and the resultant policy-judgements is so often the focus of controversy and concern in food safety policy-making (and in risk policy-making more generally) it seems anomalous that in the new French regime, the deliberations of expert scientific advisors are not fully open to public or peer scrutiny. The new status quo may be difficult to sustain.

Germany

In January 2001 the German Ministry of Agriculture was abolished and replaced by a new Ministry for Consumer Protection, Food and Agriculture (*Bundesministerium für Verbraucherschutz, Ernährung, und Landwirtschaft* or BMVEL). The remit of that ministry is noteworthy, because it embodies a quite different strategy from that being adopted in the UK and at the Commission. In both those jurisdictions, it was deemed essential to separate responsibility for consumer protection from responsibility for promoting farming and food industry interests. The approach adopted by the Schröder government was to integrate them, while at the same time ostensibly subordinating food and agricultural policy to the primary objective of consumer protection.

Renate Künast, the new German Minister for Consumer Protection, Food and Agriculture and member of the Green Party, characterised BSE as 'agriculture's Chernobyl'. She insisted that the BSE crisis necessitated a fundamental renewal of Germany's food and agricultural system, and of the CAP (Künast 2001). Künast has coined the expression of a 'magic hexagon' to refer to the shape of a table around which all the main stakeholders concerned with food safety policy would meet fully to reconcile their views and policies (Künast 2001). Künast's assumption appears to be that the interests of consumers come first, but given that premise, all other interests can be reconciled.

The BMVEL, under Künast, abolished the agency that had previously been responsible for providing both scientific and policy advice (the *Bundesinstitut für gesundheitlichen Verbraucherschutz und Veterinärmedizin*) and reorganised it into two separate parts. The Federal Office for Consumer Protection and Food Safety (or *Bundesamt für Verbraucherschutz und Lebensmittel Sicherheit –* BVLS) is now defined as having responsible for risk management, while the Federal Institute for Risk Assessment (*Bundesinstitut für Risikobewertung* or BfR) is supposed to provide scientific risk assessments and advice.

The arrangements in Germany differ from those in the UK, France and at the European Commission. The new institutional structure in Germany formally presumes a clear separation between scientific 'risk assessment' and 'risk management'. Unlike the position in France, however, responsibility for risk management is not simply assigned to a government ministry and ministers, but to an arms' length risk management policy-making institution that will be expected to provide ministers with policy advice, in ways that resemble the role of the FSA in the UK.

At the time of writing (December 2003), those two institutions (BVL and BfR) are so new that they have not had time to make more than a very few decisions, and it is therefore difficult to provide an analysis of their decision-making policies or processes. It is not clear, however, that the distinctions upon which the Germany regime has been structured, have the simplicity and clarity necessary to make the system sustainable. Since there is no evidence that the German government recognises a need to provide the BfR with explicit agenda-setting guidance, the presumed objectivity and social and ethical neutrality of the BfR will be vulnerable to contestation by other groups of experts within Germany that may choose to adopt different framing assumptions. Similarly, dissenting groups and scientific experts in Germany may highlight the differences between the judgements of the BfR and contrasting risk assessments developed by NCAs in other EU Member States. It is also unclear precisely what kind (or kinds) of advice the BfR will provide to the BVL. A similar question arises in relation to the advice that the BVL will provide to ministers in the German government. It remains to be seen precisely where the locus of responsibility for decision-making will actually lie, but it is also evident that the German system is structured on a set of premises that very closely approximate to orthodox interpretations of the Red Book model.

The contrast between the new institutional structures in the UK, France, Germany and at the European Commission indicates that a wide range of different tactics have been adopted as the different jurisdictions endeavour to provide legitimacy to the regulatory systems that cover their food supplies. No two are the same, yet they all purport to be based upon slightly differing interpretations of the inverse decisionist model. In all cases, the technocratic model has been discarded, but in no case is the science of risk assessment acknowledged to be sensitive to the social, political and cultural contexts from which they emerge. If the analysis in this book is correct, it is unlikely that any of those four systems will remain stable and sustainable, as and when further food safety disputes and crises arise.

Bibliography

Black, I. (2003) 'EU agrees to agricultural shakeup', *Guardian*, 27 June 2003, p. 15.

Blitz, J. and Kampfner, J. (1997) 'Ministers play down abattoir safety row', *Financial Times*, 8 March 1997, p. 5.

Brown, N. (1999) *Hansard*, 21 June 1999, Column 787, The Stationery Office, London.

Desenclos, J. C *et al.* (1996) 'Large outbreak of *Salmonella enterica* serotype paratyphi B infection caused by goat's milk cheese, France: a case finding and epidemiological study', *BMJ*, 312, 91–4.

Dressel, K. (2003) *BSE – The New Dimension of Uncertainty*. Edition Sigma, Berlin.

EFSA (2003a) *Participation of Third Parties at Meetings of the Advisory Forum*. European Food Safety Authority, Doc AF 04.0702003–5, Brussels.

EFSA (2003b) *The Tasks of the European Food Safety Authority*. European Food Safety Authority at *http://www.efsa.eu.int/tasks_en.html* 9/9/2003.

EFSA (2003c) *Questions and Answers on the European Food Safety Authority*. European Food Safety Authority at *http://www.efsa.eu.int/QandA_en.html* 9 Sept. 2003.

European Commission (1997) *Consumer Health and Food Safety*. COM(97)183final, 30 April 1997, Brussels.

European Commission (2000) *White Paper on Food Safety in the European Union*. COM(99)719, 12 January 2000; available at *http://europa.eu.int/comm/food/fs/intro/index_en.html*.

European Parliament (1997) *Report on Alleged Contraventions or Maladministration in the Implementation of Community Law in Relation to BSE, Without Prejudice to the Jurisdiction of the Community and National Courts*. Report of the Inquiry from a temporary committee into BSE, rapporteur: Manuel Medina Oi tega. 7 February DOC EN\RR\319\319544, Strasbourg.

Gonçalves, M. E. and Gonçalves, L. (1999) *BSE and the Portuguese National Action System*, Report for the BASES project and for the European Commission, DG XII, July 1999. Lisbon: Instituto Superior de Ciências do Trabalho e da Empresa.

Goulet, V. *et al.* (1995) ' Listeriosis from consumption of raw-milk cheese', *Lancet*, 345, 1581–2.

Hirsch, M., Duneton, P., Baralon, P. and Noiville, F. (1996) *L'affolante affaire de la vache folle*. Paris: Balland.

Hirsch, M. (2001) 'Food Policy in France', paper to WHO-Europe Conference on *Improved Coordination and Harmonization of National Food Safety Control Services*, held in Dublin, June 2001, available December 2003 at http://www.euro.who.int/foodsafety/Publications/mtgrpt.

HM Treasury (2000) *Public Service Agreement with the Department of Health (Food Standards Agency)* see: *http://www.hm-treasury.gov.uk/sr2000/sda/index.html*.

James, P. (1997a) *Food Standards Agency: an interim proposal*, report to T Blair, 30 April 1997.

James, P. (1997b) Speech on The Food Standards Agency to the Parliamentary Food and Health Forum, 10 June 1997.

James, P., Kemper, F. and Pascal, G. (1999) *A European Food and Public Health Authority*. European Commission DG-XXIV, DOC/99/17, 13 December. Brussels: available at http://europa.eu.int/comm/food/fs/sc/future_food_en.pdf.

Joly, P. B., Le Pape, Y., Barbier, M., Estadès, J., Lemarié, J. and Marcant, O. (1999) *Interactions between Scientific Expertise and Public Decision on TSEs in FRANCE*, Final Report of Task 1 of the BASES Project, Building a common data base on scientific research and public decision on TSEs in Europe. University of Grenoble, France.

Krebs, J. (2003) *Protecting Consumers in the Future World Market*. City Food Lecture, The Guildhall, London, 14 January 2003, p. 1.

Künast, R. (2001) 'The Magic Hexagon I', *The Ecologist*, vol 31, No 3, April 2001, pp. 48–49.

Lang, T., Millstone, E., Rayner, M. and Raven, H. (1996) *Modernising UK Food Policy: the case for reforming the Ministry of Agriculture, Fisheries and Food*, Discussion Paper 1, Centre for Food Policy, Thames Valley University, London, July 1996.

Lang, T. *et al.* (1997) *Food Standards and the State: A Fresh Start*, Discussion Paper 3, Centre for Food Policy, Thames Valley University, London, April 1997.

MAFF (1997a) *New Group to set rapid progress on Food Agency*, Press Release 148/97, 9 June 1997, London: Ministry of Agriculture, Fisheries and Food.

MAFF (1997b) *Public approve new agency for food safety*, MAFF Press Release 224/97, 30 July 1997. London: Ministry of Agriculture, Fisheries and Food.

MAFF (1998) *The Food Standards Agency: a force for change*, White Paper to Parliament, Jan 1998, Cm 3830. London: Ministry of Agriculture, Fisheries and Food.

MAFF (1999) *The Food Standards Agency: Consultation on Draft Legislation*. CM 4249, 27 January 1999, London: Ministry of Agriculture, Fisheries and Food.

Rooker, J. and Jowell, T., (1997) Statement to Stakeholders' Meeting, Department of Health, London, 14 October 1997.

Rooker, J. (1999) *Hansard*, 21 June 1999, Column 831. The Stationery Office, London.

Strang, G. (1995) *The Labour Party's Basic Objectives for Food Policy*, speech given to the Environmental Health Congress of the Chartered Institute of Environmental Health, September 1995, p. 1 para. 3.

Trichopoulou, A., Millstone, E., Lang, T., Eames, M., Barling, D., and van Zwanenberg, P. (2000) *European Policy on Food Safety*, report to the European Parliament's Scientific and Technological Options Assessment Programme (STOA), June 2000, European Parliament document number PE 292.026/Fin.St. available at *http://www.europarl.eu.int/dg4/stoa/en/publi/default.htm*.

Chapter 10

Summary and conclusions

The aims of this book have been organised around three main questions, namely: how was BSE policy decided, how can policy-making processes of that kind be understood and how should policy-making institutions and procedures be changed to avoid any repetition of the failures that characterised the BSE saga? The evidence we have assembled, and the analysis we have provided, shows how BSE policy, and a seemingly scientific narrative, were constructed by the authorities and how and why they eventually disintegrated. We have explained that the BSE policy and the risk narratives disseminated by the British government, at least prior to March 1996, were in our view profoundly misleading and comprehensively flawed. Our account of the BSE saga shows, moreover, that MAFF's policy agenda, and its consequent attempt to represent BSE solely as a veterinary problem, to reassure consumers that British beef was unproblematically safe, failed for both institutional and scientific reasons.

One reason why policy imploded in March 1996 is because, without any encouragement from MAFF, the Department of Health had invested in an institution, namely the CJD Surveillance Unit, and in scientists who were employed to act as epidemiological antennae. The BSE policy narrative and regime that MAFF established at the end of the 1980s might well still be in place if that epidemiological surveillance work had not been done, and if it had not been done sufficiently carefully for the CJD Surveillance Unit scientists to have been in a position to tell SEAC and the Chief Medical Officer (CMO) in early 1996 about new evidence that had emerged indicating that a new variant of CJD had been found, which was sufficiently distinctive for it probably to be a consequence of consuming foodstuffs contaminated with the BSE pathogen.

The existence and competent operation of the CJD Surveillance Unit was therefore a critical institutional condition for the collapse of MAFF's BSE policy and narrative at the end of the third week of March 1996. A crucial scientific condition, however, was that the mean incubation period for what came to be known at first as new variant-CJD (or nvCJD), and later as variant-CJD (or vCJD) was relatively short. If the average incubation period of vCJD had, as a matter of fact, turned out to be some 10 years longer it is entirely possible that MAFF's antecedent BSE policy and narrative would still be the UK government's official position, and nothing resembling the crisis of March 1996 might yet have occurred.

In the event, in the early months of 1996, the senior staff at the CJD Surveillance Unit felt able to take their concerns about the apparent emergence of a new and worrying variant of CJD in the UK to SEAC and the CMO despite the fact that the evidence available to them did not prove that the novel phenomenon that they had identified was causally related to BSE. SEAC's response to the information provided by the CJD Surveillance Unit was also important. SEAC members were, in the event, willing to tell Ministers that their BSE policy, and its underlying representation of the science, were unsustainable even though the evidence available to them fell short of causal proof. They collectively deemed a relatively modest portion of strong circumstantial evidence to provide sufficient grounds for advising Ministers to change their policies and narratives. In the end, therefore, and in spite of MAFF's unremitting efforts, it was scientific evidence and scientific experts that brought about the disintegration of the policy regime and narrative that MAFF had energetically constructed, and it took some courage on the part of those experts to take a stand against the prevailing orthodoxy.

The central theme of MAFF's narrative had been that there was no evidence that BSE posed any risk to human health. In early 1996, the findings of the CJD Surveillance Unit's epidemiologists directly contradicted that narrative, and those findings could not be concealed or spun into insignificance. Under those conditions, the policy had to change. Prior to those developments, there had been evidence that could not readily be reconciled with MAFF's narrative of reassurance, but that prior evidence (though accumulating) had been indirect. What the CJD Surveillance Unit provided in early 1996 was sufficiently direct evidence to torpedo MAFF's claims. Our analysis has therefore enabled us to explain not just how and why BSE polices were constructed, but also how and why they disintegrated.

Analytical reflections

The evidence and analysis provided in the previous chapters indicates that neither technocratic nor decisionist accounts of the relationship between science and policy provide sufficient conceptual resources with which to comprehend the complexities of real science-based risk policy decision-making. In Chapter 2, we suggested that a co-evolutionary model of the role of science in policy-making represented an important advance on technocratic and decisionist models because it highlighted the fact that scientific representations of the natural world cannot be presumed to be constructed independently of their historical, socio-economic and political contexts. Prior to the BSE saga, almost all of the empirical evidence about the social construction of official UK representations of risk was, by necessity, inferential and indirect. The detailed historical record of BSE policy-making, made available as a consequence of the Phillips Inquiry, has provided more direct evidence than had ever previously been accessible. The evidence shows that the ways in which BSE, and the risks it posed, were addressed, investigated, interpreted and represented were not independent of social and political influences; on the contrary, they were exquisitely sensitive to those influences.

Our argument, as far as science policy theory is concerned, is not that a co-evolutionary model is the correct model, or even a correct model, but rather that it represents a significant advance on previous models. It represents an advance, for example, because it abandons the pretence that science can be readily separated from its political context simply by assigning responsibility for providing risk assessment to institutions or groups that are labelled as scientific.

Although a co-evolutionary model indicates that science and politics can and often do interact, it does not provide more than an outline of an account of how those interactions occur. The historical details of the BSE saga enable us to illuminate, in greater detail than has previously been possible, the mechanisms through which science and politics have interacted and can interact. In this chapter we will provide a generalisable account of the key features of those mechanisms.

That analysis enables us to draw prescriptive conclusions, because we will not just chronicle the ways in which science and politics interacted but provide a diagnosis of the sources and extent of the pathological features of those interactions. Since BSE represented a failure in (ostensibly) science-based policy-making, and since the ways in which the science was misunderstood and mis-represented substantially contributed to that failure, and even made the policy failure significantly worse than it might otherwise had been, the question of what went wrong, and how can we avoid repeating those mistakes, becomes especially important.

We are not just arguing that the distinction, or boundary, between science and politics was drawn in different ways by different people, or that the boundary was contestable and contested. Our analysis is far more specific and less agnostic as between competing accounts. We have shown that repeatedly, official judgements about the putative risks from BSE that were unambiguously political were represented as if they were scientific, and as if they had been fully justified by robust scientific evidence and advice. We argue that science was invoked to try to provide a justification for, and a masquerade with which to disguise, flawed policy judgements. The evidence that was available in the late 1980s could have been more readily reconciled with a supposition that BSE could pose a risk to human health than with the government's preferred narrative, namely that it was unproblematically safe. In the 1990s, evidence (such as the spread of TSEs to cats) that was even harder to reconcile with the government's narrative emerged, yet the insistence with which MAFF reiterated its narrative increased rather diminished.

The official narrative eventually disintegrated in part because key groups (such as abattoir workers and officials in MAFF and the veterinary services) took the official narrative at face value, and acted as if the narrative were true. Without any claim to hindsight, or the ability to forecast the future of the BSE and vCJD epidemics, we believe it is clear that (prior to March 1996) MAFF insisted on adopting, and reiterating the least well supported of all the hypotheses available to it. It is therefore vital to understand how and why MAFF adopted that course of action, and how it managed to get away with doing so for so long and with such catastrophic consequences.

The next section of this chapter will therefore provide a distillation of, and generalisation from, the BSE case and specify some key structural and procedural lessons for science-based risk policy-making in general. Our prescriptive analysis will not, by itself, indicate what the UK government's (or any other jurisdiction's) policy on BSE, or on any other risk policy issue, should have been, or should now be. It will, however, indicate the main structural, procedural and substantive features of what a legitimate system for deciding such policy issues could be like. The subsequent section will examine the extent to which the key lessons of the BSE saga have been learnt by the new institutional regimes in the UK and neighbouring jurisdictions. We will therefore explore the gap between current practices and what the foregoing analysis suggests are the minimum conditions for the future avoidance of the types of pathologies exemplified by the BSE saga.

How science interacted with its political context

We have documented in considerable detail the routine and systematic misrepresentation of a co-evolutionary system of decision-making with technocratic and decisionist narratives. MAFF's repeated claim to the effect that policy was based on and only on sound science was a rhetorical cover for a set of covert political and commercial judgements masquerading as if they were scientific. That tactic was, furthermore, pivotal to the pathology of the policy-making regime. We have argued that some of those who articulated that narrative most emphatically were amongst those best placed to realise how misleading it was.

We are not suggesting that Ministers, officials and their advisors never believed their own rhetoric or that they never assumed that a technocratic model was correct. We recognise moreover that the institutional structures and procedures within which Ministers, officials and advisors operated were influenced by technocratic traditions. But, as we believe the preceding chapters have shown, the BSE saga was in large part the product of a series of strategic and tactical decisions to invoke technocratic narratives to conceal and misrepresent the character of the underlying processes and transactions. Technocratic idioms and procedures in part allowed British Ministers and officials to claim that policy was primarily, or even exclusively, concerned with the protection of public and veterinary health whilst in practice a set of entirely different economic, commercial and political considerations were dominant. On all but a handful of occasions, aspirations to maintain stable levels of demand for British beef in domestic and export markets, and not to increase commercial costs or public expenditures, were dominant considerations. They were only dominant because they were concealed, and we say misrepresentations of science were used to conceal them.

One possible interpretation of the account we have provided could be to try to represent it as corresponding to an inversion of the Red Book model of the sort represented by Figure 2.4 in Chapter 2. The Red Book is often glossed as a three-stage linear process: science comes first in the risk assessment phase, second risk management policy decisions are taken in the light of the science-based risk assessment, and thirdly and finally risk communication messages are devised and disseminated. If the order of that model were inverted, it could be used to represent UK BSE policy-making, at least prior to March 1996.

One could argue that MAFF first decided what its risk-communication narrative would be, namely one that was consistently reassuring, and then developed risk management measures to reinforce that narrative of reassurance, and then endeavoured to construct a scientific account of BSE that supported and reinforced the risk management regime and the narrative of reassurance. Rather than BSE being science-based policy-making it might be characterised as 'policy-based evidence-making', to invoke an expression coined by James Crabtree of the Work Foundation. Processes of that kind did sometimes occur, but that account would, by itself, be an oversimplification.

A complex set of reciprocal interactions between the various elements of policy-making became entangled with each other and evolved in ways that, in the long run, were unsustainable and counterproductive. As Moran has suggested, the relationship between MAFF and its industrial clientele was not so much a matter of regulatory capture, it was rather a type of symbiotic interdependence, although we would characterise it as a pathological type (Moran 2001). Despite MAFF's best efforts to constrain science within the straight-jacket of a narrative that asserted complete safety and secure certainty, the scientific community and the emerging evidence could not be successfully managed by MAFF. Moreover, MAFF's attempt to remain fixed within that narrative deprived the institution of its ability to learn from scientific developments or to adapt its policies. The institution tied itself into paralysing knots, and therefore cannot be accurately represented by any simple linear model. Furthermore, even though the provision of a narrative of reassurance was a crucial element in MAFF's BSE policy regime, it was a means to an end and not an end in itself. An inverted Red Book model would therefore only serve to highlight some aspects of the BSE saga, but not capture its complexity.

The key features of our analysis will be highlighted by providing an analytical summary of the different kinds of interactions between science and policy that we have documented in the historical chapters. A useful distinction can be made between policy considerations that influenced the nature of the institutional processes and practices within which scientific activities took place, and those that directly influenced the cognitive aspects of science, i.e. peoples' beliefs about, and representations of, risk. The two are, of course, often related. A decision about whether or not to convene an expert group to study BSE is not in itself a scientific decision, nor does it directly influence scientific claims, but it may have significant indirect consequences for what institutions and individuals subsequently come to know and believe about the disease.

A distinction can also be drawn between three distinct phases during which social and political considerations interacted with science, namely those that occurred upstream, mid-stream and downstream. Upstream issues are those in which policy considerations were deployed, or rather could be deployed, prior (logically or temporally) to the detailed investigations and deliberations of scientists. Midstream issues, by contrast, are those in which policy considerations were, or could be, deployed during the process of scientific deliberation and investigation, whilst downstream issues are those in which policy considerations were, or could be, deployed subsequent to a process of detailed scientific deliberation.

Even though, for analytical purposes, we are differentiating between the upstream, mid-stream and downstream, and between policy influences on the processes within which scientific activities occur and on the scientific activities themselves, we are not suggesting that these phases and sites of interaction are unrelated or disconnected, or that in practice they can always be clearly distinguished. In the BSE saga, upstream issues about, for example, the composition of an advisory committee and the kinds of questions it should be asked were often decided by the same institution, division and even personnel as those responsible for downstream representations of the grounds upon which policies had been decided. It is therefore not surprising that organisations try to ensure that the various streams are framed and managed in a consistent manner, and part of what the historical chapters in this book have done is to indicate the extent to which those attempts were successful.

Upstream interactions of science and politics

Upstream interactions between science and politics occurred partly because social considerations shaped the institutional context – the structures, procedures and practices – within which scientific investigations and deliberations took place. This section first summarises key features of that institutional context. MAFF's institutional context was partly a reflection of the historical culture of UK policy-making but also a product of a series of more tangible decisions and commitments about how policy processes ought to operate. Those decisions and commitments are identified below, and an indication provided as to how they influenced understandings of BSE.

Secrecy and the dissemination of information

In their very earliest interactions, politics compromised the science, and it did so primarily by deliberately imposing a policy of secrecy. When BSE first emerged, CVL staff immediately recognised that knowledge of a new scrapie-like disease might have adverse implications for trade in cattle, and a policy of confidentiality was adopted from the outset. That was the response of a scientific institution that was not just sensitive to the political and economic implications of its judgements, but fully subordinated to the policies and agenda of its political masters.

The behaviour of the CVL scientists in 1986 was, nonetheless, understandable. Under the terms of their contracts of employment, publishing or otherwise disclosing any information about BSE (even its mere existence) without the explicit prior consent of their superiors would have been unlawful. CVL staff were MAFF civil servants who owed their loyalty to their department, to which scientific knowledge, truth and the public interest were bound to be subordinated. The provisions of the Official Secrets Act implied that all departmental information had to be kept secret unless and until disclosure was officially authorised. Confidentiality, and subordinating decisions about disclosure to senior officials and to Ministers, was fully internalised in the culture of all governmental institutions in the UK.

When MAFF officials and Ministers learnt about BSE, they too insisted, at least until late 1987, on the policy of secrecy that their subordinates had dutifully adopted. BSE was seen, first and foremost, as a threat to the commercial interests of the meat industry and to the political reputation of the Department. Consequently both domestic and overseas consumers were kept in the dark about BSE, but so too was the Department of Health. Most members of the scientific and medical communities did not even learn about the existence of BSE until the spring of 1988, some 15 months after MAFF was first alerted. The minimum conditions for a proper response from the scientific community to BSE (as a new disease) were knowingly and deliberately prevented from being met. It is hard to diagnose, recognise, report or conduct research into something not known to exist.

Although information about BSE began to be disseminated beyond the official veterinary community after October 1987, MAFF continued to try to control and restrict the flows and representations of information about the disease until its abolition in 2001. Earlier chapters have documented numerous examples where access to information was restricted but in this context two are worth particular emphasis.

First, knowledge about the nature and extent of the possible risks from BSE, and the resulting policies, were highly dependent on accurate epidemiological information about the disease. Yet, the policy assumption that access to information about BSE must be tightly controlled by MAFF for non-scientific policy reasons was so deeply entrenched that it took until 1998, and the threat of a public rebuke from the President of the Royal Society, before MAFF would allow one of the country's most highly regarded teams of epidemiologists (but even then not the rest of the scientific community or the general public) to gain access to sufficient data to enable them to start to develop predictive models of the epidemics of BSE and variant-CJD.

Second, MAFF chose to put enormous weight on its representation of the conclusions of its advisory committees, but in several crucial respects those committees were working in the dark. When SEAC was asked to advise on slaughterhouse practices it was not told about concerns and anecdotal evidence relating to carcass splitting and cross contamination that were being raised by the meat industry, abattoir inspectors, officials and Ministers. Failing to provide the broader scientific community, and the general public, with adequate and appropriate information was bad enough, but not to provide that information to your own selected official experts, when MAFF knew that the information would be important to SEAC, was in our view pathological, unforgivable and anti-scientific.

Research strategies

We have found no direct evidence to show that MAFF deliberately chose not to invest in lines of research that might have produced results that could undermine its policy. There is, however, plenty of evidence showing that MAFF did not consider BSE research to be a high priority. Because senior MAFF officials and ministers insisted that they had secure knowledge to show that BSE was perfectly safe, they had few incentives to invest in research to diminish incidental residual uncertainties. MAFF was especially reluctant to fund research by any of its many critics or by institutions or individuals over which it would have been hard to exercise control.

In Chapter 6 we showed how a number of policy-relevant and policy-sensitive research questions were not addressed until several years into the BSE saga, some not until after March 1996. In this context one is worthy of emphasis, namely the lack of a centralised and computerised cattle-tagging and record-keeping system. Such a system was recommended on numerous occasions, promised several times by MAFF but it was not delivered until 1998, after the European Commission had insisted on such a system as a precondition for lifting the export ban on UK beef. A centralised database would not only have been vital for tracing the antecedents and descendants of BSE clinical cases, in case evidence of vertical transmission were to emerge, but also as a condition for conducting adequate epidemiological research into BSE. MAFF failure to require and create such a system substantially diminished the opportunities for scientists to improve their understanding of BSE.

The involvement of external experts

The fact that, as we believe appears from the proceeding chapters, the protection of public health was not the primary goal of MAFF's BSE policy made an enormous difference to the ways in which decisions were taken by Ministers and senior officials about whether or not, when and how to involve external scientific advisors in policy-making. Those decisions, in turn, had important consequences for the development of policy.

In the UK, for the first eighteen months of the BSE saga, MAFF did not seek any external scientific advice about BSE, formal or otherwise. The policy of concealing the disease, and of not just allowing but requiring diseased animals to enter the human food chain, was not based on scientific evidence or advice, but on a decision to avoid consulting or involving scientific advisors.

From mid-1988 onwards, only very few external scientists were asked to advise MAFF on BSE policy, usually as members of one of the government's three key advisory committees. Prior to 1995, when MAFF's control over the composition of SEAC weakened, the majority of advisory scientists had been animal health specialists. Some ostensibly 'external' advisors were indirectly or formerly employed by MAFF and at least one was acting as a paid consultant on BSE to the meat and pet food industries. MAFF officials acknowledged that it was important to choose members of advisory committees carefully in order to provide scientific credence to their findings and recommendations (Hollis 1998). Prior to 1995 none of the government's external advisors was active in TSE research. Scientists with responsibility for, or specialist knowledge of, public health, especially staff at the Public Health Laboratory Service, were excluded from official deliberations on the possible risks from BSE partly because their involvement would have given the impression that the government was concerned about possible risks to public health (Phillips *et al.* 2000, vol. 11, para. 4.28).

Reliance on a small number of advisors from a narrow range of disciplinary backgrounds meant that only some types of uncertainties would be recognised or acknowledged. For example, none of the members of the Southwood Working Party appeared to recognise that, even if BSE had resulted from exposure to an unmodified scrapie agent, it might not behave in the same way as the scrapie agent once present in a new host. The Southwood Working Party failed to acknowledge that possibility, even though it was widely appreciated within the TSE research community.

The Southwood Working Party, the Tyrell Committee and SEAC became the principal sources of external advice to MAFF, but the department sometimes sought advice from those committees when it did not need to. For example, in the late 1980s MAFF officials, including senior scientific civil servants, were well aware that no-one knew whether or not BSE would infect human beings. Nonetheless, MAFF officials used the Southwood Working Party to persuade Ministers to exclude the carcasses of clinically diseased cattle from the food chain, but otherwise to provide a seemingly scientific endorsement for the department's policy decisions on BSE that had already been taken, which entailed continued human exposure to the BSE pathogen from asymptomatic animals. Subsequently, SEAC was often asked, in effect, to legitimate policy decisions that MAFF Ministers and/or officials had already taken.

On the other hand, MAFF sometimes avoided seeking advice from the scientific advisory committees on topics when it might have been helpful. For example, decisions about the scope of the SBO ban were made without the benefit of any external advisors. There were a few occasions when advisors were asked for their opinion on the merits of including or excluding particular types of tissues from the SBO ban, but only because animal health officials in MAFF had been unable to obtain support for their proposals from colleagues at the Department of Health and from other branches of MAFF.

MAFF's failure to involve external expert advisors on issues where they could have been useful, and their involvement on issues for which scientific advice was unnecessary, entailed that decision-makers were less well-informed than they should have been and contributed to delaying decisions by MAFF. Several of the consequences of those practices are summarised below. The historical evidence adduced in Chapters 4–7 strongly suggests, however, that those practices were only sustainable because of the opacity of the policy-making system. If policy-making processes had been transparent, it would have been far harder for the department to use external experts to provide a narrative of legitimation for policy decisions that had already been taken.

Setting the agendas for scientific deliberations

The evidence we have adduced shows not just that scientific advisory committees are sensitive to the political, economic and social context in which they are operating, but it also shows the specific assumptions that framed and defined the kinds of issues that the advisory committees were expected to address and, more importantly perhaps, the reports that they issued. The Southwood Working Party was not expected to provide what would now be called a risk assessment of BSE. It was expected to provide and endorse a peculiarly narrow and convoluted narrative. That narrative was a curious blend of scientific and policy considerations of MAFF and the Department of Health's own making.

Chapter 5 explained that the terms of reference given to the Southwood Working Party were couched in exceptionally broad (and vague) terms, but that in practice officials tried to ensure, *perforce* discreetly, that the scope of the Working Party's deliberations were narrowly circumscribed and carefully managed. For example, officials persuaded the committee not to provide any advice concerning the economically sensitive issues of possible risks to (and from) non-ruminant mammals (such as pigs) or the export of contaminated animal feed-stuffs, even though, for sound scientific reasons, both were issues of concern to Southwood and his colleagues. Since the formal scope of the committee's remit had not excluded the issues on which it reluctantly agreed not to advise, MAFF officials were able to represent those omissions as indicating there were no scientific grounds for concern or action, even though those officials knew that the absence of advice on those matters represented a reluctant decision to acquiesce with the policies that MAFF had already chosen.

After Southwood and his colleagues had reported, neither the Tyrell Committee nor SEAC were ever asked to provide a comprehensive assessment of the risks that BSE might pose. Instead, SEAC was routinely asked to advise on narrow and fragmented questions, along the lines of: 'Does this new study or item of evidence on its own compel us to change the regulations concerning, or our understanding about, the safety of British beef?' If SEAC had been asked, for example, what impact the weight of evidence from the entire range of available information had on its assessment of any risks that BSE might pose, radically different answers might have been provided. The one occasion on which anything approximating to what would now be called a 'risk assessment' was requested came in 1990 when SEAC was asked to make a statement on the safety of beef, but in that context SEAC was effectively asked to endorse and reinforce statements on the safety of British beef that had already been made by ministers and senior officials.

MAFF's senior policy officials with responsibility for BSE were repeatedly reluctant to develop or request a comprehensive assessment of the possible risks from BSE, even from the Department's own internal scientific staff. During the first 18 months of the BSE saga, before the Southwood Working Party had been established, MAFF made no systematic attempt to assess the possible risks from BSE. In 1989, after MAFF learnt that the pet food industry had attempted quantitatively to estimate the risks from its products, the Head of MAFF's Food Science Division recommended explicitly that a quantitative risk assessment exercise on human foodstuffs should *not* be conducted because it might indicate that there were significant risks, which would in turn necessitate restrictions that were inconsistent with the government's policy objectives. We say that those deliberations, and their outcomes, show that MAFF saw science as little more than a tactical tool that could and should serve strategic ends. Scientific advice was not seen or used to provide an independent benchmark against which to compare policy options.

At the European Commission, risk managers also attempted to discourage scientific officials from assessing the risks posed by BSE. In September 1990, for example, the Commission's Scientific Veterinary Committee wanted to re-examine a previous Council decision on BSE but the Agriculture Commissioner instructed the Director General for Agriculture to 'stop any meeting' (European Parliament 1997, Annex 20). Furthermore, officials from DG-VI told the Standing Veterinary Committee a few weeks later that: 'It is necessary to keep cool so as not to provoke unfavourable market responses. Do not talk about BSE any more. This item should not appear on the agenda' (ibid., Annex 22).

Articulating policy objectives and policy options

One important set of factors that can influence the scope of any scientific deliberations is the particular range of policy objectives that are known, or believed, to be under consideration. Although decisions about which particular policies to adopt, in light of a scientific assessment, are what we categorise as downstream issues, prior decisions about the range of possible policy options and the overall objectives of policy can, and frequently do, influence the agenda of scientific advisors.

Scientific advisors were often not told explicitly about the government's policy objectives and options. Instead, they either guessed or shared an implicit understanding with officials. Members of the Southwood Working Party understood that restrictions on subclinically infected animals were not then considered politically feasible. That understanding of the constraints on the range of available policy options influenced the working party's selection and interpretation of the evidence, even without overt or conspicuous pressure from officials. Consequently, the Southwood Working Party's report paid very little attention to the risks from subclinical infection. Anxiety, on the part of Southwood and colleagues, about the possibility of disturbing Ministers' political equilibrium seems to have been sufficient to provoke an act of self-censorship that could not be discerned even from a careful reading of its report.

In circumstances where advisors simply guess the range of feasible policy options, or are only told discreetly, third parties may fail to recognise the constraints on the scope of the advice from a scientific committee and may assume that a far broader range of issues had been considered than was actually the case. For example, even some Ministers in MAFF believed that there was no scientific case for controls on asymptomatic animals rather than recognising that the Working Party had self-censored its evidently genuine concerns. Unless the actual objectives of policy-makers are openly and explicitly acknowledged, and some indication is provided concerning the range of policy options that are available and those that are under consideration, it is all too easy for key assumptions informing scientific advisors to be misunderstood and/or misrepresented.

The problem in the BSE saga was not, however, just that the policy objectives and options were not articulated. Sometimes scientific advisors were actively inhibited from providing relevant information and advice. MAFF's policy goal of always reassuring domestic and international consumers was never going to be consistent with the provisions of accurate depictions of the possible risks and their attendant uncertainties. Southwood and his colleagues internalised the goal of providing reassurance in several different ways. The Working Party's anxiety not to cause alarm entailed that its conclusion – that risks to humans was remote – was perversely dependent on the assumption that the committee's recommendations had already been implemented. Unfortunately many policy-makers were unaware of that assumption and consequently compliance with regulatory controls were not viewed as vital, with obvious problems for both compliance and enforcement.

Similar complications also occurred in Brussels. At the European Commission officials from the internal market and the agriculture Directorates-General sometimes sought to discreetly influence the deliberations and conclusions of their expert scientific advisory committees. In September 1990, for example, officials from DG-VI told the Standing Veterinary Committee that 'the BSE affair must be minimised by using disinformation' (European Parliament 1997, Annex 22, p. 99). In 1994, the head of DG-VI wrote to the German Federal Ministry of Health asking it to reprimand two German participants of the SVC and to ask them to refrain from issuing dissenting scientific opinions that were inconsistent with the proposals of the Commission (ibid., Annex 25, p. 111). Regulatory regimes in which the policy objectives are not genuinely and primarily orientated to the protection of public health may simply not be compatible with the production of robust scientific advice about risks to health.

Mid-stream interactions of science and politics

The concept of 'mid-stream' interactions between science and politics is used here to refer to those interactions that take place during processes of scientific deliberation and analysis. They include, for example, decisions and assumptions about which kinds of knowledge claims are taken for granted during scientific analysis and which kinds are critically investigated, and about which types of uncertainty to investigate, ignore or highlight.

Boundaries between assumed and critically examined knowledge claims

All scientific deliberations about risk need to presume a boundary between beliefs and knowledge claims that are assumed to be correct and the knowledge claims and evidence that are subject to a critical assessment. Where that boundary is located may depend on intellectual judgements, which may be in turn be influenced both by policy considerations and by issues of a entirely practical kind – for example, the availability of resources. The precise location of such boundaries can have important consequences for what is considered to be valid knowledge.

For example, the Southwood Working Party's important conclusion that it was 'most unlikely that BSE will have any implications for human health' was based on a rationale that was not its own. John Wilesmith, the CVL's veterinary epidemiologist, had written a paper in which he had concluded, on the basis of the available epidemiological data, that it was highly likely that the BSE agent was simply 'scrapie in cattle', and moreover a version of scrapie that had not altered in passing to cattle. The Southwood Working Party simply took Wilesmith's narrative at face value, and allowed his text to be reproduced in and as theirs, despite not having reviewed his arguments critically, and without having seen the data or even being allowed access to it, despite recognising that it might be an unreliable claim. Unfortunately, the Southwood Working Party's Report, which recycled and seemed to endorse Wilesmith's account, was routinely treated by numerous Ministers and public officials as if it had been conclusive and definitive, even after new evidence emerged that was inconsistent with the narrative and its underlying rationale.

Assumptions about compliance and enforcement

Risks are not purely physical phenomena, since their occurrence can depend on particular sets of social actions and practices. Scientific judgements about risks therefore typically have to make assumptions about, or analyses of, the extent of compliance with, and enforcement of, regulations. When SEAC advised on slaughterhouse practices the committee was careful to point out that its conclusions were dependent on the assumption that regulations could and would be properly enforced, even though in practice officials subsequently ignored that caveat. By contrast, the Southwood Working Party's advice that the risks to humans from BSE were 'remote' assumed not only that the controls on the food chain and pharmaceutical production system they had recommended would be properly enforced but also, as we have pointed out, that they had already been introduced. Not surprisingly, the timely introduction, proper compliance with and enforcement of regulatory controls was not consequently viewed as vital by many in the trade.

Representations of scientific knowledge

Perhaps the most important mid-stream issue over which science and politics interacted during the BSE saga was when advisory scientists had to decide how scientific knowledge about the risks should be represented, both to the public in general and to those within the policy-making institutions. Scientists were invariably faced with choices about which kinds of issues to focus on and which kinds uncertainties and data gaps to acknowledge and highlight and which to downplay.

In Chapter 5 we showed how numerous unacknowledged assumptions played a crucial role in the construction of the Southwood Working Party's published account of the possible risks from BSE, and how the selection of those assumptions was influenced by powerful but discreet policy factors. A willingness to avoid providing Ministers with unwelcome advice, and a concern to avoid alarming the public, lead the Working Party to conceal some of the uncertainties and many of their own doubts and to provide an optimistic and reassuring narrative. By recommending minimal restrictions, and then providing reassurance, the Working Party gave the mistaken impression that there was a clear threshold between the risks that were being actively controlled, and the remainder that did not need to be controlled. In the absence of any quantitative estimation of possible risks, the only way to understand the outcome of the Working Party's deliberations is as a combination of a small amount of science and a substantial amount of political considerations, misrepresented in a technocratic idiom. It is notable that the principal criticism of the Working Party in the report of the Phillip's Inquiry was that by understating their concerns about the risks and the uncertainties, and by understating their doubts about the safety of BSE, members of the Working Party endorsed a report that failed to sensitise the government to the need regularly to review and reassess those risks.

In many jurisdictions, the conclusions of scientific advisory committees are routinely depicted as consensual, presumably on the grounds that evidence that scientists disagree amongst themselves might undermine the authority of their advice. That practice inevitably fails to acknowledge competing judgements about how uncertainties should be interpreted. In July 1994, for example, two members of the European Commission's Scientific Advisory Committee dissented from a majority view about the risks of British beef and argued that muscle from animals incubating BSE might contain the infective agent and that therefore all meat from British cattle should be excluded from the human food chain (Scientific Veterinary Committee 1994).

Downstream interactions of science and politics

Since the inverted decisionist model, encapsulated in what we term the 'Red Book model', has become the new orthodoxy, the existence and legitimacy of downstream non-scientific considerations in science-based policy decision-making has become widely acknowledged. Many of those who accept that some downstream inputs are relevant and indispensable may nevertheless underestimate the complexity, subtlety and importance of the ways in which, for example, scientific advice is communicated and science is interpreted for policy. During the BSE saga, many of what we consider to be 'downstream' issues were in practice relocated or reassigned to the midstream stage, in the UK and in most other jurisdictions. In particular, advisory scientists were expected to deploy their own political judgements, or to incorporate officials' political judgements into decisions that were then subsequently represented as scientific.

Representing the advice of the scientists by policy-makers

Expert advisors were not the only actors involved in articulating assessments of the possible risks posed by BSE. Just as importantly, senior officials and Ministers were responsible for communicating the advice from their own internal and external scientific advisors to others within official institutions and to the public in general. As the Phillips Inquiry concluded, MAFF's communication strategy was one of 'sedation' (Phillips *et al.* 2000, vol. 1, para. 1179, p. 233). The absence of direct evidence of risk was routinely represented by senior officials within MAFF as if it provided direct evidence of the absence of any risk. Known uncertainties were almost always discounted or understated. The advice that was being received was consistently represented as reassuring, certain, secure and sufficient.

In particular, from the publication of the report of the Southwood Working Party in 1989 until March 1996, UK Ministers and senior officials endeavoured to represent the Southwood report not as an early and rudimentary representation of available evidence and understandings, but as if it had provided a final and conclusive judgement. We have also argued that senior MAFF officials also took full advantage of numerous opportunities to conceal from their Ministers, junior colleagues and the general public the limitations officials had discreetly placed on the scope of the Working Party's deliberations. The absence of any remarks on issues that fell outside the Working Party's remit was routinely portrayed as demonstrating the absence of any scientific concerns.

Unfortunately, presumably because officials assumed that dissemination of the truth would undermine the Department's political and economic goals, we say they not only provided an optimistic gloss on the available evidence, but occasionally also tried to distort more fundamentally the scientific understandings and representations of the risks that BSE might pose. We believe the attempts by senior officials to distort and misrepresent science began right at the start. In mid-1987, MAFF's CVO told CVL scientists that they could only release details of BSE to the professional veterinary community if scrapie was not mentioned; a restriction that CVL scientists refused to adopt on the grounds that it was scientifically indefensible. In public, senior scientifically trained officials also sometimes made public statements that could not be sustained, even by an optimistic reading of the available evidence, for example, about the complete absence of any infectivity in the food supply. We believe such claims were not simply less precautionary than the evidence suggested; they were profoundly unscientific.

Risk managers from the UK also sometimes sought to alter the conclusions of European advisory committees. For example, in November 1989, the EU's

Scientific Advisory Committee concluded that meat from countries with BSE 'is not considered to be a (significant) danger to public health.' A British note of that meeting pointed out that

> By contact with Mr Marchant in Brussels [the Commission official responsible for convening the meeting and an ex-MAFF employee] we are attempting to have [the word 'significant'] removed since it is inconsistent with the present and accepted scientific data.

(Bradley 2000)

By June 1990, at another crucially important meeting of the Scientific Advisory Committee, the word 'significant' had been dropped (Scientific Veterinary Committee 1990).

Scientists within CVL and MAFF occasionally sent clear signals indicating to Ministers that they should not claim that British beef was perfectly safe, and that the tissues permitted in the human food chain might contain the BSE pathogen, but Ministers either did not receive those messages or would not accept the advice. In several instances, as with CVL's advice about the potential risks from mechanically recovered meat and the risks of sheep contracting BSE in 1989, or SEAC advice on the safety of beef in 1990, it appears senior agriculture officials failed to convey to Ministers the true picture that was being painted by the scientists. On other occasions the evidence appears to have been simply insufficient to support the statements of senior officials, as for example when MAFF's CVO told Ministers in 1989 that residual levels of the BSE agent in tissues not included in the SBO ban would be insignificant or that the emergence of a feline TSE in 1990 was of little consequence. MAFF Ministers made the mistake of taking at face value the narratives that their senior officials were providing.

Decisions in MAFF about how to represent risks, both internally and externally, were driven by prior policy commitments to provide reassurance to customers that British beef, milk and dairy products were entirely safe, and to avoid harming the beef industry, rather than to minimise the risk to the public, and science was subordinated to that purpose. Both MAFF and the European Commission succumbed to a form of inflexible rigor mortis because any acknowledgement of uncertainty of possible risks would have been seen, correctly, as a thin but irresistible end of a substantial wedge. Consequently, officials vigorously resisted proposals to introduce what they knew would be practical and cheap risk-reducing measures.

Interpreting science for policy

The UK Government's three BSE expert advisory committees were expected not only to advise on the nature of the possible risks from BSE but also to provide specific policy recommendations. That was arguably their main task and part of what we have documented has been the strategies adopted by officials to influence the process, thereby ensuring that MAFF's policy objectives were recycled through the scientific advice that it engineered. The Southwood Working Party was convened by the CMO to persuade ministers marginally to shift to a new policy of excluding overtly diseased cattle from the food chain and, in the event, that was the only major policy change that it recommended. By the time SEAC had been established, all the key regulations were in place and the primary role of the committee was to advise on the *policy* implications of *new* evidence. That was a task that the committee understandably found difficult though, more often than not, it was willing to defer to the preferred response of MAFF officials.

It would be an oversimplification, which we have not made, to suggest that MAFF simply decided what policy advice it wanted to receive and then tried to ensure that, as far as possible, it obtained the advice that it already knew that it wanted to receive. Scientists have rarely been putty in the hands of ministers and senior officials. On the other hand, expert scientific advisors always knew the dominant and preferred policy framework within which they were being asked for their advice. Although the committees did not always comply exactly with the government's preferred policy intentions, their advice rarely deviated significantly from the dominant policy framework.

For most of the duration of the BSE saga, the authorities (both in the UK and in other jurisdictions) successfully followed a policy of risk reduction, not risk elimination. In practice the benchmark used by policy-makers to decide the level down to which risks were to be reduced were those that provided sufficient reassurance to stabilise the market for beef and to protect Ministerial reputations. The role of expert advisors was, when seen from the point of view of MAFF, to represent that cusp as if it were scientifically justified and as if it was independent of political and economic considerations.

The practice of asking scientific experts to make downstream evaluative policy decisions may have provided a shield, or set of shields, behind which Ministers and officials could hide – especially when those decisions were misrepresented as scientifically legitimated – but it was problematic. Clearly, scientists did not have the mandate to make judgements about the social acceptability of a risk, even if all they were doing in practice was covertly endorsing and defending official and Ministerial judgments on those matters. In any case, scientists did not usually possess the requisite expertise to make downstream trade-offs between the possible risks, costs, practicalities and benefits of various policy options. Committee members typically knew little about the practices or economics of the meat industry, and reliance on the committees to make or endorse policies often resulted in poor decisions. For example, the Southwood Working Party failed to recommend controls on, or raise concerns about, the practice of producing and using mechanically recovered meat, but then its members probably did not even know that such a process existed.

Representing the basis for policy decisions

We argue that the true nature of, and grounds for, policy decisions were routinely misrepresented by Ministers, senior officials and in some cases by members of the government's advisory committees. Usually, this was achieved by representing policy as based solely on scientific considerations, thus providing the impression that political decisions about the acceptability of risk were just scientific judgements about the extent to which risks existed. That tactic was not always easy to disguise. For example, the Southwood Working Party possessed, and could provide, no scientific rationale for its judgement that overtly diseased animals were deemed sufficiently risky to be excluded from the human food chain while subclinically infected animals, that were presumed to be contaminated with the BSE pathogen but not yet exhibiting symptoms of BSE, were deemed to be acceptably safe. Their reasoning was crucially dependent on non-scientific policy considerations, as critics in 1989 were quick to point out, though the precise nature of those considerations could not be discerned by reading their report.

Most of the time, however, the real grounds for the government's policy decisions on BSE were successfully disguised. UK BSE policy would not have been politically or scientifically sustainable if that had been otherwise. One problem was that it was not just the public who were unaware of the policy choices that had been exercised, and who were therefore unable to exercise their own judgements about whether to expose themselves and their families to a possible risk. Many in the core policy community were also unaware of the full spectrum of policy choices available or of the selections that had been made. It was consequently often hard for Ministers and key officials to appreciate the scope for, or the strength of the case for, exercising precaution, or for those responsible for implementing and enforcing regulations to appreciate their importance.

We also believe British members of the European Commission's Veterinary Committees (which consisted predominantly of scientifically trained officials from the Member States) did not always accurately represent the grounds for their decisions within the committee meetings in an attempt to avoid broader Community-wide restrictions on the export of British beef. For example, in September 1989, British members of the Standing Veterinary Committee

(SVC) told their continental European colleagues that '[t]he action taken [in the UK] to slaughter and destroy suspect animals and their milk was purely precautionary to ensure that public confidence was maintained' (Lawrence 1990). That was not true. The Southwood Working Party had advised the UK government to remove clinically affected animals on clear public health grounds (Phillips *et al.* 2000, vol. 1, para. 252).

To cut an extremely long story as short as possible, and to couch our conclusions in general terms, we have shown how the context in which scientific deliberations about risks occur can influence, amongst other things:

+ which experts are invited, involved and excluded
+ which questions are asked and which avoided or discounted
+ which scientific claims are scrutinised and which uncritically accepted
+ which research topics and questions are commissioned and which avoided
+ which data are collected and which omitted or discounted
+ which data are revealed and which concealed
+ which interpretations of the data are considered and which ignored or discounted
+ which interpretations of the evidence and advice are accepted and which rejected
+ which uncertainties and data gaps are acknowledged and which ignored or discounted, and
+ which policies are endorsed and which questioned or undermined.

The types of linkages between science and politics that have been documented in the BSE saga, can and do occur in numerous other domains too. What is special about BSE is not the existence of such linkages, but our ability to document them.

General lessons for science-based risk policy-making

We have concluded that the ways in which science-based policy decisions on BSE were taken were inadequate, inappropriate and unsustainable. Much of our analysis has focused on explaining why that was the case. We have tried to illustrate how, in practice, scientific and non-scientific considerations interacted and why the ways in which those interactions occurred undermined democratic accountability and prevented science from playing a constructive or legitimate role in policy-making. Our analysis does not imply that science and non-scientific considerations can readily be separated into two separate institutions that can be entirely independent of each other. It implies rather that scientific and policy deliberations routinely and necessarily interact, and that those interactions can be legitimate scientifically and democratically but only under certain conditions. The questions therefore are: what are those conditions, and how can science be deployed in policy decision-making processes in ways that are properly democratic without being anti-scientific, and rigorously scientific without being anti-democratic? Our view is that there at least three types of conditions for such legitimacy namely structural, procedural and substantive.

Separating regulation from sponsorship

There are inevitable and generally irreconcilable tensions, within any government, between the promotion of particular industrial and commercial sectors on the one hand and their regulation on the other. The traditional British practice of locating responsibility for regulating a particular sector within the same institution that has responsibility for sponsoring that sector is rarely a sensible way to manage those conflicts. In the BSE saga, the fact that responsibility for regulation lay primarily with ministers of agriculture entailed that the protection of public health was routinely subordinated to goals of commercial and industrial sponsorship. The same institutional arrangement helps to explain why, in the UK and at the European Commission, BSE was perceived primarily as a problem of animal health, trade and consumer confidence, but not a public health problem, at least until March 1996.

The key point, however, is not just that locating responsibility for the control of BSE within a department responsible for sponsoring commercial interests meant that the policies adopted were insufficient adequately to protect public health from the possible risks of BSE. In addition, those institutional structures compromised the ability of scientific evidence, expertise and understanding to enlighten policy deliberations. Science was not used in MAFF to illuminate the possible consequences of adopting a range of different possible courses of action, it was recruited primarily to reinforce a policy trajectory that had already been chosen (at least prior to March 1996).

If, in late 1986 and 1987, the scientific agenda of MAFF's Central Veterinary Laboratory had been solely public health-orientated, it might not have responded to the discovery of BSE by keeping information about the disease secret. A scientific institution that was focused on the protection and promotion of public health might have placed the limited information it had gathered in the public domain and would thereby have informed the scientific and veterinary community and the broader community too, enabling all social groups to consider the existence and possible significance of BSE.

If MAFF's agenda had been genuinely public health-orientated it would have invested and commissioned numerous lines of research that were crucial to reducing the main policy-relevant uncertainties. It might have attempted to perform or commission adequate and regularly updated risk assessments. It might have encouraged the broader scientific community to assist in diminishing the key uncertainties as rapidly as possible and in identifying the possible risks posed by BSE. It might also have shared all relevant information with its expert advisors, and it might have tolerated disagreements amongst its advisors, recognising that dissent and disagreement are vital mechanisms by which learning and the testing of ideas takes place. It might have avoided deploying inaccurate and misleading accounts of the available scientific evidence. If the principal objective of BSE policy had been to protect public health, it would have been far more straightforward for scientific evidence and judgments to be developed in a sound, prudent and responsible fashion.

Public interest science?

All too frequently, as we have shown, expert scientific advisors dealing with public health policy-making internalised, and sometimes even represented, political and economic interests and agendas that were at best tangential to, and at worst antithetical to, the protection of public health. They did so moreover while representing their deliberations and judgements as if they constituted unproblematically sound science.

To diminish the likelihood that official expert advisors will covertly be enrolled into the chosen policy agendas of risk managers, and of other vested interests, there is a powerful case for locating them and their secretariats in institutions that are separate from the policy-making departments that will request and receive their advice. The lines of accountability of expert advisors, and the officials that provide their secretariats, should not be solely to the departments requesting and receiving their advice. They should therefore be institutionally separated from those departments, with their own independent terms of reference, and lines of accountability.

In recent years, moreover, public policy-makers have been trying to change academic cultures by providing researchers with incentives to collaborate with 'users' of research, which is predominantly interpreted as referring to the private sector. It has, moreover, become increasingly difficult to obtain funding for research to investigate potential risks from commercial products. As a consequence, public policy-makers have difficulty in recruiting expert advisors that have the protection of public and environmental health at the centre of their intellectual agendas, and who have not been compromised by their links to, or collaborations with, parts of the private sector.

Transparency

If BSE policy-making in the UK, at least prior to March 1996, had been governed by a comprehensive freedom of information regime, MAFF's policy would have been seen to be scientifically unsustainable and consequently it would have been politically unsustainable. The pivotal claim in the Southwood report that the risks to human health from BSE were remote was constructed by MAFF officials for reasons that were substantially more political than scientific. The claim was scientifically problematic, involving as it did numerous over-optimistic assumptions about the behaviour of the BSE pathogen.

If the available evidence about, and knowledge of, BSE and other TSEs had all been in the public domain then any group of expert advisors, either within the civil service or in ostensibly independent bodies, would have been unable to endorse a regime that repeatedly asserted secure knowledge of complete safety. If, moreover, the expert advisors had conducted their deliberations in public rather than in private, their representation of the science and the risks would not have been able to rely on so many non-scientific assumptions. Transparency of evidence and process would have deprived their advice of any legitimacy it might otherwise have been able to claim. When uncertainties become explicit, political choices become conspicuous and undeniable, and responsibility for making those political choices could shift from appointed expert advisors to elected representatives that are subject to some form of democratic accountability.

The concept of transparency is important, though its meaning and interpretation are contested. From 1986 to 1996 the UK government routinely insisted that it was being entirely open with the scientific evidence about BSE. The kind of transparency which we envisage is rather more exacting and comprehensive than obtained during that era. For policy-making processes to achieve both scientific and democratic legitimacy all the available scientific evidence needs to be in the public domain, from the point at which it is received by the policy-making institution. There are no longer any scientific or technological reasons for not making all such information publicly accessible; electronic files can be published on an institution's web site within a few moments of being received.

The traditional practice in the UK, at the European Commission and most European states, was only to publish some, but never all, of the available information, and even then only once policies had been decided. The selection and interpretation of the available evidence was routinely tailored to suit the policy that had been decided, and any suggestions that the evidence might have supported alternative policy options, as well or even better, were conspicuous by their overwhelming absence.

The kind of transparency that our analysis suggests will be important would reveal both the extent and limitation of prevailing knowledge. It should also ensure full disclosure about the existence of expert advisory committees and their recruitment, membership, remit and possible conflicts of interest. The ways in which expert advisors select and interpret evidence should be revealed rather than concealed, and so too should be such framing and policy guidance as policy-makers provide. Under those conditions the relationships between scientific and non-scientific considerations should become easier to discern and harder to conceal or misrepresent. Experts need to be accountable to their professional peers and to the broader society, and nothing can help confer legitimacy on their contributions to policy-making more than their demonstrating that they have nothing to hide. The scope of the rules of transparency should also extend to research decision-making, because stakeholders have an interest in knowing the steps that are being taken to diminish the policy-relevant uncertainties.

Expert scientific advisors have everything to gain, and nothing to lose, from conducting all their meetings and deliberations in public. Nothing else could more effectively confer scientific and democratic legitimacy onto their deliberations and advice. Were they to do so, it would however transform their relationships with, and the responsibilities of, civil servants and government ministers; but those transformation should improve the scientific legitimacy of the advice available to policy-makers, and contribute to conferring greater democratic legitimacy on their decisions.

Articulating the objectives of policy and the scope of the requested advice

When expert committees were asked by policy-makers for their advice about the existence and consequences of risks, members of those committees have typically been well aware of the policy constraints within which their advice had been sought and in which it will be used. The subsequent reports of the advisory committees have, however, usually been presented in ways that concealed those constraints and assumptions, and implied that the experts' advice had been constructed in isolation of, and abstraction from, their contexts. The current arrangement of just labelling advisers as 'independent' and presuming or pretending that their deliberations and judgements are socially and politically neutral is insufficient, especially while those delibera-tions remain insufficiently transparent.

If the kinds of mistakes that characterised the conduct of BSE policy-making are not to be repeated, advisory scientists, and others, will need to know explicitly what the objectives of policy are, what courses of action are under consideration, and which might be implemented. Scientific deliberations on risks cannot deliver useful relevant advice on decision-making in a policy vacuum. If scientists are to comment usefully on possible risks, and policy responses to those risks, they need to consider, and give advice on, what is known (and not known) about the likely consequences of following, or failing to follow, alternative possible courses of action. They therefore need explicitly to know which policy goals are being sought and which options are under consideration. Ministers and senior officials may no longer be able to pretend that they are merely following the advice of scientific experts and are not responsible for any of the key judgements or decisions. The solution is not to pretend that experts deliberate in a vacuum or that scientists are indifferent to any and all competing social interests and values, but rather to show that those considerations are being dealt with in an open, accountable, systematic and legitimate fashion.

Decisions about the scope of advice and the particular questions that advisors will be expected to assess, should therefore be explicit rather than implicit or provided discreetly or left to the committee members themselves to second guess. Although the scope of a risk assessment may in practice need to be negotiated between policy-makers, scientists and other stakeholders, responsibility for deciding those agenda-setting issues should rest with those who are subject to democratic accountability. Expert advisors could then be expected to indicate how their deliberations have taken account of the risk assessment policy guidance with which they should be provided. Scientific advisors may be at liberty to extend the scope of their deliberations, but if they were to do so they could be expected to provide an explanation of how and why they have done so. Under those conditions, the scientific and non-scientific strands of risk appraisal and policy decision-making could be disentangled to the maximum extent possible, and the relationship between them clarified and legitimated.

Recognising and reporting uncertain and incomplete knowledge

Regulatory policy-makers typically need to make decisions in circumstances where scientific knowledge is uncertain, incomplete and disputed. Yet, the output of most regulatory agencies and their expert scientific advisory committees have historically been replete with discussions of risks and evidence from which discussions of scientific uncertainty were almost entirely absent, or present only selectively and in homeopathic doses. The impression has typically been that consensus has been arrived at within expert committees even when there had been undisclosed disagreements about what the available evidence indicated and about how much more evidence to request. It has been even rarer for regulatory agencies or their committees to acknowledge that they might be ignorant about key aspects of possible risks. That practice has enabled policy-makers and their advisors to pretend that no adverse effects could be anticipated.

For policy-makers, the task of having to choose how to respond to uncertain risks will never be entirely straightforward, but it could be more tractable if decision-makers were better informed. One condition for being well informed would be to oblige scientific civil servants and external expert advisors to draw the policy-makers' attention to the full range of policy-relevant uncertainties. If MAFF policy-makers had reached decisions in a scientifically and democratically legitimate way they would also have needed to acknowledge the uncertainties, and acknowledged that their judgements concerned the extent to which, and the ways in which, precaution could and would be exercised.

The Phillips Inquiry has rightly recommended that uncertainties should be explicitly identified by expert committees (Phillips *et al.* 2000, vol. 1, para. 1290). One reason why uncertainties were often not fully acknowledged in BSE policy-making was because the advisory committees were expected to provide prescriptive policy recommendations. A frank discussion of uncertainties would have undermined the apparent authority of the committee's policy recommendations. If advisors were to confine their comments to scientific matters, and avoid making prescriptive policy recommendations, then the incentives to conceal the uncertainties would be significantly diminished.

Although many of the uncertainties concerning BSE were recognised, at least privately, by external advisors and by MAFF scientists, that was not always the case. By obtaining advice from a broad range of different parts of the scientific community, and from other stakeholder groups, the likelihood that policy-makers would recognise key policy-relevant uncertainties would be significantly increased. One tactic for encouraging the explicit recognition of uncertainties (and for guarding against official misrepresentations of evidence and advice) would be to commission more than one expert group to conduct a particular category of risk assessment. A plurality of sources of advice can help to make scientific uncertainties explicit and can encourage policy-makers and their expert advisors to be frank about the ways in which they construct and represent their assessments of risk. Furthermore, where competing risk assessments are juxtaposed the underlying differences in framing conditions are more likely to be evident than if they are considered individually. Diversity probably complicates the procedure by which closure is reached in policy-making, but it can contribute to conferring scientific and democratic legitimacy on policies which would not otherwise attain such legitimacy.

Coupling science with policy: the provision of plural and conditional advice

By long tradition, stretching back at least 50 years, policy-makers have routinely expected their expert advisory committees to provide them with discussions of evidence and conclusions about risks as if they were definitive, and with advice on specific policies and courses of action, even though the policy-makers themselves have routinely failed to provide their expert advisers with explicit guidance concerning their policy objectives and the scope and parameters within which the experts were expected to develop their advice. Risk assessment policies and other framing conditions have been highly influential, though typically invisible. For many years, scientists who had been selected to join official expert committee acquiesced in, or colluded with, that arrangement. The BSE saga demonstrates that scientists would frequently internalise the ambiguities between, and the tensions amongst, the policy objectives that ministers were expected to meet. Consequently they provided advice that was tailored to suit the policy agendas, while portraying that advice as politically neutral. Those arrangements provided Ministers with spuriously scientific shields behind which they could hide – as they endeavoured to insist that their policy decisions had been scientifically legitimated, and that the only kind of legitimation that policies could have, or needed, was scientific.

Scientific considerations can never, by themselves, entail specific judgements about what levels of risk, and which levels of uncertainty, are acceptable – that is always a social and political judgement. Consequently, whenever scientific advisers provided policy-makers with 'prescriptive' and 'monolithic' (Stirling 2003) advice those advisors had made policy judgements that were not, and could not have been, legitimated by the scientific evidence and understandings available to them, and opportunities will remain for policy-makers to use experts to shield themselves from taking responsibility for policy-decisions.

The provision of what Stirling has called 'plural and conditional' advice (Stirling 2003) would help ensure that the different roles of scientific advisors and policy-makers are clearly and appropriately differentiated, and that what we have called upstream, midstream and downstream policy judgements are rendered transparent and subject to social choice. Plural advice, instead of providing a single estimate of the existence, and likely significance, of a risk, would consist of a range of alternative risk scenarios. It may involve making explicit the uncertainties and assumptions inherent in alternative reasonings. Conditional advice would mean that expert advisors would provide a commentary on the range of alternative possible courses of action that policy-makers might adopt, each predicated on a set of explicitly articulated assumptions which a scientific committee is neither competent nor mandated to decide. That advice would indicate what was, and was not, known about the possible and/or likely consequences of following, or failing to follow, alternative possible courses of action, but it would be the responsibility of policy-makers to identify and justify particular policies and courses of action. It is policy-makers who should be responsible for deciding which options to adopt, and they should be held accountable for their decisions, by reference to their choices and rankings of competing social, economic and political objectives and interests.

Summary

If both policy-makers and expert advisors acknowledge that non-scientific considerations invariably exert some influence on their deliberations and advice, and a genuinely transparent regime of freedom of information were operating, the conditions should be in place for policies to be made in ways that could be both scientifically and democratically accountable and legitimate.

A suitable structural and procedural arrangement would be one in which policy-makers who are responsible for risk management decision-making provide their risk expert advisors with explicit risk assessment policy guidance. That guidance would have both a procedural and a substantive element. It would include scoping guidance on the minimum limits of their agenda, i.e. which issues they should consider and which kinds of risks they should assess. It would include an indication of the range of possible policy measure that were under consideration, and provide explicit guidance on how to interpret and respond to uncertainties. It could direct the advisors not, in the first place, to recommend specific policy measures, but rather to advise on what was known, and not known, about the consequences of following, or failing to follow, the range of different policy options. The expert advisors, and the broader communities from which they are drawn, could also be provided with procedural guidance on how their deliberations can and should be accountable and legitimate. Under those conditions, politics would not masquerade as science, and scientific advisors should be able to make an effective, appropriate and scientifically legitimate contribution to policy-making and to the protection of environmental and public health.

To what extent have the lessons from the BSE saga been learnt?

The impact of the BSE saga, and especially the crisis of March 1996, has been considerable, not only in the UK but also at the European Commission and in the policy-making regimes of most of our continental neighbours. In the UK, at the European Commission and in the policy-making regimes of France and Germany antecedent institutions have been abolished and new ones established. The discourse and rhetoric in terms of which policy-making is officially described has also changed. Technocratic idioms are invoked far less frequently; the new preferred official discourse, often but not always, invokes the rhetoric of the 'Red Book version' of Inverted Decisionism. Before March 1996 the concepts of 'risk assessment' and 'risk management' were used very sparingly in the official narratives of risk appraisal and decision-making bodies of the UK and the EU. The crucial question therefore is: to what extent have the underlying policy-making processes changed? Have they learned all the lessons of the BSE saga, or only some of them? How have the rhetorics changed, and do the new practices match the new rhetorics?

In all of these jurisdictions, policy-making processes have become more open than they were, but since there were very opaque it is not always easy to establish how far the underlying practices have changed. In many European jurisdictions, but especially in France, the new rhetoric has frequently claimed that policy-making processes are now (or are in the process of becoming) 'transparent', and that expert advisors are now 'independent'. The ways in which those key terms are being interpreted is not always easy to discern. We are rarely told what it is that will be, or should be, transparent nor what or who is supposed to be independent of whom. That lack of clarity is reflected in a lack of uniformity.

Of the jurisdictions that we will be discussing – the UK, the European Commission, France and Germany – no two have established similar structures. They are interpreting the lessons of the food safety policy crises of the end of the twentieth century differently, but none of them have fully taken on board the lessons indicated above. Perhaps not surprisingly, they have learnt the relatively easy lessons rather than the harder ones.

All of these administrations have explicitly acknowledged that science alone can not decide food safety policies, nor risk policies more generally. Not everyone is always reliably 'on message', but institutions have been reformed in ways that recognise that non-scientific considerations make an indispensable contribution to policy-making, at least downstream. In each of the jurisdictions, there is a recognition that policy-makers need advice from scientific experts, but also that 'other legitimate factors' apart from scientific ones have to contribute to policy-making deliberations. None of these administrations, however, explicitly and consistently acknowledge that non-scientific considerations can, and frequently do, influence the framing, conduct and outcome of scientific risk assessments. In all three EU Member States and at the European Commission some officials have indicated that they recognise that scientific assessments of the existence and potential significance of risks typically do reflect their social and policy contexts, but such co-evolutionary views are unorthodox and have yet to be accepted and endorsed by the main policy-making institutions and authorities.

The British Government has not wholly endorsed a Red Book model, or any other particular model, but there has been some recognition in UK official circles that regulators need to find out how much risks matter to whom and why, before departments articulate their regulatory responses (ILGRA 1998; RCEP 1998, p. 105). A Cabinet Office paper in 2002 even suggested that departments should involve the public in framing key issues and discussing possible policy solutions (Cabinet Office 2002, Recommendation 38b, p. 86). Despite those comments that imply some appreciation of the ways in which scientific deliberations are framed by risk assessment policies, the Prime Minister has continued to articulate a technocratic approach to risk policy-making.

Taking advantage of his first opportunity to ask questions as a backbencher in the House of Commons, Michael Meacher (a former Environment Minister) asked if:

> The Prime Minister [was] aware that there have been no human feeding trials in either the United States or the United Kingdom to establish the health or biochemical effects of consuming GM foods? Does he agree that until such tests are carried out, an important option for the Government when they are reaching a decision later this year is the exercise of the precautionary principle? Does he agree with that, and will he ensure that it is taken on board very seriously?
>
> (Meacher 2003)

In reply the PM said:

> I certainly think it is important for us to take on board all the issues relating to GM food. The only thing I have said, and I say it again, is that it is important for the whole debate to the conducted on the basis of scientific evidence, not on the basis of preju-dice . . . I would just point out to the House that the biotech industry in this country is an immensely important industry, important for the future of that industry that they recognise that the decisions the government takes are going to be based on proper scientific evidence . . . I do worry that there are voices here and in the rest of Europe that are not prepared to give enough consideration to the potential benefits as well as to the potential downsides of this . . . for the future both of our country and other countries it is important that this is conducted on proper scientific grounds.
>
> (Blair 2003a)

The PM's comments were replete with ambiguities. First he indicated that all the issues needed to be addressed, and that all kinds of considerations need to be taken into account, but then insisted that 'the whole debate' had to be conducted 'on the basis of scientific evidence', as if there was sufficient evidence on all the scientific issues, and as if all the issues were fundamentally scientific ones. He then insisted that decisions should not be made on the basis of prejudice, but then promptly displayed the prejudices that informed his own approach to policy-making. More importantly, in this context, the PM implied that he understood, or at any rate was trying to represent, policy-making within the narrow confines of either a technocratic or a decisionist model, he was implicitly rejecting any suggestion that upstream and midstream assumptions should or could influence the scientific deliberations of expert advisors.

Tony Blair reiterated that position on 22 October 2003, when he was again questioned about genetically modified crops immediately after the results of a set of Farm Scale Trials had been published. He insisted: 'We will proceed only according to science' (Blair 2003b). That suggests that while his grasp of the complexities of science-based risk policy-making may be oversimplified, his rhetoric is fairly consistent.

At the European Commission and in Germany, policy-making has ostensibly been restructured in stricter conformity with the Red Book model. New institutions have been created with a remit to provide scientific risk assessments, while separate bodies take responsibility for risk management policy-making. The arrangements in France are slightly more complex and hybrid, but in none of these jurisdictions are scientific expert advisors being provided with explicit risk assessment policy guidance by policy-makers. Such guidance as has been provided has been fragmentary and contingent on political difficulties.

Separating regulation from sponsorship

In three of the four jurisdictions, namely the UK, France, and the European Commission, new institutional arrangements have been established that have relocated responsibility for the protection of consumer interests and public health from food-borne risks in institutions that are not also expected to promote the economic interests of the food, farming and chemical industries. That was one of the main reasons for creating the FSA, the EFSA and AFSSA.

In Germany the pattern of reform has been significantly different. Prior to the BSE crisis of autumn 2000, responsibility for BSE policy was shared between the health and agriculture ministries, with the health ministry taking the lead on issues of consumer protection. The German government, under its policy of *Agrarwende* (or agricultural turn-around) abolished the former Federal Ministry of Food, Agriculture and Forestry, took responsibility for consumer protection away from the Federal Ministry of Health (BMG) and created a new Federal Ministry of Consumer Protection, Food, and

Agriculture (BMVEL) in January 2001 with responsibility for both consumer protection and the economic welfare of the German farming sector.

Even though the new British FSA and the European Commission's EFSA are supposed to put consumers first, and shed their predecessors' concerns for the commercial interests of farmers and the food industry, there are indications that the process of cultural change has been incomplete. In many contexts, the FSA and EFSA have represented their remits as entirely consumer-orientated, but some comments suggest that the reality diverges from the rhetoric, and resembles rather the *status quo ante*. One example emerged in the context of discussions about the potential cancer risks from a food contaminant called acrylamide.

Acrylamide is a contaminent of some cooked foodstuffs, especially those fried or roasted at high temperatures. Acrylamide has been characterised by the International Agency for Research on Cancer (IARC) as a 'probably human carcinogen' and by the European Commission's Scientific Committee for Food as a 'genotoxic carcinogen', which means that acrylamide is potentially very dangerous because as little as one molecule of the compound might be sufficient to trigger the development of a tumour. Consequently it would not be scientifically legitimate, without a great deal more information, to assume that there was a threshold of consumption below which the risks from acrylamide were negligible.

Acrylamide is not being deliberately added to foods, but some may be entering the food chain as an unintended contaminant and some may be formed during cooking. The fact that acrylamide is present in our food supply came as an unwelcome shock to the regulatory authorities. Its presence was uncovered as a by-product of an investigation into a cause célèbre in Sweden. In 1997, while constructing a tunnel at Hallandsåsen contractors used an unsuitable material as grouting between the wall and ceiling tiles. The grout contained acrylamide and water from the surrounding strata leached some acrylamide into the fluid that drained from the tunnel, which contaminated some of the construction workers as well as some of the neighbouring fields. Several tunnel workers and local cattle were found to have been contaminated and poisoned by the acrylamide (Sweden's National Food Administration 2002). The novel form of cattle pathology was initially suspected to be a variant of BSE.

Swedish scientists wanted to estimate the magnitude of the difference between the levels of acrylamide in the blood of those occupationally exposed to acrylamide in the tunnel with a control group drawn from the general public. They found unexpectedly high levels of acrylamide in the blood samples taken from the control group, and consequently started testing food and water to try to establish the source(s) of that contamination. The results showed far higher levels of acrylamide in food products than had been anticipated. Those findings caused a severe ripple of anxiety not just in Sweden but in many countries, and especially so in the food safety regulatory institutions.

The response of the German authorities was to test food products in their own jurisdiction, and to publish the results with advice to German consumers to modify their eating and cooking habits, to avoid the most highly contaminated kinds of products (BfR 2002). Most other European jurisdictions have chosen to handle this challenge quite differently.

The UK FSA's initial response was not to draw public attention to the risks that acrylamide and the contaminated products might pose, but to recruit the government's Central Science Laboratory (CSL) in York to check the Swedish and German results. By 17 May 2002 the results from CSL confirmed the Swedish and German figures. The FSA's policy response has been described by Tim Lang, the UK's only professor of food policy, as 'back to 1984', by which he meant that the assumptions and practices of the FSA were similar to those that could have been expected from MAFF 20 years earlier (personal communication, June 2003).

The FSA officials clearly understood that, since IARC categorised acrylamide as a genotoxic carcinogen, there could be no scientific legitimacy for assuming a threshold level of exposure below which the risks could be discounted (Lützow 2003). The FSA did not respond by banning commercial products contaminated with acrylamide, but instead articulated a policy narrative recommending that 'levels in food should be as low as reasonably achievable' (FSA *Draft Acrylamide consultation paper*, 30/05/03, p. 2). The expression 'reasonably achievable' is notoriously vague, because there can be, and are, very different perceptions of what is reasonable. For example, the perceptions of food manufacturers may not coincide with those of consumer groups. The evidence suggested, moreover, that FSA officials shared the perceptions of the producers rather than those of consumers.

The FSA, and subsequently the embryonic EFSA, focused on the fact that, during cooking, the rate of acrylamide formation seems to increase with temperature. One option therefore could have been to recommend that foods should be cooked at lower temperatures. FSA officials were reluctant to issue advice of that kind to householders, apparently because they feared that undercooking perishable foods such as meat, fish or dairy products could risk increasing microbiological risks. Advice on lowering, or instructions to lower, cooking temperatures in industrial processes would have been far less problematic because industrial processors typically have far more accurate information and controls on processing temperatures than domestic cooks, but no such advice or instructions were given to either industrial or domestic cooks.

The only advice that the FSA provided directly to consumers was simply to reiterate its general guidelines on healthy eating, emphasising the desirability of eating at least five portions of fruit and vegetables a day to ensure a sufficient level of protective nutrients such as Vitamins C and E. If the FSA was putting consumers first it might have advised the general public that, while it was not possible to estimate the scale of the risks that acrylamide might pose, consumers could diminish the risks that they were taking by eating less of the kinds of foods, especially fried and roasted foods, that contained the highest levels of acrylamide. No such advice was, however, issued by the FSA nor by the EFSA.

At a meeting between the FSA's Chemical Safety and Toxicology Division and representatives of consumer groups, a consumer representative:

> Asked why the Agency awaited further research before issuing precautionary advice to consumers. He had expected firmer advice given that acrylamide is a genotoxic carcinogen . . . The Chairman replied by saying it was difficult to advise people what not to eat, when it wasn't known for sure how acrylamide was forming in food and what amounts were present in which foodstuffs.

> (FSA 2002c, para. 3.v)

FSA officials asserted that the Agency had adopted a precautionary approach because no regulatory action was being taken until the scientific uncertainties had been significantly diminished. That was, however, an idiosyncratic interpretation of the concept of precaution.

FSA officials cited an FAO/WHO consultation that suggested 'that a great deal more scientific work was needed before a fuller risk assessment for acrylamide and further advice to consumers' (FSA 2002c, para. 3.iii). The FSA was acknowledging some of the uncertainties, as grounds for not taking regulatory action, but that approach was characteristic of MAFF's traditional culture. Officials also suggested that since there was no reason to suppose that the risks from acrylamide were new, they were in effect already accepted, and were therefore acceptable. Consumers however readily distinguish between the risks that they take knowingly, and those of which they are unaware (MacGregor and Slovic 1986).

On 28 March 2003, a meeting was organised by the Dutch government's agency (the *Voedsel en Waren Autoriteit* or VWA) in collaboration with the FSA, to which a draft White Paper on acrylamide was presented. The document had been jointly prepared not just by the British and Dutch authorities but also with representatives of Europe's food industry, but without a single consumer representative. The food industry was represented then (and at preparatory meetings) by the EU-wide CIAA (Confédération des Industries

AgroAlimentaires), which is the main Brussels-based trade association for European food companies and by ILSI (or the International Life Sciences Institute) which is a pseudo-scientific organisation of some of the most powerful food and chemical companies. The minutes of the meeting held in Brussels on 28 March 2003 indicate that it was agreed that: 'It is essential to create mutual trust between industry and regulators where this does not exist and to encourage sharing of information' (FSA and EFSA 2003). The fact that that comment was omitted from the subsequent paper for the EFSA's Advisory Forum on 4 July 2003 was also significant.

For organisations, in this case the FSA, the EFSA and the VWA, that are supposed to be putting consumers first and distancing themselves from the food industry, that comment is seriously problematic. It is the kind of comment that was routinely made in the 1970s in the context of the secretive and collusive non-statutory Pesticides Safety Precaution Scheme that was discussed in Chapter 3; in the context of an FSA/EFSA document in 2003 it was inappropriate and revealing. Maybe Lang was over-optimistic and the FSA's and EFSA's response to the possible risks from acrylamide was more like 1974 than 1984.

An alternative hypothesis might be that the comment was inaccurately minuted or unrepresentative of the general culture of these institutions. Without the kind of transparency for which we have argued, neither of those hypotheses can be directly examined. It does suggest, however, that locating responsibility for controlling risks in new institutions labelled as 'putting consumers first' may be a necessary for changing an institutionalised policy-making culture, but it may not be sufficient. The rhetoric of institutionally separating regulation from sponsorship is widely endorsed, but in practice the *status quo ante* has not been entirely displaced.

Coupling science with policy: are risk assessment policies explicitly articulated?

In Germany and at the European Commission, where the reformed institutions have ostensibly been structured along orthodox Red Book lines, risk assessment policies have not been explicitly articulated by those responsible for risk management policy-making, or by any other officials. If they had been explicitly articulated officially that act of articulation would have undermined and contradicted the assumptions upon which the institutional structures were being based. Consequently the BfR and EFSA have been established, with responsibility for providing scientific risk assessments of food-borne risks, with virtually no explicit risk assessment policy guidance. The BfR has been told that the scope of its responsibilities includes plant protection products (i.e. pesticides), additives to animal feeds, chemicals, biocides, novel foods and additives and genetically modified organisms but beyond setting out those categories, no further guidance has been provided concerning, for example, which kinds of risks to include and which if any to discount. The graphic representation of the relationship of the BfR to the BVL and BMVEL provided by the Ministry itself indicates that while the BfR is supposed to provide advice to both the BVL and BMVEL, the BMVEL provides the BfR with nothing whatsoever while the BVL should provide only 'data' (BMVEL 2001).

The relationship between DG-SANCO at the European Commission and the EFSA has not been represented graphically by the Commission, but it has been represented, and seems to be understood by the participants themselves, in terms analogous to those in Germany between the BfR and the BMVEL. Consequently, both the BfR and EFSA have full responsibility for delivering risk assessments, but they must do so in circumstances in which their risk assessment policies either remain implicit, or are conveyed by risk managers and other stakeholder interest groups discreetly or covertly, or they are left to the chosen expert advisors to decide for themselves. They might even remain unacknowledged and therefore would be presumed uncritically.

The approach in the UK is a slightly fuzzy hybrid of several of the models. The British government has provided the Food Standards Agency, and in particular its Board, with some upstream framing policy guidance. Unlike the EFSA and BfR it has not been entirely pushed in at the deep end, and left to fend for itself. The 1998 White Paper on the FSA stipulated, and Ministers have subsequently reiterated, guidance to the effect that the FSA should:

> Have protection of the public as its essential aim. It will be open and transparent in the way it works and will consult fully with all the interest groups affected by its activities. Its guiding principles will be laid down by law. They are designed to ensure that the Agency exercises its very considerable powers sensibly and responsibly, without compromising its duty to make protection of public health its first priority.
>
> (MAFF 1998, para. 1.3)

The 1998 White Paper on the Food Standards Agency included a set of 'Guiding Principles'. They stipulated that:

1 The essential aim of the Agency is the protection of public health in relation to food.

2 The Agency's assessments of food standards and safety will be unbiased and based on the best available scientific advice, provided by experts invited in their own right to give independent advice.

3 The Agency will make decisions and take action on the basis that:
  - the Agency's decisions and actions should be proportionate to the risk; pay due regard to costs as well as benefits to those affected by them; and avoid over-regulation;
  - the Agency should act independently of specific sectoral interests.

4 The Agency will strive to ensure that the general public have adequate, clearly presented information in order to allow them to make informed choices. In doing this, the Agency will aim to avoid raising unjustified alarm.

5 The Agency's decision-making processes will be open, transparent and consultative, in order that interested parties, including representatives of the public:
  - have an opportunity to make their views known;
  - can see the basis on which decisions have been taken;
  - are able to reach an informed judgement about the quality of the Agency's processes and decisions.

6 Before taking action, the Agency will consult widely, including representatives of those who would be affected, unless the need for urgent action to protect public health makes this impossible.

7 In its decisions and actions, the Agency will aim to achieve clarity and consistency of approach.

8 The Agency's decisions and actions will take full account of the obligations of the UK under domestic and international law.

9 The Agency will aim for efficiency and economy in delivering an effective operation (MAFF 1998, p. 5).

In relation to science, evidence, expertise and advisors, however, guidance was provided in only microscopic doses. The FSA is supposed to base its judgements on the best available scientific evidence and advice, and to guided by the precautionary assumption that

> Where there are uncertainties about the scientific evidence, an element of political judgement is inevitably involved in reaching decisions on the best course of action. Where there is a risk of serious damage to public health, lack of full scientific certainty should not be used as a reason for postponing cost effective measures to reduce the health risks.

> (MAFF 1998, para 2.7)

It is not obvious that the FSA's response to acrylamide has been consistent with that element of the guidance. In that particular case, a lack of scientific certainty was invoked by the FSA as grounds for investing in further studies, and for postponing regulatory decisions.

The FSA has however provided its scientific advisory committees with some detailed procedural guidance. The FSA Board's guidelines for its scientific advisory committees are intended to bring about increased transparency and to demonstrate the scientific legitimacy of any advice that is provided. Analogous guidance has not yet been provided in France, Germany or by the EFSA or by DG-SANCO. The FSA Board, however, has not provided its expert advisory committees with any risk assessment policy guidance, but rather represents the deliberations of its scientific advisors as being entirely independent of policy considerations and judgements.

Procedural guidance to scientific committees

In the UK, the Board of the FSA has provided its scientific advisory committees with some up-stream framing guidance, but that has been procedural rather than substantive. The FSA Board recognised that it had to transform the ways in which its expert advisory committees operated. The Board therefore established a working party (chaired by John Krebs) to review the role and conduct of the FSA's scientific committees. After a year's deliberation and consultation, a report went to the Board in April 2002; it provided a bold and refreshing set of procedural recommendations that were promptly adopted by the Board (Food Standards Agency 2002a). The guidance that the Board provided was however entirely procedural; it did not indicate which risks should be included in the purview of the committees but it did indicate the steps it wants its committees to follow when they gather and interpret evidence and especially when they provide advice.

Some of the most important guidelines concern the implementation of the FSA policy of openness and transparency. The FSA policy now stipulates that: '. . . all committees should move as quickly as possible to a position where they conduct as much of their business as possible in open sessions' (FSA 2002a, para. 66). The FSA Board itself meets mostly in public sessions, although financial and managerial issues are discussed in closed meetings, and on those occasions 'technical briefings' are also provided (Krebs, 10 July 2003). FSA policy now also stipulates that:

> Data used as the basis for risk assessments and other committee opinions should be made freely available, within the constraints of confidentiality . . . at as early a stage in the process as possible . . . Whenever time permits committees should issue a draft opinion for public consultation before offering their final advice.

> (FSA 2002a, paras 64–65)

On the issue of 'confidentiality' the FSA recommends: 'that each committee should have clear guidelines to define what material can justifiably be regarded as confidential' (FSA 2002a, para. 68). It is not clear why the FSA Board recommended that each advisory committee should decide for itself which data it will treat as confidential rather than observing an agency-wide policy of full disclosure in the public interest. Unless all relevant information is in the public domain it is hard to see how the FSA's decisions will gain credibility or democratic legitimacy.

Perhaps more importantly, the policy is that:

> Chairs of advisory committees . . . [should ensure] . . . that no view is ignored or over-looked, and that unorthodox and contrary scientific views are considered . . . [and should ensure] that the proceedings of the committee, if necessary including minority opinions, are properly documented . . . so that *there is a clear audit trail showing how the committee reached its decisions.* . . . [and] . . . that committee decisions should include an explanation of where differences of opinions have arisen during discussions and why conclusions have been reached, even if alternative opinions were expressed. They should also explain *any* assumptions and uncertainties that are inherent in their conclusions.

> (FSA 2002a, paras 88–89, emphasis added)

If those guidelines were to be strictly observed, it would represent a considerable change from traditional British policy-making practices. Their implementation would entail that, amongst other things, the uncertainties and gaps in the scientific basis of policy-making will be revealed and the available science will be shown to be uncertain, equivocal and insecure. It will also reveal many of the non-scientific considerations that, for the most part, account for disagreements amongst the scientists.

If expert advisors were fully to follow those guidelines, they would fundamentally transform policy-making regimes, and not just in the UK. Once all the evidence and reasoning were in the public domain in the UK, policy protagonists and analysts in other jurisdictions could (and almost certainly would) use the information obtained from the UK to deconstruct decision-making in their own regimes. Transparency can be contagious. Policy-makers would no longer be able to hide behind their experts, and the role of non-scientific considerations in the upstream, midstream and downstream phases of the policy-making process will become increasingly evident.

In those circumstances, it will be far harder for scientific considerations to be represented as if they were decisive, and scientific advisors can be expected increasingly to provide plural and conditional advice. The locus of policy decision-making will then shift to those that have democratic authority and legitimacy. The scientific and democratic legitimacy of advice from scientists will be enhanced by confining it to matters of their scientific competence, and away from judgements about the social acceptability, or unacceptability, of risks and uncertainties. If the different but proper roles of scientific advisors and policy-makers were clearly and appropriately identified and differentiated, then both groups could be properly, but separately, accountable for their judgements and decisions.

Although the European Commission has not conspicuously tried to provide the EFSA with up-stream framing assumptions, the European Parliament has in effect done so, at least in respect of GM crops. From 1990 until 2001, the EU-wide policy regime on GM crops policy-making was governed by a *Directive on the Deliberate Release into the Environment of Genetically Modified Organisms* (EC Directive 90/200). Under the provisions of that Directive, all Member States had to assess risks from GMOs before GM crops could lawfully be cultivated, either experimentally or commercially. The Directive was worded sufficiently vaguely that the risk assessments carried out in different countries could, and did, differ in their scope and breadth. Some countries, including the UK, interpreted its scope relatively narrowly, and focused only on short-term and direct effects, while others extended and broadened their scope to include long-term and indirect effects.

In the context of the public policy debates about the safety and acceptability of foods in general, and GM foods in particular, at the end of the 1990s and the start of this decade, EU Member States agreed that the policies of Member States should converge and that environmental protection and public acceptability of agricultural biotechnology could only be achieved and reconciled if the scope of risk assessments was consistently sufficiently broad to command democratic consent. The decision to stipulate, as the new Directive (2001/18) does, that risk assessments of the environmental release of GM crops should include long-term and indirect effects was taken by the European Parliament, rather than by the Commission or the Council of Ministers.

One consequence of revising the 1990 Directive in 2001 was that, in the UK, an argument could effectively be made that unless the Farm Scale Trials of GM crops, or something very much like them, occurred any proposal to consent to the commercial cultivation of GM crops might be successfully challenge in the British courts and at the European Court of Justice. The grounds for such a challenge would be that the antecedent risk assessments had not adequately considered the likely indirect or long-term effects of cultivation. The consequences of the change from 90/220 to 2001/18 provides a concrete illustration of the point that 'risk assessment policy' and upstream framing assumptions about the scope of scientific deliberations are not irrelevant abstractions but pivotal issues of contemporary policy.

Coupling science with policy: the provision of plural and conditional advice

The kinds of advice from their expert scientific advisors that the new agencies and institutions expect and receive vary quite markedly. In Germany, in the context of the debate about acrylamide that erupted shortly after the BfR and BVL had been established, the BfR published not just data on estimated levels of contamination in particular kinds and brands of food products, it also recommend that a specific regulatory and legislative changes should be made. This provoked a dispute and friction between the BfR on the one hand and the BVL and BMVEL on the other (Spoek 2003). Officials in BVL insisted that the BfR should have confined itself to providing estimates of the concentrations of the contaminant and of the risks that those concentrations might pose, and not ventured into the risk management territory that properly belonged to the BVL. Furthermore, the view of the BVL was that the BfR should not have issued any publications without allowing the BVL to check and agree them first.

Our analysis suggests that the kinds of friction that emerged in that case were not a form of random noise, but a systematic consequence of a poorly designed, and inadequately thought through, institutional structure. Officials in the BVL want the actions of the BfR to conform to a set of restrictions for which nobody has taken explicit responsibility by articulating (even less legitimating) upstream risk assessment policy guidelines. Our argument is not just that the division of labour envisaged by the BVL officials was unrealistic or inappropriate, but rather that it was implicit in ways that were always likely to be problematic.

The role of expert scientific advisory committees within EU Member States at the EFSA are likely to remain problematic because a great deal of ambiguity remains about which kind of advice is being, and will be, sought. In relation to acrylamide, the BVL wanted the BfR to provide only plural and conditional advice, and not monolithic and prescriptive advice, but on that occasion the BfR chose to be prescriptive. The position at the European Commission remains embryonic and vague. Neither DG-SANCO officials or staff at the EFSA have provided any clarifications on the pivotal question of the kinds of advice that DG-SANCO expects the EFSA to provide. Traditional practice, exemplified by all the advice embodied in the forty four reports of the Scientific Committee for Food that have emerged since 1975, has been for the scientific advisory committee to provide monolithic and prescriptive policy advice, rather than conditional comments on the possible consequences of adopting a plurality of alternative policy options.

Even though it would be premature to predict how the EFSA's newly reconstituted expert advisory committee will conduct, interpret and report on their deliberations, there is no evidence that DG-SANCO has indicated to the EFSA that it should strictly confine its advice to non-prescriptive judgements. When a senior official at DG-SANCO commented that the Commission wanted the EFSA to be 'independent but not out of control' it implied that DG-SANCO wanted the EFSA to take some responsibility for policy formulation without the Commission having to provide any explicit risk-assessment policy guidance.

In France, the terms of reference under which AFSSA operates have also been couched in vague and imprecise terms. The approach taken by senior AFSSA officials has been to respond to requests for advice from ministers and senior officials in a variety of ways that are being decided on a case-by-case basis. There have been several cases where AFSSA concluded that the grounds were sufficiently robust and unambiguous for it to provide the French government with monolithic prescriptive policy advice, but in other circumstances AFSSA has been more reticent. In the context of what came to be called (by the British mass media at any rate) the UK–French Beef war, AFSSA was asked to assess the risks and acceptability of British beef that might be exported to France under the terms of the Date-Based Export Scheme. AFSSA responded by commenting on the inconclusive character of the evidence available to it, and consequently declined to provide specific policy advice. AFSSA found that the kind of comments it had provided were not exactly what Ministers had wanted. They had wanted AFSSA to recommend that the policy of continuing to exclude British beef should remain in place, even though the European Commission had deemed it to be acceptably safe.

In the UK several ambiguities also remain on this matter. Many of the expert scientific committee that advise the FSA, such as the Advisory Committee on Novel Foods and Processes, continue to provide the kind of prescriptive monolithic advice to the Board of the FSA that they used to provide to MAFF. On the other hand, in circumstances where significant uncertainties are explicitly acknowledged, some committees have only provided the Board of the FSA with advice that has been plural and conditional. For example, in the context of the Review of BSE Controls, SEAC indicated some of what was and was not known but declined to made specific policy judgements. In the context of the 2002–2003 review of the Over Thirty Months Scheme, DNV (the firm of consultants that advised the Board of the FSA) indicated what the likely consequences of alternative policy options might be, without recommending for or against any of the options. Similarly, when in December 2001 the FSA considered the possible risks that could arise because of the use of sheep intestines as sausage casings, two separate quantitative estimates of the extra risks that might be posed were considered (FSA 2002b §45; DNV 2001).

Although the FSA has provided its expert advisory committees with some detailed procedural guidance, that guidance provided no indication as to which kinds of advice the FSA wants or expects, or the conditions under which prescriptive or non-prescriptive advice might be appropriate. Despite the ambiguities in the terms of reference of the FSA, and the role of its Board, it has become clear that the Minister for Public Health, as well as the Secretary of State at the Department of Health, expect the FSA Board to deliver monolithic and prescriptive policy advice to ministers, so that the Department needs to take responsibility for little more than the application of a rubber stamp.

Transparency

One of the strongest claims made on behalf of all the new institutions is that they were to be 'transparent', but the precise meaning of that term remains unclear. There is some clarity in the sense that in all cases the new bodies and procedures will be less opaque than the institutions and processes that they have replaced. On the other hand it remains to be seen just how much of which kinds of information will be placed in the public domain, and at which stages in the policy-making process.

For contingent historical reasons, the process of providing some clarity to the competing interpretations of 'transparency' is evolving rather slowly. The BSE crisis of March 1996 came as a severe shock to the policy-making system, and the debates about the risks and acceptability of GM foods show that those shocks continue to reverberate. The creation of new food safety advisory institutions has provoked industrial companies into rethinking their innovative strategies and their tactics for dealing with regulatory institutions. Many food and chemical companies are behaving cautiously and waiting to see how their competitors and regulators will behave. Before they approach one of the new institutions with a request for consent to market a new product or process, and before trying to assemble dossiers of data and analyses, they are waiting to see how those institutions respond to requests from other companies. Rather than finding out the hard way that their dossiers are insufficient, they have been hoping that their competitors will serve as guinea pigs for the new processes.

There are some indications, moreover, that several of the new institutions are waiting to see how their counterparts in other jurisdictions will behave when confronted by requests for marketing consent, before making their own judgements. As a consequence the food safety regulatory processes of western Europe are in a relatively quiet interlude. Neither companies nor agencies are keen to take specific initiatives unless and until they can see how each other conduct themselves in the new reformed environment. The numbers of petitions for consent to introduce new food additives, pesticides, veterinary medicines or industrial processes have fallen sharply in recent years. Consequently it has not yet been possible fully to test the commitments of the new bodies to openness and transparency.

The EFSA has not yet made any significant decisions, or assessed any significant risks, and so it is not yet possible to tell how open the EFSA and its advisory committee will be with the data they receive. Will they perpetuate the *status quo ante* and continue to keep data confidential on behalf of food and chemical companies, or will they ensure that much, or even all, of the data are publicly accessible? Will those data be available before decisions are taken and advice is given, or only once the deliberative and decision-making processes have been completed? It is too soon to tell.

We know relatively little about the transparency policies that the BfR, BVL and BVMEL will adopt in Germany, but the example of acrylamide provides some clues. In that case the BfR published estimates of concentrations of the genotoxic contaminant in several named branded products, and indicated that the risks from the contamination might be non-trivial. It is not clear how far the resulting friction between the BfR and the BVL was a consequence of the release of those figures without prior agreement by the BVL or because the BfR supplemented the data with a specific policy recommendation. What is clear, however, was that, from the BVL's point of view, the BfR had either been overly transparent in publishing the figures, or at any rate that it had published prematurely without providing the BVL with an opportunity to comment, and maybe even to conclude its policy deliberations. One plausible hypothesis is that the BVL and BfR were in agreement about what the policy should be, but the BVL wanted to take credit for the decision, rather than letting the BfR do so. In any case, this example reinforces the impression that structuring institutions in accordance with a Red Book model does not enable all the frictions to be avoided, nor can it guarantee that institutions always see full transparency as in their own interests.

Since the UK Food Standards Agency is not receiving large quantities of new data about novel ingredients and processes, it is difficult to be sure how open the FSA will become. The guidance that the FSA Board has provided to its scientific committees remains slightly difficult to interpret. The Board instructed its committees to change their practice by holding some of their meetings in public. How far that will go, remains to be seen. If the only meetings that are held in public are the ones at which important and controversial decisions are not taken, the advice of the committees from closed meetings will be seen as less than fully legitimate. If meetings are held in public, while some of the information being discussed at those meetings remains undisclosed, legitimacy will also be compromised. Pressure for comprehensive accountability may in due course oblige the FSA and its expert advisory committees always to meet in public, and only to discuss publicly available information. SEAC, the Spongiform Encephalopathy Advisory Committee, has adopted the practice of holding most, if not all, of its meetings in public but the same cannot be said of all the FSA's other advisory committees.

The FSA Board does, however, hold almost the entirety of its meetings in public. Those meetings are broadcast live on the Internet, and the papers upon which the Board reaches its decisions are all public documents. Transparency of that kind provides the unprecedented conditions under which it has become possible to discern how scientific and political considerations interact in the deliberations and decision-making of the Board.

The position is France is slightly curious. When AFSSA reaches a decision, and issues a judgement and its advice, it publishes a detailed account of its deliberations and explains why it adopted its interpretation of the evidence it cites, but AFSSA does not routinely publish the reports it receives from its expert advisors, and data are kept confidential until the agency has completed its deliberations and announced its conclusions. Members of AFSSA advisory committees also do not always have full access to the data that they are expected to consider, and not all the data reach the public domain. Those routines and practices inhibit numerous forms of accountability and prevent many stakeholders from participating in scientific and policy deliberations with AFSSA.

In the UK, France and at the European Commission, expert advisors are not yet obliged to be entirely transparent about any and all conflicts of interest they might have. At the European Commission, advisors declare the topics on the agenda on which they have a conflict of interest, but they are not expected to reveal the identity of the firm(s) concerned. In Germany the rules indicate that such conflicts of interest should be declared and detailed, but it is not yet possible to estimate the extent to which those rules are being complied with, or what the consequences of full compliance might be.

Transparency is a difficult policy to implement, but as the experience of the USA has shown, as Freedom of Information policies have evolved, once the rhetoric has been adopted and once a policy of transparency has been articulated, the pressure towards exhaustive disclosure inevitably accumulates.

Recognising and reporting uncertain and incomplete knowledge

All the relevant new institutions in all four jurisdictions acknowledge, in general terms, the existence and significance of uncertainties – at least in the science of risk assessments, and sometimes in the estimation of benefits too. On the other hand, in all documented cases, only some of the uncertainties have been taken into account, not all of them.

In the acrylamide case, the UK and EU authorities emphasised the scientific uncertainties when arguing that any imposition of restrictions would be premature. In Germany the BfR acknowledged the same uncertainties, but interpreted their implications for policy quite differently. In France, AFSSA cited some of the uncertainties in its assessment of the risks that might arise as a consequence of importing UK beef under the Date-Based Export Scheme, but drew less attention to the uncertainties in estimates of the risks from BSE in French herds.

In the debate in the UK about the relative costs and benefits of organic produce when compared to mainstream produce, it has been said that the FSA understated the uncertainties in estimates of the risks from pesticides and veterinary medicines, while proponents of organic food and farming have understated the uncertainties in their estimates of the benefits that accrue from producing food organically and from eating the resultant produce. Policy-makers on the Board of the FSA are not providing members of their expert advisory committees with incentives to highlight the uncertainties fully but only to do so partially and selectively.

In the context of the discussion in the UK in 2003 about the proposed reforms of the Over Thirty Months Scheme (or OTMS), that banned the sale of meat from older cattle, the FSA Board was provided with estimates of the likely consequences (both economic and to public health) of adopting several alternative courses of action, and some of the attendant uncertainties (DNV Consulting 2002; FSA 2003b). The FSA Board was given to understand by their advisors that, even on the most pessimistic reading of their estimates of the possible extra risks that might arise as a consequence of allowing meat from older animals to enter to human food chain, the extra infectivity would be vanishingly slight. In that case, however, the advisors only drew attention to the uncertainties within the model that they chose to use. They did not high-light the fact that several alternative models were available, and consequently the uncertainties inherent in the differences between the predictions of those competing models were not acknowledged.

While UK Health Ministers have otherwise left responsibility for food safety policy-making with the FSA Board, on that occasion Ministers did take responsibility for a policy decision. The FSA Board was not able to decide on its own that the OTMS should be ended, because implementing that decision required other changes to be implemented by other departments, especially DEFRA. In the event, despite a recommendation from the FSA Board in July 2003 that the OTMS should be phased out, ministers adopted a more precautionary approach; they referred the issue back to the FSA (FSA 2004). Ministers had at least two reasons for caution, apart from the obvious one that they did not wish to be represented as diminishing public confidence in the safety of British beef.

In May 2004 two significant sets of information emerged both of which suggested that the FSA, and its expert advisors, might have been overoptimistic in their assessments of the likely consequences of ending the ban on cattle over 30 months of age, and replacing it with a post mortem testing regime. First:

> A retrospective check of records at fresh meat abattoirs by the Meat Hygiene Service (MHS) uncovered a significant level of failure by the MHS, over a two year period, to ensure that . . . cattle were tested.
>
> (FSA 2004, p. 6, para. 13)

FSA officials were obliged to acknowledge that the 'risk assessments carried out [in 2002 and 2003] for the OTM rule review [did] not take into account the possibility that testing failures may occur' (FSA 2004, p. 7 para. 17). Second:

> The final results of a retrospective survey of tonsils and appendices, removed during routine surgery, were published. These tissues were examined for evidence of accumulation of prion protein that is indicative of likely infection with the vCJD agent. Three appendices were found to give a positive result in a total of over 12,000 sampled that were tested.
>
> (FSA 2004, p. 10, para. 30)

In the light of that new information, SEAC and FSA staff revised their estimates of the possible consequences of ending the OTMS by 'using a more comprehensive statistical method' and concluded that the resultant risks might be at least 10 times the size of the risks that they had estimated one year earlier (FSA 2004, pp. 11–12, paras 34–37). While the most recent estimates of the possible consequences of ending the OTMS suggest the risks might be slight, it remains the case that in 2004 SEAC and the FSA acknowledged uncertainties of which it had either not previously been aware, or which it had not previously acknowledged. It also acknowledged more forcibly than before that 'risk assessment was limited by the paucity of data and significant uncertainties remained' (FSA 2004, p. 11, para. 35). That example showed that in 2003 both SEAC and the FSA had under-reported some of the uncertainties with which they had been struggling, and had chosen to make relatively optimistic assumptions, especially about rates of industrial compliance with regulatory requirements, even though experience suggested that those assumptions were unrealistic.

While the evidence of a link between vCJD and the BSE pathogen is very strong, a causal link has not been proven (Collinge *et al.* 1996). In several other respects, however, the science of BSE remains gravely uncertain. For example, at the time of writing, the number of cases of BSE in animals born after the ban on feeding MBM to cattle was reinforced was not falling as rapidly as

SEAC had predicted. It is not possible to be sure whether that anomaly is a consequence of intensified active surveillance or because BSE is being spread through some vector(s) other than animal feedstuffs. Members of SEAC and the TSE research community more widely are uncertain whether BSE has spread to sheep flocks, and consequently whether the pathogen may be infecting sheep meat. More generally, too little is known about the extent to which the muscle tissue of subclinically infected cattle contains the BSE pathogen, and if so at what kinds of levels. Those three particular sets of uncertainties have, from time to time, been officially and publicly acknowledged by SEAC or by government officials, but it is harder to discern why those uncertainties have, in effect, been discounted.

Enabling public interest science

The new food safety policy-making institutions are relatively young, and have not yet made significant steps forward in promoting new institutionalised forms of public interest science. They have slowly started to redirect their research programmes in ways that provide some in the professional research community with incentives to increase the proportion of their time devoted to public interest science, but institutional initiatives have yet to emerge. In the UK, in the months leading up to the creation of the FSA, some in MAFF and the UK research community were suggesting that MAFF seemed keener on signing long-term contracts for research projects than had been MAFF's practice in the preceding few years. Some interpreted that change charitably as MAFF trying to relieve the FSA of some complex challenges of research policy-making that might otherwise have arisen, while less charitable interpretations suggested that MAFF was keen to tie-up the FSA's research budget for several years to come.

On the issue of the extent to which the secretariats of expert advisory committees are located in the policy institutions for which advice is provided, the pattern is mixed. In the UK and France, the FSA and AFSSA provide the secretariats to committees that advice them. In Germany, the BfR is distinct and separated from the BVL, and at the Commission the EFSA has been established to separate it from DG-SANCO, yet both the Commission officials at DG-SANCO and policy-makers in BVLS and BVEL seem to want their advisors to be 'independent but not out of control'.

Scientific and democratic legitimacy

Since none of the new institutional regimes are fully transparenct, and none are fully accountable, the extent of the legitimacy of their deliberations and judgements is hard to estimate. Moreover, as none of them involve the explicit provision of risk assessment policy by risk managers, and since in many cases policy decisions are being taken by appointed officials rather than by elected representatives, none of the new regimes have yet developed and implemented fully legitimated structures and processes. That entails that it would be premature to assume that the kinds of problems that characterised much of the BSE saga will not reoccur.

Bibliography

BfR (2002) Acrylamide in foods serious problem or exaggerated risk? 28 Nov 2002, Bundesinstitut für Risikobewertung available at http://www.bfr.bund.de/cms/detail.php?template=internet_en_index_js.

Blair, T. (2003a) Hansard, 18 June 2003, The Stationery Office London.

Blair, T. (2003b) Hansard, 22 October 2003, Column 643 ,The Stationery Office, London.

BMVEL (2001) *Bericht der Arbeitsgruppe Reorganisation des gesundheitlichen Verbraucherschutzes* [Task Force Report] 14 December 2001.

Bradley, R. (2000) Extended report of meeting with representatives of community institutions or of major governments Scientific Veterinary Committee, YB 89/11.28/5.1, in Phillips *et al.* 2000, Disc 2.

Cabinet Office (2002) *Risk: Improving government's capability to handle risk and uncertainty, Strategy Unit Report,* available at http://www.number-10.gov.uk/SU/RISK/risk/report/index.html December 2003.

Collinge, J., Sidle, K.C.L., Meads, J., Ironside, J., Hill, A.F. (1996) 'Molecular analysis of prion strain variation and the aetiology of 'new variant' CJD', *Nature,* **383,** 685–90.

DNV Consulting (2002) *Assessment of the Risk of Exposure to the BSE Agent Through the Use of Natural Sausage Casings* (for the European Natural Sausage Casings Association). DNV (Det Norske Veritas) Consulting, London.

European Commission (1990) Directive 90/220/EEC of 23 April 1990 on the deliberate release into the environment of genetically modified organisms, *Official Journal of the European Union,* No. L117 p. 15, 1990/05/08.

European Parliament (1997) *Report on Alleged Contravention or Maladministration in the Implementation of Community Law in Relation to BSE, Without Prejudice to the Jurisdiction of the Community and National Courts.* Doc_EN\RR\319\319579 A4–0020/97A/Annexes.

European Union (2001) *Directive 2001/18/EC of the European parliament and of the council on the deliberate release into the environment of genetically modified organisms and repealing Council Directive 90/220/EEC.* Brussels, 2001.

Food Standards Agency (2002a) *Report on the Review of Scientific Committees,* 15 April 2002, available from http://www.food.gov.uk/news/newsarchive/58746.

Food Standards Agency (2002b) *BSE and Sheep: Report of the Core Stakeholder Group,* May 2002; available from http: //www.food.gov.uk/foodindustry-consultations/completed/uk/bsesheepstakeholder report.

Food Standards Agency (2002c) Minutes of Chemical Safety and Toxicology meeting with Representative of Consumer Organisations, 15 October 2002.

FSA (2003a) 'Acrylamide in Food', 23/05/03, Annex 1, para. 2.

FSA (2003b) FSA Paper to the Board on the OTM Rule, 10 July 2003, Annex 3.

FSA and EFSA (2003) Outcome of the acrylamide workshop held in Brussels on
March 28, 2003, Annex 3: document for White Paper on acrylamide: Presented to
EFSA Advisory Forum, 4 July 2003, p. 6.

Food Standards Agency (2004) FSA Board Meeting, Paper 04/07/06, Agenda Item 6,
6 July 2004.

Hollis, G. (1998) BSE Inquiry – Hearing Day 38, 29 June 1998, pp. 78–9.

ILGRA (Inter-Departmental Liaison Group on Risk Assessment, Risk Assessment and Risk
Management) (1998) *Improving Policy and Practice within Government Departments.*
Sudbury: HSE Books.

Krebs, J. (2003) Statement at Food Standards Agency Board Public Meeting, Kensington
Town Hall, London 10 July 2003.

Lawrence, A. (1990) Public Health SVC 13 September: BSE, Minute dated 15 September
1990, *BSE Inquiry Year Book* document Reference No. 89/09.15/5.1, indexed in Phillips
et al. 2000, Disc 2.

Lützow, M. (2003) FAO/WHO Consultation on Health Implications of Acrylamide in Food,
16 April 2003. UN Food and Agriculture Organization, Rome.

MAFF (1998) *The Food Standards Agency: a force for change.* Report to Parliament, Cm
3830, January 1998. Ministry of Agriculture, Fisheries and Food, London.

MacGregor, D. G. and Slovic, P. (1986) 'Perceived acceptability of risk analysis as a
decision-making approach', *Risk Analysis,* 6, 245–56.

Meacher, M. (2003) Hansard, 18 June 2003, Column 349. The Stationery Office,
London.

Moran, M. (2001) 'Not steering by drowning: policy catastrophes and the regulatory state',
Political Quarterly, 414–27.

Phillips, Bridgeman J. and Ferguson-Smith, M. (2000) *The BSE Inquiry: Report: evidence
and supporting papers of the Inquiry into the emergence and identification of Bovine
Spongiform Encephalopathy (BSE) and variant Creutzfeldt-Jakob Disease (vCJD)
and the action taken in response to it up to 20 March 1996.* London: The Stationery
Office.

RCEP (Royal Commission on Environmental Pollution) (1998) London: Royal
Commission on Environmental Pollution, The Stationery Office, London.

Russell, J. (2002) 'Could these foods be giving us cancer?', *Guardian,* 15 August 2002.

Scientific Veterinary Committee (1990) Joint meeting of Animal and Public Health
sections of the Scientific Veterinary Committee, Brussels, 6 June 1990,
YB 90/06.06/12.7, indexed in Phillips *et al.* 2000, Disc 2.

Scientific Veterinary Committee (1994) *Report on Bovine Spongiform Encepahalopathy
(BSE),* 11 July 1994, DG-VI, European Commission, Brussels.

Spoek, A. (2003) 'Uneasy Divorce' or 'Joint Custody'? The separation of risk assessment and
risk management in food policy, SPRU, 2003, MSc thesis, University of Sussex, Brighton.

Stirling, A. (2003) Risk, uncertainty and precaution: some instrumental implications from the
social sciences. In F. Berkhout, M. Leach and I. Scoones (eds) *Negotiating Environmental
Change: new perspectives from social science.* Edward Elgar, Cheltenham, UK.

Sweden's National Food Administration (2002) *Acrylamide in Heat-Processed
Foods,* 26 April 2002, available from www.mindfully.org/Food/
Acrylamide-Heat-Processed-Foods26apr02.htm 28 July 2003.

Wynne, B. (1992) 'Uncertainty and environmental learning: reconceiving science and
policy in the preventative paradigm', *Global Environmental Change,* 2 (2), 111–27.

Bibliography

Abraham, J. (1993) 'Scientific standards and institutional interests: carcinogenic risk assessment of benoxaprofen in the UK and US', *Social Studies of Science*, **23**, 387–444.

ACARD (Advisory Council for Applied Research and Development) (1982) *The Food Industry and Technology*. London: HMSO, Cabinet Office, London.

Acheson, D. (1988) Letter dated 20 March 1988 to Sir Richard Southwood, *BSE Inquiry Year Book* Reference No. 88/4.20/1.1–1.2, in Phillips *et al.* 2000.

Acheson, D. (1998) Witness Statement No. 251a, in Phillips *et al.* 2000.

Adam Smith Institute (1988) *A Change of Government*, London.

AEBC (2001) *Crops on Trial*. Agriculture and Environment Biotechnology Commission, September 2001, London.

Albert, R.E. (1994) 'Carcinogen risk assessment in the U. S. Environmental Protection Agency', *Critical Reviews in Toxicology*, **24** (1), 75–85.

Anderson, R. (1998) Statement to BSE Inquiry No. 9c, annex 1, in Phillips *et al.* 2000.

Andrews, D. (1988) Bovine Spongiform Encephalopathy (BSE), Memo dated 24 February 1988, *BSE Inquiry Year Book* Reference No. 88/2.24/2.2.

Andrews, D. (1988a) Confidential – Bovine Spongiform Encephalopathy (BSE), Memo dated 31 March 1988, *BSE Inquiry Year Book* Reference No. 88/3.31/5.1–5.2.

Andrews, D. (1988b) Letter to Sir Richard Southwood dated 12 July 1988, *BSE Inquiry Year Book* Reference No. 88/7.12/2.1.

Anon (1988) Note of a meeting on Bovine Spongiform Encephalopathy 17 March 1988 Venue, DHSS, Richmond Terrace, Whitehall. *BSE Inquiry Year Book* Reference No. 88\03.17\8.1–8.3, in Phillips *et al.* 2000.

Anon (1988) Working Party on Bovine Spongiform Encephalopathy (BSE) Note of a Meeting Held on 10 November in Room 37D at the Department of Zoology, South Parks Road, Oxford. *BSE Inquiry Year Book* Reference No. 88\11.10\2.1–2.6, in Phillips *et al.* 2000.

Anon (1989a) Meat Imports into the Federal Republic of Germany from the United Kingdom, Telex Message, *BSE Inquiry Year Book* No. 89/08.21/8.1, in Phillips *et al.* 2000.

Anon (1989b) Bovine Spongiform Encephalopathy: risk to animal and public health. A resume of the private experts, opinions expressed at an EC meeting on 6 November 1989 in Brussels. *BSE Inquiry Year Book* No. YB 89/11.6/6.2, in Phillips *et al.* 2000.

Anon (1989c) 'The Food Bill', *Which?*, November 1989, 536–7.

Anon (1997) *The Economist*, 22 February 1997, p. 25.

Anon (1996) *Guardian*, 26 March 1996, p. 1.

Arnold, N. (1990) 'Are you ready for the Food safety Act?', *Catering*, August, 10.

Barbier, M. and Janet, C. (1999) *BSE and the Swiss National Action System*, Report for the BASES project and for the European Commission, DG XII, July 1999. Université Pierre Mendès France: INRA, Economie et Sociologie Rurales.

Barclay, C. (1996) *Bovine Spongiform Encephalopathy*, Commons Library Research Paper No 96/62.

Barnes, B., Bloor, D. and Henry, J. (1996) *Scientific Knowledge: a sociological analysis.* London: Athlone Press.

Barnett, L. M. (1985) *British Food Policy in the First World War.* London: Allen and Unwin.

Bates, J. A. R. (1978) 'The control of pesticides in the United Kingdom', *Biotrop, Special Publication,* 7, 165–79.

Bernstein, M. H. (1955) *Regulating Business by Independent Commission.* Princeton, NJ: Princeton University Press.

Beveridge, W. (1928) *Food Control.* Oxford: Clarendon Press.

BfR (2002) Acrylamide in foods serious problem or exaggerated risk? 28 Nov 2002, Bundesinstitut für Risikobewertung available at http://www.bfr.bund.de/cms/detail.php?template = internet_en_index_js.

Bidstrup, P. L. (1950) 'Poisoning by organic insecticides', *BMJ,* 548–51.

BIFHS-USA Guide British Isles Research, 2003, http://www.rootsweb.com/∼bifhsusa/admhist.html

Black, I. (2003) 'EU agrees to agricultural shakeup', *Guardian,* 27 June 2003, p. 15.

Blair, T. (2003a) *Hansard,* 18 June 2003.

Blair, T. (2003b) *Hansard,* 22 October 2003, Column 643.

Blitz, J. and Kampfner, J. (1997) 'Ministers play down abattoir safety row', *Financial Times,* 8 March 1997, p. 5.

BMA (1939) *Nutrition and Public Health: proceedings of a national conference on the wider aspects of nutrition.* London: British Medical Association.

BMVEL (2001) *Bericht der Arbeitsgruppe Reorganisation des gesundheitlichen Verbraucherschutzes* [Task Force Report], 14 December 2001.

Bowles, C. (1987) Bat rabies and bovine spongiform encephalopathy (BSE), Minute from C. Bowles dated 23 July 1987, *BSE Inquiry Year Book* Reference No. YB 87/7/23/2.1.

Boyd Orr, J. (1936) *Food, Health and Income: a report on a survey of adequacy of diet in relation to income.* London: Macmillan.

Bradley, R. (1987) BSE Article, *BSE Inquiry Year Book* Reference No. 87/12.10/5.1–5.6.

Bradley, R. (1988) BSE research projects, Minute dated 19 July 1988 to W. A. Watson. *BSE Inquiry Year Book* Reference No. 88\07.19\2.1–2.2, in Phillips *et al.* 2000.

Bradley, R. (1988) BSE research projects, Minute dated 19 July 1988 to W. A. Watson, *BSE Inquiry Year Book* Reference No. 88\07.19\2.1–2.2, in Phillips *et al.* 2000.

Bradley, R. (1989) 'BSE: Disposal of brains and spinal cords from aged-cull cattle and sheep', Minute dated 12 April 1989 to A. J. Lawrence, *BSE Inquiry Year Book* Reference No. 89\04.12\1.1–1.5 in Phillips *et al.* 2000.

Bradley, R. (1989) Extended report of meeting with representatives of community institutions or of major governments, Scientific Veterinary Committee, YB 89/11.28/5.1, in Phillips *et al.* 2000.

Bradley, R. (2000) Extended report of meeting with representatives of community institutions or of major governments. Scientific Veterinary Committee, YB 89/11.28/5.1, in Phillips *et al.,* 2000, Disc 2.

Brickman, R., Jasanoff, S. and Ilgen, T. (1985) *Controlling Chemicals: The Politics of Regulation in Europe and the USA.* Ithaca: Cornell University Press.

Brown, N. (1999) *Hansard,* 21 June 1999, Column 787.

BSE Inquiry (1988) Transcript, oral hearings, Day 43, 7 July 1998, pp. 124–5, in Phillips *et al.* 2000.

BSE Inquiry (1998) Transcript, 6 November 1998, in Phillips *et al.* 2000.

BSE Inquiry (1999a) The Central Veterinary Laboratory 1985–1989, Revised Factual Account No. 4, para. 234.

BSE Inquiry (1999b) Revised Factual Account No 5. 'The Early Days'.

BSE Inquiry Transcripts, in Phillips *et al.* 2000.

Bufton, M. (2001) 'Coronary heart disease versus BSE: characterising official British expert advisory committees', *Science and Public Policy*, **28** (5), 381–8.

Burnett, J. (1979) *Plenty and Want: a social history of diet in England from 1815 to the present day*. London: Scolar Press.

Butler, D. and Butler, D. (2000) *Twentieth Century British Political Facts*. Macmillan.

Byrne, D. (2000) See, for example, comments of Commissioner David Byrne in European Commission (2000) *Food Law from farm to table – Creating a European food authority*, 8 November 2000, Doc. IP/00/1270, Brussels.

Cabinet Office (2002) *Risk: Improving government's capability to handle risk and uncertainty, Strategy Unit Report*, available at http://www.number-10.gov.uk/SU/RISK/risk/report/index.html December 2003

Cannon, G. (1987) *The Politics of Food*. London: Century.

Capstick, C. (1990) Secretary's Meeting with CMO – Friday 22 June 1990, Minute dated 20 June 1990. *BSE Inquiry Year Book* Reference No. YB90/6.20/15.1, in Phillips *et al.* 2000.

Carter, N. (2001) *The Politics of the Environment: ideas activism, policy*. Cambridge University Press.

Castleman, B. I. and Ziem, G. E. (1998) 'Corporate influences on threshold limit values', *American Journal of Industrial Medicine*, **13**, 531–9.

CEC (2000) *Science, society and the citizen in Europe*, SEC (2000) 1973, Brussels: Commission of the European Communities.

Channel 4 Television (1994) *Dispatches: BSE – the human link*. Broadcast on 25 January 1994.

Cockburn, C. (1989) BSE: Use of offals in meat products, Minute, *BSE Inquiry Year Book* Reference No. 89/06.02/51–5.10, in Phillips *et al.* 2000.

Codex Alimentarius Commission (2001) *Draft Working Principles for Risk Analysis in the Framework of the Codex*, 2001, CL 001/24-GP CX/GP 02/3.

Coller, F. H. (1925) *A State Trading Adventure: an account of the Ministry of Food, 1917–21*. Oxford: Oxford University Press.

Collinge, J., Sidle, K. C.L., Meads, J., Ironside, J. and Hill, A. F. (1996) 'Molecular analysis of prion strain variation and the aetiology of 'new variant' CJD' *Nature*, **383**, 685–90.

Colquhoun, J. W. (1976) *MAFF, Food Quality and Safety: a century of progress*, p. 19. HMSO.

Commission of the European Communities (2000) *White Paper on Food Safety*, COM(1999) 719 final. 12 January 2000, Brussels.

Cooper, A. F. (1989) *British Agricultural Policy 1912–36: a study in conservative politics*. Manchester: Manchester University Press.

Corbally, M. (1990) Letter to Animal Health Division of MAFF, from Institute of Environmental Health Officers, 1 February 1990.

Court of Auditors (2001) 'Special Report No 14/2001, Follow up to Special Report No 19/98 on BSE', *Official Journal of the European Communities*, C 324/1 20 November.

Cowen, J. R. (1988) Bovine spongiform encephalopathy, Minute dated 26 February 1988, *BSE Inquiry Year Book* Reference No. 88/2.26/3.1–3.3, in Phillips *et al.* 2000.

Crouch, D. (1988) *A Political Sociology of Toxicology*, unpublished DPhil thesis, University of Sussex, Brighton.

Cruickshank, A. (1998) Statement to the BSE Inquiry No 75, in Phillips *et al.* 2000.

Cruickshank, A. R. (1988) Bovine Spongiform Encephalopathy, Memo, *BSE Inquiry Year Book* Reference No. YB88/2.16/1.1.

Dawson, A. (1987) Bovine Spongiform Encephalopathy (BSE), Minute from Dr Ann Dawson, dated 7 March 1988, *BSE Inquiry Year Book* 88/3.7/6.1–6.2.

Dealler, S. and Lacey, R. W. (1991) 'Transmissible spongiform encephalopathies: The threat of BSE to man – a reply to K. C. Taylor', *Food Microbiology*, **8**, 259–62.

Dealler, S. (1996) *Lethal Legacy*. London: Bloomsbury Publishing.

Deer, B. (1985) 'The stark lessons of a scrapheap hospital', *Sunday Times*, 19 May 1985.

DEFRA (2001) *Government expands BSE testing programme*, News Release 233/01, 13 November 2001.

Department of Education and Science (1967) *Review of the Present Safety Arrangements for the Use of Toxic Chemicals in Agriculture and Food Storage*, Report by the Advisory Committee on Pesticides and Other Toxic Chemicals. London: HMSO.

Desenclos, J. C. *et al.* (1996) 'Large outbreak of *Salmonella enterica* serotype paratyphi B infection caused by goat's milk cheese, France: a case finding and epidemiological study', *BMJ*, **312**, 91–4.

Dewey, P. E. (1989) *British Agriculture in the First World War*. London: Routledge.

Dickens, C. (1854) *Hard Times*. London: Hazell Watson and Viney (1868 corrected edn.)

Dickinson, A. G. (1976) 'Scrapie in sheep and goats'. In R. H. Kimberlin (ed.) *Slow Virus Diseases of Animals and Man*. Amsterdam, Oxford and New York: North Holland and Elsevier.

DNV Consulting (2002) *Assessment of the Risk of Exposure to the BSE Agent Through the Use of Natural Sausage Casings* (for the European Natural Sausage Casings Association).

Dressel, K. (1999) *BSE and the German National Action System*, Report for the BASES project and for the European Commission, DG XII, July 1999. Munich: Institut für Soziologie der Ludwig-Maximilians, Munich University.

Dressel, K. (2003) *BSE – The New Dimension of Uncertainty*. Sigma Press.

Durkheim, E. (1912) *The Elementary Forms of Religious Life*.

Efron, E. (1984) *The Apolcalyptics: how environmental politics controls what we know about cancer*. New York: Simon and Schuster.

EFSA (2003a) *Participation of Third Parties at Meetings of the Advisory Forum*. European Food Safety Authority, Doc AF 04.0702003–5.

EFSA (2003b) *The Tasks of the European Food Safety Authority*. European Food Safety Authority at http://www.efsa.eu.int/tasks_en.html 9/9/2003.

EFSA (2003c) *Questions and Answers on the European Food Safety Authority*. European Food Safety Authority at http://www.efsa.eu.int/QandA_en.html 9/9/2003.

Epstein, S. S. (1978) *The Politics of Cancer*. Sierra Club Books,

Erlichman, J. (1987) 'Food watchdog denies conflict of interest', *Guardian*, 20 July 1987, p. 4.

Erlichman, J. (1989) 'German ban on "suspect" UK beef is confirmed', *Guardian*, 7 November 1989, p. 2.

Erlichman, J. (1990) 'NFU seeks independent food agency', *Guardian*, 3 July 1990, p. 4.

European Commission (1996) Commission Decision 96/239/EC.

European Commission (1997) *Consumer Health and Food Safety*, COM(97)183final, 30 April 1997.

European Commission (2000) *White Paper on Food Safety in the European Union*, COM(99)719, 12 January 2000; available at *http://europa.eu.int/comm/food/fs/intro/index_en.html*.

European Commission (2002) *Report on the monitoring and testing of bovine animals for the presence of Bovine Spongiform Encephalopathy (BSE) in 2001.* Brussels: European Community.

European Commission (1990) Directive 90/220/EEC of 23 April 1990 on the deliberate release into the environment of genetically modified organisms, *Official Journal,* No L117 p. 15, 1990/05/08.

European Parliament (1997) *Report on Alleged Contraventions or Maladministration in the Implementation of Community Law in Relation to BSE, Without Prejudice to the Jurisdiction of the Community and National Courts.* Report of the Inquiry from a temporary committee into BSE, rapporteur: Manuel Medina Ortega. 7 February DOC EN\RR\319\319544, Strasbourg.

European Parliament (1997) *Report on Alleged Contraventions or Maladministration in the Implementation of Community Law in Relation to BSE, Without Prejudice to the Jurisdiction of the Community and National Courts.* Doc_EN\RR\319\319579 A4–0020/97A/Annexes.

European Parliament (1997a) *Report on Alleged Contraventions or Maladministration in the Implementation of Community Law in Relation to BSE.* Part A, PE220.544/fin./A, 7 February 1997. European Parliament.

European Parliament (1997b) *Report on Alleged Contravention or Maladministration in the Implementation of Community law in Relation to BSE.* Part A – Annexes, PE220.544/fin./Ann, 7 February 1997. European Parliament.

European Parliament (1997c) *Report on Alleged Contravention or Maladministration in the Implementation of Community Law in Relation to BSE.* Part B – Work of the Committee on Inquiry and Basic Data, PE220.544/fin./B, 7 February 1997. European Parliament.

Evans, D. (1988) Parliamentary Secretary (Commons)'s meeting on BSE, Friday 27 May 1988, Minute dated 2 June 1988. *BSE Inquiry Year Book* Reference No. 88/6.2/3.1–3.3, in Phillips *et al.* 2000.

FAO (2001) Press Release 01/41, 21 June 2001, 'FAO: More Than 30 countries have taken action on BSE, but more needs to be done.', available at: http://www.fao.org/ waicent/ois/press_ne/presseng/2001/pren0141.htm.

Ferguson-Smith, M. (2001) 'A sorry tale of BSE blunders', *The Times Higher Educational Supplement,* 2 November 2001, p. 21.

Filby, F. A. (1934) *A History of Food Adulteration and Analysis.* London: Allen and Unwin.

Food Safety Advisory Committee (1989) *Bovine Spongiform Encephalopathy, Report to the Minister for Health and the Minister for Agriculture and Food.* December 1989, Republic of Ireland.

Food Standards Agency (2002a) *Report on the Review of Scientific Committees,* 15 April 2002. available from http://www.food.gov.uk/news/newsarchive/58746

Food Standards Agency (2002b) *BSE and Sheep: Report of the Core Stakeholder Group.* May 2002; available from http://www.food.gov.uk/foodindustry/consultations/ completed_consultations/completeduk/bsesheepstakeholderreport.

Food Standards Agency (2002c) *Minutes of Chemical Safety and Toxicology meeting with Representative of Consumer Organisations,* 15 October 2002.

FSA and EFSA (2003) *Outcome of the acrylamide workshop held in Brussels on March 28, 2003,* Annex 3: document for White Paper on acrylamide: Presented to EFSA Advisory Forum, 4 July 2003, p. 6.

FSA (2003) *Research Projects MO3*, at http://www.food.gov.uk/science/research/
   meat_hygiene_research/m03programme/m03projilist/
FSA (2003a) 'Acrylamide in Food', 23/05/03, Annex 1, para. 2.
FSA (2003b) FSA Paper to the Board on the OTM Rule, 10 July 2003, Annex 3.
Food Standards Agency (2004) FSA Board Meeting, Paper 04/07/06, Agenda Item 6,
   6 July 2004.
Funtowicz, S. and Ravetz, J. (1993) 'Science for the post-normal age', *Futures* 25, S. 739–55.
Gajdusek, D. C. (1985) Unconventional viruses causing subacute spongiform
   encephalopathies. In B. N. Fields *et al.* (eds) *Virology*. New York: Raven Press.
Gallagher, J. (1987) 'Bovine spongiform encephalopathy – confidentiality', J. Gallagher,
   letter to Richard Cawthorne, MAFF, dated 19 June 1987, YB 87/06.19/6.1.
Gerhardt, C. J. (ed.) (1890) *Die philosophischen Schriften von Gottfried Wilhelm
   Leibniz*, vol. 7. Berlin.
Gibbs, C. J., Gajdusek, D. C., and Amyx, H. (1979) Strain variation in the viruses of
   Creutzfeldt-Jakob disease and kuru. In S. B. Prusiner and W. J. Hadlow (eds) *Slow
   Transmissible Diseases of the Nervous System*, vol 2, pp. 87–110. New York: Academic
   Press.
Gilbert, D. G. R. (1987) *Pesticide Safety Policy and Control Arrangements in Britain*,
   Unpublished PhD thesis, University of London.
Giles, R. F. (1976) 'The development of food legislation in the UK'. In MAFF 1976,
   pp. 4–21.
Gillespie, B., Eva, D. and Johnson, R. (1979) 'Carcinogenic risk assessment in the
   United States and Great Britain: The case of Aldrin/Dieldrin', *Social Studies of
   Science*, **9**, 265–301.
Goffman, E. (1974) *Frame Analysis: an essay on the organization of experience*. New York:
   Harper and Row; reprinted 1986, Boston, MA: Northeastern University Press.
Gonçalves, M. E. and Gonçalves, L. (1999) *BSE and the Portuguese National Action System*,
   Report for the BASES project and for the European Commission, DG XII, July 1999.
   Lisbon: Instituto Superior de Ciências do Trabalho e da Empresa.
Goulet, V. *et al.* (1995) 'Listeriosis from consumption of raw-milk cheese', *Lancet*,
   345, 1581–2.
Griffin, J. M. *et al.* (1997) 'Bovine spongiform encephalopathy in the Republic of
   Ireland', *Irish Veterinary Journal*, **50** (10), 593–600.
Griffiths, M. J. (1990) 'BSE: splitting heads', Minute dated 2 May 1990 to M. Hill, MAFF.
   BSE Inquiry Year Book Reference No. 90\05.02\1.1–1.2, in Phillips *et al.* 2000.
Gummer, J. (1990) *Hansard* 21 May 1990, vol. 173, No. 110, Column 82.
Gummer, J. (1990) *Hansard*, 8 June 1990, Column 906.
Gummett, P. (1980) *Scientists in Whitehall*. Manchester: Manchester University Press.
Habermas, J. (1971) 'The scientization of politics and public opinion', first published in
   Technik und Wissenschaft als Ideologie, Suhrkamp Verlag 1968, and translated in
   English in *Toward a Rational Society*, Beacon Press, 1971, pp. 62–80.
Hadlow, W. J., Kennedy, R. C. and Race, R. E. (1982) 'Natural infection of Suffolk Sheep
   with scrapie virus', *The Journal of Infectious Diseases*, **146** (5), 657–64.
Haine, D. B. (1988) Bovine Spongiform Encephalopathy: Secretary's Meeting with
   Sir R Southwood and the CMO, Minute dated 24 May 1988. *BSE Inquiry Year Book*
   Reference No. 88/5.24/2.1, in Phillips *et al.* 2000.
Haine, D. B. (1988) Minute to the Private Secretary of Mr Thompson, dated 29 February
   1988, *BSE Inquiry Year Book* Reference No. YB 88/2.29/4.1.

Hammond (1951) *Food – Volume I: The Growth of Policy.* London: HMSO.

Hammond (1954) *Food and Agriculture in Britain: 1939–45*, Stanford University Press.

Hanssen, M. (1984) *E for Additives: the complete E number guide.* Wellingborough: Thorsens.

Hencke, D. (1979) 'Rolling back the frontiers of government', *Guardian*, 3 Sept 1979, p. 4.

Hirsch, M. (2001) 'Food Policy in France', paper to WHO-Europe Conference on *Improved Coordination and Harmonization of National Food Safety Control Services*, held in Dublin, June 2001, available December 2003 at *http://www.euro.who.int/foodsafety/Publications/mtgrpt*

Hirsch, M., Duneton, P., Baralon, P. and Noiville, F. (1996) *L'affolante affaire de la vache folle.* Paris: Balland.

HM Treasury (2000) Public Service Agreement with the Department of Health (Food Standards Agency) see: *http://www.hm-treasury.gov.uk/sr2000/sda/index.html*

Hogg, D. (1996) *Hansard*, 3 April 1996, Column 407.

Hollis, G. (1998) Comments to BSE public inquiry. Transcript, day 38 (29 June 1998): 80–81; available: *http://www.bse.org.uk*

Holt, T. A. and Phillips, J. (1988) 'Bovine spongiform encephalopathy', *BMJ*, **296**, 1581–2.

Hornsby, M. (1989) 'German action a restraint of trade', *The Times*, 2 November 1989, p. 2.

House of Commons (1815) *Report from the Committee of the House of Commons on the Laws relating to the Manufacture, Sale and Assize of Bread (1815): Minutes of Evidence*, reprinted in *The Pamphleteer*, Vol. VI, 1815, p. 162; cited in Burnett 1979.

House of Commons (1987) *The Effects of Pesticides on Human Health*, vol. III, Second special report of the Agriculture Committee, Session 1986–87. London: HMSO.

House of Commons (1996) Agriculture and Health Select Committees Report.

House of Lords (2000) Science and Technology Committee, Third Report, HL 38, *Science and Society*, February 2000. London: The Stationery Office.

http://www.fao.org/livestock/AGAP/FRG/Feedsafety/ffsp2.htm (1 March, 2002)

Huff, J. (2002) 'IARC monographs, industry influence, and upgrading, downgrading, and undergrading chemicals', *International Journal of Occupational and Environmental Health*, **8** (3), 249–70.

ILGRA (1998) *InterDepartmental Liaison Group on Risk Assessment, Risk Assessment and Risk Management: Improving policy and practice within government departments.* Sudbury: HSE Books.

ILGRA (1998) *Risk Communication. A Guide to Regulatory Practice*, Interdepartmental Liaison Group on Risk Assessment, Health and Safety Executive. London.

Inquiry Secretariat (1999) Information provided by Sir Richard Southwood, Sir Anthony Epstein, Dr William Martin and Lord Walton. Statement of Information No. 483, in Phillips *et al.* 2000.

Interagency Regulatory Liaison Group (1979) 'Scientific bases for identification of potential carcinogens and estimation of risks: report of the Interagency Liaison Group, Work Group on Risk Assessment', *Journal of the National Cancer Institute*, **63** (1), 241–68.

Irwin, A. (1995) *Citizen Science: a study of people, expertise and sustainable development.* London: Routledge.

Isaacs, D. and Fitzgerald, D. (1999) 'Seven alternatives to evidence-based medicine', *BMJ*, **319**, p. 1618.

Jacobson, M. F. (1972) *Eater's Digest.* New York: Doubleday.

James, P. (1997a) *Food Standards Agency: an interim proposal*, report to T. Blair, 30 April 1997.

James, P. (1997b) Speech on *The Food Standards Agency* to the Parliamentary Food and Health Forum, 10 June 1997.

James, P., Kemper, F. and Pascal, G. (1999) *A European Food and Public Health Authority*, European Commission DG-XXIV, DOC/99/17, Brussels, 13 December 1999 available at http://europa.eu.int/comm/food/fs/sc/future_food_en.pdf.

Jasanoff, S. (1987a) 'Contested boundaries in policy-relevant science', *Social Studies of Science*, 17, 195–230.

Jasanoff, S. (1987b) Cultural aspects of risk assessment in Britain and the United States. In B. B. Johnson and V. T. Covello (eds) *The Social and Cultural Construction of Risk: Essays on Risk Selection and Perception*, pp. 359–97. Dordrecht and Boston: D. Reidel.

Jasanoff, S. (1990) *The Fifth Branch: science advisors as policy-makers.* Harvard University Press.

Jasanoff, S. and Wynne, B.(1998) Science and decision-making. In S. Rayner and E. L. Malone (eds) *Human Choices and Climate Change: Volume 1 – the societal framework.* Ohio: Battelle Press.

Joly, P. B., Le Pape, Y., Barbier, M., Estades, J., Lemarié, J. and Marcant, O. (1999) *BSE and the French National Action System.* Report for the BASES project and for the European Commission, DG XII, July 1999, INRA, Economie et Sociologie Rurales, Université Pierre Mendès France available at *http://www.grenoble.inra.fr/Docs/pub/A1999/ BASEFRA.pdf*

Joly, P. B., Le Pape, Y., Barbier, M., Estades, J., Lemarié, J. and Marcant, O. (1999) *Interactions between Scientific Expertise and Public Decision on TSEs in FRANCE.* Final Report of Task 1 of the BASES Project, Building a common data base on scientific research and public decision on TSEs in Europe.

Krebs, J. (2003), *Protecting Consumers in the Future World Market*, City Food Lecture, The Guildhall, London 14 January 2003, p. 1.

Künast, R. (2001) 'The magic hexagon', *The Ecologist*, vol. 31, No 3 April pp. 48–49.

Lacey, R. (1987) interview given to BBC Television, 15 April 1997.

Lang, T., Lobstein, T. and Miller, M. (1989) *Food Legislation: time to grasp the nettle*, London Food Commission, October 1989.

Lang, T. (1997) Going public: food campaigns during the 1980s and early 1990s. In D. F. Smith (ed.) *Nutrition in Britain: science, scientists and politics in the twentieth century.* Lonmdon: Routledge.

Lang, T. *et al.* (1988) *Food Adulteration and how to Fight it.* London: Unwin.

Lang, T. *et al.* (1997) *Food Standards and the State: A Fresh Start*, Discussion Paper 3, Centre for Food Policy, Thames Valley University, April 1997.

Lang, T., Millstone, E., Rayner, M. and Raven, H. (1996) *Modernising UK Food Policy: the case for reforming the Ministry of Agriculture, Fisheries and Food*, Discussion Paper 1, Centre for Food Policy, Thames Valley University, July 1996.

Lang, T. (1999) 'The complexities of globalization: the UK as a case study of tensions with the food system and the challenges to food policy', *Agriculture and Human Values*, 16, 169–85.

Lawrence, A. (1989) BSE, Minute dated 29 March 1989. *BSE Inquiry Year Book* Reference No. YB 89/3.29/3.1, in Phillips *et al.* 2000.

Lawrence, A. (1989a) BSE: The Southwood Report, Minute dated 7 February 1989, *BSE Inquiry Year Book* Reference No. 89/2.7/1.1, in Phillips *et al.* 2000.

Lawrence, A. (1989b) BSE: Exports of meat and bonemeal to other Member States, Minute dated 3 July 1989, *BSE Inquiry Year Book* Reference No. 89/7.03/5.1–5.2, in Phillips *et al.* 2000.

Lawrence, A. (1989a) Standing Veterinary Committee (SVC) Meeting on 5 September: BSE, Memo to Mr Lebrecht, MAFF, *BSE Inquiry Year Book* Reference No.89/9.6/9.3, in Phillips *et al.* 2000.

Lawrence, A. (1989b) Public health SVC 13 September: BSE, *BSE Inquiry Year Book* Reference No. YB 89/09.15/5.1, in Phillips *et al.* 2000.

Lawrence, A. (1989c) BSE – SVC meeting on 24 October, Memo, *BSE Inquiry Year Book* Reference No. 89/10.25/6, in Phillips *et al.* 2000.

Lawrence, A. (1998) Statement No. 76 to the BSE Inquiry, in Phillips *et al.* 2000.

Lawrence, A. (1990) Public Health SVC 13 September: BSE, Minute dated 15 September 1990, *BSE Inquiry Year Book* Reference No. 89/09.15/5.1, indexed in Phillips *et al.*, 2000, Disc 2

Lawrence, A. (1990a) SVC 7 March, *BSE Inquiry Year Book* Reference No. 90/3.8/1.1, in Phillips *et al.* 2000.

Lawrence, A. (1990b) BSE: Standing Veterinary Committee Meeting on 13th March, *BSE Inquiry Year Book* Reference No. 90/03.14/9.1, in Phillips *et al.* 2000.

Lawton, F. J. (1976) In MAFF, *Food Quality and Safety: a century of progress*, p. 14. HMSO.

Le Gros Clarke, F. and Titmuss, R. M. (1939) *Our Food Problem and its Relation to our National Defences*. Harmondsworth: Penguin Books.

Lebrecht, A. J. (1989) Minister's Meeting with UKASTA: 2 October 1989, minute datated 4 October 1989. *BSE Inquiry Year Book* Reference No. YB 89/10.04/5.1–5.2, in Phillips *et al.* 2000.

Leibnitz, G. W. (1666) Dissertio de arte combinatoria. In C. J. Gerhardt (ed.) *Die philosophischen Schriften von Gottfried Wilhelm Leibniz*, vol. 7, 1890, p. 200. Berlin: Weidmann.

Levidow, L., Carr, S., Wield, D. and von Schomberg, R. (1997) 'European biotechnology regulation: framing the risk assessment of a herbicide-tolerant crop', *Science, Technology and Human Values*, **22**, 472–505.

Linton, M. (1988) 'Think tank urges Mrs Thatcher to abolish four ministries', *Guardian*, 28 March 1988, p. 3.

LFC (1985) *Consumer Protection and Food Legislation*, The London Food Commission.

London Food News (1985) No 1, Spring 1985 p. 1.

Lowson, R. (1989) Briefing for Incoming Ministers – Animal Health, minute dated 25 July 1989. *BSE Inquiry Year Book* Reference No. 89\07.25\5.1–5.5, in Phillips *et al.* 2000.

Lowson, R. (1990) BSE: paper on the safety of beef. *BSE Inquiry Year Book* Reference No. 90\07.13\5.1–5.13.

Lowson, R. (1990) BSE: Note for the Prime Minister, dated 26 January 1990. *BSE Inquiry Year Book* Reference No. 90/01.26/13.1–13.6, in Phillips *et al.* 2000.

Lowson, R. (1990) BSE: Standing Veterinary Committee (SVC), *BSE Inquiry Year Book* No. 90/1.18/1.1, in Phillips *et al.* 2000.

Lützow (2003) FAO/WHO Consultation on Health Implications of Acrylamide in Food, 16 April 2003.

MacGregor, D. G. and Slovic, P. (1986) 'Perceived acceptability of risk analysis as a decision-making approach', *Risk Analysis*, **6**, 245–56.

MacGregor, J. (1998) Statement to the BSE Inquiry No 302, in Phillips *et al.* 2000.

MacIntyre, D., Hunt, L. and Arthur, C. (1996) 'Ministers admit possible link between mad cow disease and human deaths', *Independent*, 21 March 1996, p. 1.

MAFF (1976) *Food Quality and Safety: a century of progress*. HMSO.

MAFF (1980) Proposed Processing Order: Consultation Paper, 16 April 1980, cited in Barclay, C. (1996) *Bovine Spongiform Encephalopathy and Agriculture* House of Commons Library Research Paper 96/62, Section II B, p. 13.

MAFF (1989a), Press Release 375/89, Ministry of Agriculture, Fisheries and Food, 25 September 1989.

MAFF (1989b) Press Release 379/89, Ministry of Agriculture, Fisheries and Food, 29 September 1989.

MAFF (1989c) *Food Safety – protecting the consumer*. London: HMSO.

MAFF (1990) *The Food Safety Act 1990 and you: a guide for the food industry*. London: HMSO.

MAFF (1990a) *British Beef Is Safe, Gummer*, News Release 185/90, 15 May 1990, London: Ministry of Agriculture Fisheries and Food.

MAFF (1990a) *Government Action on BSE*, News Release FF 1/90, 9 January 1990, London: Ministry of Agriculture Fisheries and Food.

MAFF (1990b) *Bovine Spongiform Encephalopathy (BSE)*, News Release 184/90, 15 May 1990, London: Ministry of Agriculture Fisheries and Food.

MAFF (1990b) *News Release 184/90*, 15 May 1990, London, Ministry of Agriculture Fisheries and Food.

MAFF (1993) Press Release No 350/93, 21 October 1993.

MAFF (1996) *Food Biotechnology must not be over-regulated says Douglas Hogg*, Press Release 76/96, 5 March 1996, London: Ministry of Agriculture, Fisheries and Food.

MAFF (1997a) *New Group to set rapid progress on Food Agency*, Press Release 148/97, 9 June 1997, London: Ministry of Agriculture, Fisheries and Food.

MAFF (1997b) *Public approve new agency for food safety*, MAFF Press Release 224/97, 30 July 1997/

MAFF (1998) *The Food Standards Agency: a force for change*, Report to Parliament, Cm 3830, January 1998.

MAFF (1998) *The Food Standards Agency: a force for change*, White Paper to Parliament, Jan 1998, Cm 3830.

MAFF (1999) *The Food Standards Agency: Consultation on Draft Legislation*, CM 4249, 27 January 1999, London: Stationery Office.

MAFF/DoH (1988) Draft Report of the Expert Working Party on Bovine Spongiform Encephalopathy *BSE Inquiry Year Book* Reference No. 88/12.22/3.1–3.58, in Phillips *et al.* 2000.

MAFF/DoH (1989) *Report of the Working Party on Bovine Spongiform Encephalopathy*. London: Ministry of Agriculture Fisheries and Food/Department of Health.

MAFF/DoH (1990) Consultative Committee on Research into Spongiform Encephalopathies, *The 'Tyrell Report'.* Interim report.

Marsh, R. F., Burger, D. and Hanson, R. P. (1969) 'Transmissible mink encephalopathy: behaviour of the disease agent in mink', *American Journal of Veterinary Research*, **30**, 1637–43.

Martin, W. B. (1989) Letter to Sir Richard Southwood, dated 16 January 1989, *BSE Inquiry Year Book* Reference No. 89/1.16/1.1, in Phillips *et al.* 2000.

Martin, W. B. (1998) Involvement with scrapie as Scientific Director of the Moredun Research Institute, The BSE Inquiry, Statement No. 5.

Meacher, M. (2003) *Hansard*, 18 June 2003, Column 349. The Stationery Office, London.

Meldrum, K. (1989) Confidential – sensitive issues in the animal health sector, *BSE Inquiry Year Book* Reference No. 89/1.10/7.1–7.4, in Phillips *et al.* 2000.

Meldrum, K. (1992) *Radio Times*, 31 May 1992.

Meldrum, K. (1998) Statement No. 184 to BSE Inquiry.

Mellanby, E. (1951) 'The chemical manipulation of food', *BMJ*, October 13, 863–86.

Metters, J. S. (1989) BSE: Action proposed by MAFF Ministers on bovine offal, minute dated 9 June 1989. *BSE Inquiry Year Book* Reference No. 89/6.9/5.1–5.4, in Phillips *et al.* 2000.

Millstone. E. (1984) 'Food additives: a technology out of control?', *New Scientist*,

Millstone, E., Brunner, E. and Mayer, S. (1999) 'Beyond substantial equivalence', *Nature*, **401**, 525–6.

Ministry of Agriculture Fisheries and Food/Department of Health (1989) *Report of the Working Party on Bovine Spongiform Encephalopathy*, 3 February.

Moran, M. (2001) 'Not steering by drowning: policy catastrophes and the regulatory state', *Political Quarterly*, 414–27.

Mounts, G. J. (1980) 'OSHA Standards: the burden of proof', *Monthly Labor Review*, **103** (9), 53–6.

Nelkin, D. (1971) *Nuclear Power and its Critics: the Cayuga Lake controversy*. Cornell University Press.

Nelkin, D. (ed.) (1979) *Controversies: the politics of technical decision making*. Sage Publications.

Nettleton, P. (1989) 'Only science can decide food safety, MPs told', *Guardian*, 30 June 1989, p. 6.

Neyer, J. (2000) 'The regulation of risks and the power of the people: lessons from the BSE crisis', *European Integration Online Papers*, 4 (6) http://netec.mcc.ac.uk/WoPEc/data/Articles/erpeiopxxp0049.html

O'Donoghue, K. (1996) BSE, minute dated 15 March 1996. *BSE Inquiry Year Book* Reference No. 96/3.15/2.1–2.4, in Phillips *et al.* 2000.

Office Internationale des Epizooties (2003) see data at *http://www.oie.int/eng/info/ en_esbmonde.htm*

Ordish, G. (1952) *Untaken Harvest: man's loss of crops from pest, weed, and disease: an introductory study*. London: Constable.

Owen, E. (1988) Bovine Spongiform Encephalopathy (BSE) – Emergency Order, Minute dated 10 June 1988. *BSE Inquiry Year Book* Reference No.88/6.10/8.1, in Phillips *et al.* 2000.

Packer, R. (1996) Draft minute for the Minister to send to [The Prime Minister], *BSE Inquiry Year Book* Reference No. 96/3.18/8.1–8.6).

Palmer, J. and Myers, P. (1990) 'EC court action likely on beef', *Guardian*, 5 June 1990, p. 1.

Pattison, I. H. and Millson, G. C. (1960) 'Further observations on the experimental production of scrapie in goats and sheep', *Journal of Comparative Pathology*, **70**, 182–93.

Pattison, I. H. and Millson, G. C. (1962) 'Distribution of the scrapie agent in the tissues of experimentally inoculated goats', *Journal of Comparative Pathology*, **72**, 233–44.

Paulus, I. (1974) *The Search for Pure Food: a sociology of legislation in Britain*. London: Martin Robertson.

Pearce, F. (1996) 'Ministers HOSTILE to advice on BSE', *New Scientist*, 30 March, p. 4.

Penman (1995) 'Top scientists adds to BSE warnings', *Independent*, 4 December 1995, p. 4.

Pennington, H. (2003) *When Food Kills: BSE, e.coli, and disaster science*. Oxford: Oxford University Press.

Phillips, Bridgeman J. and Ferguson-Smith, M. (2000) *The BSE Inquiry: Report: evidence and supporting papers of the Inquiry into the emergence and identification of Bovine Spongiform Encephalopathy (BSE) and variant Creutzfeldt-Jakob Disease (vCJD) and the action taken in response to it up to 20 March 1996*. London: The Stationery Office.

Pickles, H. (1988a) The transmission of bovine spongiform encephalopathy. *BSE Inquiry Year Book* Reference No. 88\11.07\1.2–1.5, in Phillips *et al.* 2000.

Pickles, H. (1988b) Bovine Spongiform Encephalopathy, Minute dated 11 November 1988. *BSE Inquiry Year Book* Reference No. 88/11.11/1.1/1.2, in Phillips *et al.* 2000.

Pickles, H. (1988c) Bovine spongiform encephalopathy: first Meeting of Working Party Minutes dated 20 June 1988. *BSE Inquiry Year Book* Reference No. 88/6.20/3.1, in Phillips *et al.* 2000.

Pickles, H. (1989) Letter to Sir Richard Southwood, dated 17 January 1989, *BSE Inquiry Year Book* Reference No. 89/1/17/1.1–1.2, in Phillips *et al.* 2000.

Pickles, H. (1990a), 'Bovine Spongiform Encephalopathy', minute dated 1 June 1990. *BSE Inquiry Year Book* Reference No.YB 90/6.01/3.1–3.2.

Pickles, H. (1990b) Safety of beef, draft dated 15 June 1990, *BSE Inquiry Year Book* Reference No. 90/6.15/19.1.

Pickles, H. (1998) Statement to the BSE Inquiry No 115, in Phillips *et al.* 2000.

Prentice, (1990) *The Times*, 22 January 1990.

PRO MAF 130/61, Public Records Office, Ministry of Agriculture and Fisheries, file 130/61.

PRO, MH 55/1069, Public Records Office, Ministry of Health, file 55/1069.

Ratcliffe, E. (1994) BSE: Parliamentary Secretary's meeting with German delegation: 26 May 1994, Minute, *BSE Inquiry Year Book* No. YB 94.5.27/5.1, in Phillips *et al.* 2000.

Rees, H. (1987) Minute dated 5 June 1987 to Parliamentary Secretary and others, Newly identified bovine neurological disorder – Bovine Spongiform Encephalopathy, *BSE Inquiry Year Book* 87\06.05\2.1–2.2.

Rees, H. (1998) BSE Inquiry transcript of oral hearings, Day 54, 10/9/1998, p. 106, in Phillips *et al.* 2000.

Rees, W. H. G. (1988) Bovine spongiform encephalopathy, submission dated 6 May 1988. *BSE Inquiry Year Book* Reference No. 88/5.6/3.1–3.22, in Phillips *et al.* 2000.

Render, T. J. (1994) BSE: Secretary's Meeting with German officials: 24 May 1994, minute to Mr Eddy, Ministry of Agriculture Fisheries and Food, dated 25 May 1994, *BSE Inquiry Year Book* Reference No. 94/5.24/7.1–7.7, in Phillips *et al.* 2000.

Report of the Committee of Inquiry on Food and Mouth Disease – 1968: Part One, 1969, Cmnd. 3999. London: HMSO.

Richmond, *et al.* (1990) *The Microbiological Safety of Food*, Report of the Committee on the Microbiological Safety of Food. London: HMSO.

Robbins, C. J. *et al.* (1983) 'Implementing the NACNE Report', *Lancet*, 1351–6.

Robbins, D. and Johnston, R. (1976) 'The role of cognitive and occupational differentiation in scientific controversies', *Social Studies of Science*, 6, 349–68.

Roe, N. (1989) 'Swallowed by the market', *Independent*, 19 June 1989, p. 21.

Rooker, J. and Jowell, T., 14 October 1997, Statement to Stakeholders' Meeting, Department of Health.

Rooker, J. (1999) *Hansard*, 21 June 1999, Column 831.

Rose, H. and Rose, S. (1969) *Science and Society*. Harmondsworth: Penguin Books.

Royal Commission on Environmental Pollution (1979) *Agriculture and Pollution*. London: HMSO.

Royal Commission on Environmental Pollution (1998) *Setting Environmental Standards*. London: HMSO

Russell, J. (2002) 'Could these foods be giving us cancer?', *Guardian*, 15 August 2002.

Schwartz, M. (2003) *How the Cows Turned Mad*, E. Schneider trans. Berkeley, CA: University of California Press.

Scientific Veterinary Committee (1990) Joint meeting of Animal and Public Health sections of the Scientific Veterinary Committee, Brussels 6 June 1990, *BSE Inquiry Year Book* Reference No. 90/06.06/12.7, indexed in Phillips *et al.* 2000, Disc 2.

Scientific Veterinary Committee (1994) *Report on Bovine Spongiform Encepahalopathy (BSE)*, 11 July 1994, DG-VI.

Sheppard, J. (1987) *The Big Chill: a report on the implications of cook-chill catering for the public services*, LFC.

Smith, M. (1990) *The Politics of Agricultural Support in Britain: the development of the agricultural policy community*. Aldershot: Gower.

Southwood, R. (1998) Statement No 1 to BSE Inquiry, in Phillips *et al.* 2000.

Southwood Working Party (1999) Witness Statement No. 1D, in Phillips *et al.* 2000.

Spoek, A. (2003) 'Uneasy Divorce' or 'Joint Custody'? The separation of risk assessment and risk management in food policy, SPRU, 2003.

Stagg, S. (1989a) Southwood Report – BSE, Letter dated 24 February 1989, *BSE Inquiry Year Book* Reference No. 89/02.24/14.1 in Phillips *et al.* 2000.

Stagg, S. (1989b) Minute on BSE: use of offals in meat products, dated 7 June 1989, *BSE Inquiry Year Book* Reference No. 89/6.07/7.1, in Phillips *et al.* 2000.

Stern, P. C. (1991) Learning through conflict: A realistic strategy for risk communication. *Policy Sciences*, **24**, 99–119.

Stigler, G. (1975) *The Citizen and the State*. University of Chicago Press.

Stirling A. (2003) Risk, uncertainty and precaution: some instrumental implications from the social sciences. In F. Berkhourt, M. Leach and I. Scoones (eds) *Negotiating Environmental Change: new perspectives from social science*. Cheltenham: Edward Elgar.

Strang, F. (1988) Bovine Spongiform Encephalopathy: Secretary's Meeting with Sir Richard Southwood and the CHO. *BSE Inquiry Year Book* Reference No. 88\05.19\4.1–4.3, in Phillips *et al.* 2000.

Strang, G. (1995) The Labour Party's Basic Objectives for food Policy, speech given to the Environmental Health Congress of the Chartered Institute of Environmental Health, September 1995, p. 1 para. 3.

Strang, W. G. G. (1996) BSE and CJD, Minute to K O'Donoghue, *BSE Inquiry Year Book* Reference No. 96/3.15/3.1–3.2 in Phillips *et al.* 2000.

Suich, J. C. (1989) BSE – Southwood Working Party, Minute dated 10 January 1989. *BSE Inquiry Year Book* Reference No. 89\1.10\3.1–3.2, in Phillips *et al.* 2000.

SVC (1990) Joint meeting of Animal and Public Health sections of the scientific veterinary committee, Brussels 6 June 1990, BSE Inquiry Document No. YB 90/06.06/12.7, in Phillips *et al.* 2000.

SVC (1994) Standing Veterinary Committee, 8 November 1994, BSE, Minute, in *BSE Inquiry Year Book* Reference No. 94/11.09/3.1.

Swann (1998) Statement No. 158 to the BSE Inquiry, in Phillips *et al.* 2000.

Sweden's National Food Administration (2002) *Acrylamide in Heat-Processed Foods*, 26 April 2002, available from www.mindfully.org/Food/Acrylamide-Heat-Processed-Foods26apr02.htm 28 July 2003

Tannahill, R. (1988) *Food in History*. Harmondsworth: Penguin Books.

Taylor, D. M. (1989) 'Bovine spongiform encephalopathy and human health', *The Veterinary Record*, **125**, 413–15.

The Specified Risk Material Order (1997) S.I. 1997/2964.

Thatcher, M. (1999) Statement No 401 to the BSE Inquiry, in Phillips *et al.* 2000.

Thompson, D. (1989) BSE – Southwood Working Party. Minute dated 19 January 1989, *BSE Inquiry Year Book* Reference No. 89/1.19/4.1, in Phillips *et al.* 2000.

Trichopoulou, A. *et al.* (2000) *European Policy on Food Safety.* Report to the STOA Programme of the European Parliament, Athens, September 2000.

Trichopoulou, A., Millstone, E., Lang, T., Eames, M., Barling, D. and van Zwanenberg, P. (2000) *European Policy on Food Safety.* Report to the European Parliament's Scientific and Technological Options Assessment Programme (STOA), June 2000, European Parliament document number PE 292.026/Fin.St. available at *http://www.europarl.eu.int/dg4/stoa/en/publi/default.htm*

Turner, J. S. (1970) *The Chemical Feast: the Ralph Nader study group report on the Food and Drug Administration.* New York: Grossman.

Tyrrell, D. (1990) Opinion on the public health implications of eating beef and the epidemic of BSE, Draft of 3 July 1990, *BSE Inquiry Year Book* Reference No. YB90\07.03\13.1–13.13, in Phillips *et al.* 2000.

US Congress (1958) Food Additive Amendments to the 1938 Federal Food, Drug and Cosmetic Act.

US Department of Agriculture (1999) *Transmissible Mink Encephalopathy,* Fact Sheet, Veterinary Services, Animal and Plant health Inspection Services, September 1999. Available at: *http://www.idfa.org/reg/bse/fstme.pdf*

US NRC (1983) *Risk Assessment in the Federal Government: Managing the Process.* Washington, DC: US National Academies Press.

US NRC (1994) *Science and Judgment in Risk Assessment.* Washington DC: Commission of the Life Sciences, US National Research Council.

van Zwanenberg, P. (1999) *BSE and the Republic of Ireland's National Action System.* Report for the BASES project and for the European Commission, DG XII, July 1999. SPRU, University of Sussex.

van Zwanenberg, P. and Millstone, E. (2000) 'Beyond skeptical relativism: evaluating the social constructions of expert risk assessments', *Science, Technology and Human Values,* **25** (3), 259–82.

van Zwanenberg, P. (1996) *Science, Pesticide Policy and Public Health: ethylene bisdithiocarbamate regulation in the UK and USA.* Unpublished DPhil, SPRU – Science and Technology Policy Research, University of Sussex.

Verrett, J. and Carper, J. (1974) *Eating May be Hazardous to Your Health.* New York: Simon and Schuster.

Walker, C. and Cannon, G. (1984) *The Food Scandal.* London: Century.

Watson, W. (1987) Minute dated 30 July 1987 'Bovine spongiform encephalopathy (BSE)', *BSE Inquiry Year Book* Reference No. YB 87/7.30/1.1–1.4.

Webb, S. and Webb, B. (1904) 'The Assize of Bread', *Economic Journal,* 14 (54), 196–218.

Webb, T. and Lang, T. (1987) *Food Irradiation: the myth and the reality.* Wellingborough: Thorsons.

Weber, M. (1958) *Gesammelte Politischen Schriften,* 2nd edn. J. C. B. Mohr, Tübingen.

Weinberg, A. (1972) 'Science and trans-science', *Minerva,* **10**, 209–22.

Weingart, P. (1999) 'Scientific expertise and political accountability: paradoxes of science in politics', *Science and Public Policy,* June, 151–61.

Wells, G. (1998) Statement No 65 to the BSE Inquiry.

Wells, G., Scott, A., Johnson, C., Gunning, R., Jeffrey, M. and Bradley, R. (1987) 'A novel progressive spongiform encephalopathy in cattle', *Veterinary Record,* **121**, 419–20.

White, L. (1926) *Introduction to the Study of Public Administration*. New York: Macmillan. Cited in Jasanoff 1990, p. 10.

Wilesmith, J. W. *et al.* (1988) 'Bovine spongiform encephalopathy: epidemiological studies', *Veterinary Record*, **123**, 638–44.

Wilesmith, J. W., Wells, G. A. H., Ryan, J. B. M., Gavier-Widen, D., Simmons, M. (1997) 'A cohort study to examine maternally-associated risk factors for bovine spongiform encephalopathy', *Veterinary Record*, **141**, 239–43.

Will, R. G. (1991) 'The spongiform encephalopathies', *Journal of Neurology Neurosurgery and Psychiatry*, **54** (9), 761–3.

Winter, M. (1996) *Rural Politics: policies for agriculture, forestry and the environment*. London: Routledge.

Wintour, P. (1996) 'Major goes to war with Europe', *Guardian*, 22 May 1996, p. 1.

Wintour, P., Bowcott, O. and Bates, S. (1996) Ministers defy beef outcry, *Guardian*, 26 March 1996, p. 1.

Woodward, L. (1962) *The Age of Reform: 1815–1870*. Oxford: Clarendon Press.

Wynne, B. (1982) *Rationality and Ritual: The Windscale Inquiry and Nuclear Decisions in Britain*, Monograph No. 3. Chalfont St Giles, UK: British Society for the History of Science.

Wynne, B. (1992) 'Uncertainty and environmental learning: reconceiving science and policy in the preventative paradigm', *Global Environmental Change*, **2** (2), 111–27.

Index

LaVergne, TN USA
21 March 2011

220960LV00002B/5/P